FOUNDATIONS OF ĀYURVEDA, VOLUME III

Principles of Holistic Living in Āyurveda

(स्वस्थ वृत्त - Svastha Vṛtta)

Vaidya (Dr.) Jessica Vellela, BAMS
Vaidya (Dr.) Prasanth Dharmarajan, PhD (Ayu)

ĀYU ACADEMY LLC

1001 S. Main St. STE 500
Kalispell, MT 59901

https://www.ayu.academy

FOUNDATIONS OF ĀYURVEDA, VOLUME III
Principles of Holistic Living in Āyurveda

Author
Vaidya (Dr.) Jessica Vellela, BAMS

Contributor
Vaidya (Dr.) Prasanth Dharmarajan, PhD (Ayu)

Third Edition

Notice - Disclaimer

Knowledge and best practices in the field of Āyurveda regularly change as new research and experience broaden the understanding of the subject. Adaptable changes with research methods, professional practice and/or management protocols may become necessary. Every effort has been made to ensure that the content provided in this publication is accurate and complete at the time of publishing. However, this is not an exhaustive treatment of the subject. No liability is assumed for losses or damages due to the information provided. Interpretation and application of information from this publication is solely the responsibility of the reader. Always consult an appropriate professional with any questions related to legal, medical or healthcare issues.

Previous editions copyrighted 2018, 2019, 2020.

ISBN: 978-1-950876-12-9

To all of our teachers,

and their teachers,

and the teachers before them

Special thanks to the

SVASTHA ĀCHĀRYA STUDENTS

for helping to make this book and

higher standards of Āyurveda a reality.

येषामेव हि भावानां संपत् संजनयेन्नरम् । तेषामेव विपद्व्याधीन्विविधान्समुदीरयेत् ॥

च. सू. २५।२९

Yeṣhāmeva hi bhāvānāṁ saṁpat saṁjanayennaram |

Teṣhāmeva vipadvyādhīnvividhānsamudīrayet ||

Cha. Sū. 25/29

"The very same foods that may be used in a wholesome manner to promote healthy growth of individuals can also be, in their unwholesome state, the specific causes for various diseases."

Contents

UNIT I

External factors that influence health

Chapter 1 : Svastha

KEY TERMS

āchāra rasayana
agni
āhāra
āhāra śhakti
asvastha
āyu
bala
bṛmhana
daśha-vidha parikṣha
deśha
dhātu sāmya
doṣha śhamana
dvādaśha-vidha parikṣha
ekādaśha-vidha parikṣha
kāla
mala kriya
nidāna
pañchakarma
prakṛti
prasanna ātma
prasanna indriya
prasanna manas
rasāyana
ṛtu
sama agni
sama dhātu
sama doṣha
sātmya
sattva
stha
sva
svastha
Svastha Vṛtta
trayopastambha
upavāsa
vikṛti
vṛtta

balance
disease
health
illness
imbalance
sickness
wellness

The study of Svastha Vṛtta is an area that deserves special attention within the science of Āyurveda. It is directly responsible for fulfilling one of the two main goals of the science, to maintain the health of the heathy (स्वस्थस्य स्वास्थ्यरक्षणम, *svasthasya svāsthya-rakṣhaṇam*, Cha. Sū. 30/26).

NIRUKTI AND PARIBHĀṢHĀ

The term *svastha* can be directly translated as health, although its original meaning carries a much deeper implication in classical literature. The word *svastha* is composed of the prefix *sva-* and the term *stha*. These indicate:

sva — own, one's own

stha — standing, staying, abiding, being situated in, existing or being in, on or among

In this context, it can also be considered "occupied with, engaged in, devoted to performing, practicing." *Svastha* literally means "being in one's own," as in one's personal, natural, and healthy normal state. The opposite of this, or *asvastha*, is considered a lack or absence of normal health.

Vṛtta is directly translated as "round, rounded, circular," and here refers to a "cycle, regimen, routine." Svastha Vṛtta is the cycle, routine or regimen that supports, maintains and improves a normal healthy state for an individual.

An appropriate healthy routine is something which adjusts with an individual's needs over the course of their lifetime. Different seasons, years, periods of development and fluctuating states of health can result in wide changes in requirements to determine appropriate routines. While general guidelines for Svastha Vṛtta exist, they are not normally meant to be interpreted as strict rules. The underlying principles, purposes and benefits should be understood and recognized to allow customizations that provide the best individualized results.

The practices and regimens of Svastha Vṛtta also contribute to fulfilling the second major goal of Āyurveda, to alleviate the disorders of the sick (आतुरस्य विकारप्रशमनं, *āturasya vikāra-praśhamanaṁ*, Cha. Sū. 30/26). In these situations, the individual's diet and habits are regulated to best support the line of management and treatment protocols. Depending on many factors that contribute to the state of the disorder, appropriate recommendations may include standard protocols for the disorder and customized rules for the unique presentation.

Ultimately, the purpose of Āyurveda is to prevent disease and provide abundant, consistent health so that individuals may pursue their life goals.

This is achieved through the proper application of the science. Charaka states that "Complete health is the best foundation for being able to work towards fulfilling one's *dharma*, *artha*, *kāma* and *mokṣhā*," (धर्मार्थकाममोक्षाणामारोग्यं मूलमुत्तमम्, *dharma-artha-kāma-mokṣhāṇām-ārogyaṁ mūlam-uttamam*, Cha. Sū. 1/15). Practicing Svastha Vṛtta appropriately is perhaps the best first step towards prevention of disease and maintenance of complete health.

Vāgbhaṭa reiterates this point at the opening of Aṣhṭāṅga Hṛdaya, mirroring Punarvasu Ātreya's position. He states:

आयुः कामयमानेन धर्मार्थसुखसाधनम् ।
आयुर्वेदोपदेशेषु विधेयः परमादरः ॥

अ. हृ. सू. १।२

Āyuḥ kāmayamānena
dharmārthasukhasādhanam |
Āyurvedopaśheṣhu vidheyaḥ
paramādaraḥ ||

AH Sū. 1/2

Āyuḥ kāmayamānena (Those who desire a long life to fulfill their) dharma, artha, sukha, sādhanam (*dharma*, *artha*, *sukha*, and *sādhanam*) Āyurveda-upaśheṣhu vidheyaḥ paramādaraḥ (should do their best to learn and carefully apply the proper methods of Āyurveda).

While Āyurveda can guide an individual to a state of complete health, it does so best when the individual is independently capable of recognizing their purpose in life and acting appropriately.

Chakrapāṇi recognizes the importance of this at the very beginning of the treatise and explains that disease prevents and prohibits an individual from realizing lifetime goals. He specifically mentions one of the goals as *upavāsa*, or the intentional restriction, limitation and control of basic desires which are not conducive to long-term health.

This is considered as one of the major signs of development of the individual towards a mature state of *manas* and *buddhi*. This has a direct impact on the individual's ability to identify that which is right or wrong for the *śharīra*, *indriya*, *manas* and *ātma*. Making correct choices for these four constitutes the basis of extending and maximizing the quality of *āyu*.

A long life and good quality of life are in fact the two basic components of the definition of Āyurveda according to Suśhruta. At the onset of his treatise he clearly states that, "The science itself is called Āyurveda because it allows one to become proficient with the knowledge of life, and how to enhance and extend life," (आयुरस्मिन् विद्यते, अनेन वाऽऽयुर्विन्दन्ति इत्यायुर्वेदः, *Āyur-asmin vidyate, anena vā''yurvindanti ityāyurvedaḥ*, Su. Sū. 1/15). The core science has always been based on longevity and the guidelines of Svastha Vṛtta are integral to this outcome.

The classical texts contain very detailed instructions on Svastha Vṛtta. However, it must be remembered that these instructions have been recorded based on long-term adaptation to life in the Indian subcontinent, which is the primary geographical region for the practice of Traditional Āyurvedic Medicine. The general and specific recommendations are customized for the people, culture and life in the Indian subcontinent.

Today, numerous countries and cultures around the globe look to Āyurveda to provide guidance on basic recommendations for diet and lifestyle activities. Accurate and reliable advice cannot simply be provided through direct classical references.

Instead, the appropriate recommendations should ideally be proposed, tested and reviewed over a sufficient period of time to draw reliable conclusions and consider the results within the context of the continuously changing local environment. The application of the science has always been intended in this manner and is succinctly described by major classical authors.

Suśhruta explains this concept as "nothing exists in the world which does not have the capacity to act as a medicine," (नानौषधीभूत, *na-ānauṣhadhī-bhūta*, Su. Sū. 41/5). The determination of what to use, when to use it, how much to use and appropriate application based on all variable factors is key in producing effective, positive health outcomes. This same logic is required to properly apply the concepts of Svastha Vṛtta.

TEST YOURSELF

Learn, review and memorize key terms from this section.

sva

---

stha

---

svastha

---

vṛtta

Svastha Vṛtta

---

upavāsa

CURRENT PERSPECTIVES ON HEALTH

Today, perspectives on health vary considerably throughout many levels of society. Perceptions of health within the general public are often quite different from definable factors measured by trained medical professionals. Adding the Āyurvedic perspective to this may further increase the complexity because the specifications of the science are unfamiliar to so many. It is important that Āyurvedic professionals be capable of communicating the distinctions of the science effectively from both classical and current perspectives.

The following sections review many commonly used terms in the health and wellness fields. These are followed by an introductory analysis of Āyurvedic terms and their comprehensive meanings. Note similarities and differences between these terms and consider whether the common English terms are capable of providing appropriate translations of the concepts.

All definitions are cited from the Merriam-Webster dictionary and include general definitions, medical definitions, and examples of their usage. Synonyms, anytonyms, word history and etymology are included to provide perspective on the long-term development of the understanding of health in the English language.

Health

\ ˈhelth also ˈheltth \ noun, often attributive

General definition	Examples
1. The condition of being sound in body, mind, or spirit a. Especially, freedom from physical disease or pain	• She is the picture of health. • We nursed him back to health.
2. The general condition of the body	• How is your mother's health? • He has continued to enjoy good health in his old age. • He's in good health these days.
3. A condition in which someone or something is thriving or doing well a. See also, well-being	• defending the health of the beloved oceans, - Peter Wilkinson
4. General condition or state	• poor economic health

Medical definition	Examples
1. the condition of an organism or one of its parts in which it performs its vital functions normally or properly a. especially: freedom from physical disease and pain	• dental health • mental health • nursed him back to health
2. the condition of an organism with respect to the performance of its vital functions especially as evaluated subjectively or non-professionally	• how is your health today

Synonyms		Antonyms
• fitness	• soundness	• illness
• healthiness	• wellness	• sickness
• heartiness	• wholeness	• unhealthiness
• robustness	• wholesomeness	• unsoundness
• sap		

First known use	History and etymology
Before the 12th century, in the meaning defined in #1	Middle English helthe, from Old English hǣlth, from hāl

Disease

\ di-ˈzēz \ noun

General definition

1. a condition of the living animal or plant body or of one of its parts that impairs normal functioning and is typically manifested by distinguishing signs and symptoms
    a. See also, sickness, malady
2. A harmful development (as in a social institution)
3. Obsolete: trouble

Examples

- He suffers from a rare genetic disease.
- a disease of the mind
- Thousands die of heart disease each year.
- sees the city's crime as a disease

Medical definition

1. an impairment of the normal state of the living animal or plant body or one of its parts that interrupts or modifies the performance of the vital functions, is typically manifested by distinguishing signs and symptoms, and is a response to environmental factors (as malnutrition, industrial hazards, or climate), to specific infective agents (as worms, bacteria, or viruses), to inherent defects of the organism (as genetic anomalies), or to combinations of these factors
    a. Called also morbus

Synonyms

- ail
- ailment
- bug
- complaint
- complication
- condition
- disorder
- distemper
- distemperature
- fever
- ill
- illness
- infirmity
- malady
- sickness
- trouble

Antonyms

- health
- wellness

First known use

14th century, in the meaning of "trouble"

History and etymology

Middle English disese, from Anglo-French desease, desaise, from des- dis- + eise ease

Wellness

\ ˈwel-nəs \ noun

General definition	Examples
1. the quality or state of being in good health especially as an actively sought goal	• Daily exercise is proven to promote wellness. • Discounted gym memberships are part of the company's employee wellness program.

Medical definition	Examples
1. the quality or state of being in good health especially as an actively sought goal	• lifestyles that promote wellness

Synonyms		Antonyms
• fitness • health • healthiness • heartiness • robustness	• sap • soundness • wholeness • holesomeness	• illness • sickness • unhealthiness • unsoundness

First known use	History and etymology
1653, in the meaning defined in #1	Middle English helthe, from Old English hǣlth, from hāl

Illness

\ ˈil-nəs \ noun

General definition	Examples
1. As defined in sickness, #2 2. an unhealthy condition of body or mind 3. Obsolete a. wickedness b. unpleasantness	• Her body was not able to defend itself against illness. • He showed no signs of illness.

Medical definition	Examples
1. an unhealthy condition of body or mind a. See also, sickness	• Hundreds of soldiers died from illness and hunger.

Synonyms	Antonyms
• indisposition • sickness • unhealthiness • unsoundness	• health • healthiness • soundness • wellness • wholeness • wholesomeness

First known use	History and etymology
circa 1500, in the meaning of "wickedness"	Middle English helthe, from Old English hǣlth, from hāl

Balance

\ ˈba-lən(t)s \ noun

General definition	Examples
1. physical equilibrium	• trouble keeping your balance on a sailboat • lost his balance and fell • a boxer kept off balance for a whole round
2. the ability to retain one's balance	• Gymnasts must have a good sense of balance.
3. stability produced by even distribution of weight on each side of the vertical axis	• when the two sides of the scale are in balance • tipped the statue off balance
4. equipoise between contrasting, opposing, or interacting elements	• … the balance we strike between security and freedom, - Earl Warren • Both parties were interviewed to provide balance in the report. • the right balance of diet and exercise
5. an aesthetically pleasing integration of elements	• achieving balance in a work of art
6. weight or force of one side in excess of another	• The balance of the evidence lay on the side of the defendant.
7. mental and emotional steadiness	• I doubt that Thoreau would be thrown off balance by the fantastic sights and sounds of the 20th century, - E. B. White
8. an instrument for weighing, such as a beam that is supported freely in the center and has two pans of equal weight suspended from its ends, or a device that uses the elasticity of a spiral spring for measuring weight or force	
9. a means of judging or deciding	• the balance of a free election
10. a counterbalancing weight, force, or influence	• The comedic character serves as a balance to the serious subject matter of the play.

Medical definition

1. an instrument for weighing
2. mental and emotional steadiness
3. the relation in physiology between the intake of a particular substance and its excretion —used with positive when the intake of a substance is greater than the body's excretion of it and with negative when the intake of a substance is less than the body's excretion of it — see nitrogen balance, water balance
4. the maintenance (as in laboratory cultures) of a population at about the same condition and level

Examples

Synonyms

- coherence
- consonance
- consonancy
- harmony
- orchestration
- proportion
- symmetry
- symphony
- unity

Antonyms

- asymmetry
- discordance
- disproportion
- disunity
- imbalance
- incoherence
- violence

First known use

13th century, in the meaning defined at #8

History and etymology

Middle English, from Anglo-French, from Vulgar Latin *bilancia, from Late Latin bilanc-, bilanx having two scalepans, from Latin bi- + lanc-, lanx plate

Imbalance

\ (ˌ)im-ˈba-lən(t)s \ noun

General definition	Examples
1. lack of balance: the state of being out of equilibrium or out of proportion	• a vitamin imbalance • racial imbalance in schools • Her depression is caused by a chemical imbalance in the brain.

Medical definition	Examples
1. lack of balance: the state of being out of equilibrium or out of proportion	
2. loss of parallel relation between the optical axes of the eyes caused by faulty action of the extrinsic muscles and often resulting in diplopia	• a vitamin imbalance • if the ductus arteriosus fails to close, a circulatory imbalance results, - E. B. Steen & Ashley Montagu
3. absence of biological equilibrium	
4. a disproportion between the number of males and females in a population	

First known use	History and etymology
circa 1890, in the meaning defined in #1	

Sickness

\ ˈsik-nəs \ noun

General definition

1. ill health
   a. See also, illness
2. a disordered, weakened, or unsound condition
3. a specific disease
4. nausea, queasiness

Examples

- He died from an unknown sickness.
- She was plagued by sickness most of her adult life.

Medical definition

1. the condition of being ill: ill health
2. a specific disease
3. nausea

Examples

Synonyms

- illness
- indisposition
- unhealthiness
- unsoundness

Antonyms

- health
- healthiness
- soundness
- wellness
- wholeness
- wholesomeness

First known use

Before the 12th century, in the meaning defined in #1

History and etymology

Equilibrium

\ ˌē-kwə-ˈli-brē-əm \ noun

General definition	Examples
1. a state of intellectual or emotional balance a. See also, poise b. a state of adjustment between opposing or divergent influences or elements	• trying to recover his equilibrium
2. a state of balance between opposing forces or actions that is either static (as in a body acted on by forces whose resultant is zero) or dynamic (as in a reversible chemical reaction when the rates of reaction in both directions are equal)	• She was plagued by sickness most of her adult life.
3. balance, definition 3	

Synonyms		Antonyms	
• balance	• equipoise	• disequilibration	• nonequilibrium
• counterpoise	• poise	• disequilibrium	• unbalance
• equilibration	• stasis	• imbalance	• healthiness

First known use	History and etymology
Early 17th century (in the sense 'well-balanced state of mind')	from Latin aequilibrium, from aequi- 'equal' + libra 'balance'

Disequilibrium

\ (ˌ)dis-ˌē-kwə-ˈli-brē-əm \ noun

General definition	Examples
1. loss or lack of equilibrium	• The condition is caused by a disequilibrium in the brain's chemistry.

Medical definition	Examples
1. sensation of impending fall or of the need to obtain external assistance for proper locomotion	

First known use	History and etymology
Early 20th century	

Normal

nor·mal | \ ˈnȯr-məl adjective

General definition	Examples
1. a) conforming to a type, standard, or regular pattern	• normal working hours • He had a normal childhood. • the effect of normal aging
b) according with, constituting, or not deviating from a norm, rule, or principle	• The normal way to pluralize a noun is by adding -s.
2. occurring naturally	• normal immunity
3. a) of, relating to, or characterized by average intelligence or development	• IQs within the normal range • symptoms of paranoia in otherwise normal persons
b) free from mental illness : mentally sound	
4. a form or state regarded as the norm	

Synonyms

- average
- common
- commonplace
- ordinary
- routine
- standard
- usual

Antonyms

- abnormal
- odd
- strange
- unusual

First known use

Adjective, circa 1696, in the meaning of perpendicular

Noun, 1728, in the meaning of relating to, or characterized by average intelligence or development

History and etymology

Adjective
borrowed from Latin normālis "made according to a carpenter's square, forming a right angle," from norma "carpenter's square" + -ālis

Noun
borrowed from New Latin normālis, noun derivative of Latin normālis "forming a right angle"

Abnormal

ab·nor·mal | \ (ˌ)ab-ˈnȯr-məl adjective

General definition	Examples
1. deviating from the normal or average	• a person with abnormal [=exceptional] strength • abnormal powers of concentration
2. unusual in an unwelcome or problematic way	• abnormal behavior • abnormal test results

Synonyms		Antonyms	
• aberrant • anomalous • atypical • exceeding	• odd • peculiar • uncommon • unusual	• common • normal	• typical • unexceptional • usual

First known use	History and etymology
Adjective, 1817, in the meaning defined above Noun, 1857, in the meaning defined	Adjective New Latin abnormis "deviating from the average" (going back to Medieval Latin, "not conforming to rule," going back to Latin, "belonging to no school of philosophy," from ab- AB- + norma "carpenter's rule, pattern") + -AL Noun Noun derivative of abnormal

The definitions of health and wellness demonstrate that the understanding of these concepts is non-specific without clear indicators or well-defined, measurable outcomes. Using English terminology, health is not considered to be measurable.

Many of the definitions attempt to explain the terms in context of their opposite state which can leave the subject unclear, ambiguous, and open to interpretation. While this allows freedom of expression and a broad field of potential scope, it also leaves opportunity for confusion and miscommunication in professional spheres.

The World Health Organization adopted a definition for health in 1948 that states "Health is a state of complete physical, mental and social well-being and not merely the absence of disease or infirmity." The bibliographic citation for this definition is the Preamble to the Constitution of WHO as adopted by the International Health Conference, New York, 19 June - 22 July 1946; signed on 22 July 1946 by the representatives of 61 States (Official Records of WHO, no. 2, p. 100) and entered into force on 7 April 1948. The definition has not been amended since 1948.

TEST YOURSELF

Learn, review and memorize key terms from this section.

health

disease

wellness

illness

balance

imbalance

sickness

normal

abnormal

ĀYURVEDA'S PERSPECTIVE ON HEALTH

Āyurveda recognizes the depth and breadth of a complete state of health through specific, measurable outcomes determined through application of the core principcles of the science. This complete state of health is termed *svastha*. Although *svastha* is often translated as health, the original term indicates a very specific meaning and scope. *Svastha* goes beyond the absence of disease and varying states of well-being. Classical literature provides guidance on understanding the scope of *svastha* from numerous angles.

General definitions of *svastha* are geared towards ease of use and application in a larger population. Detailed definitions provide specific means to assess and measure an individual's health in a personalized manner. At a high level, these include all aspects of *āyu* and their components of *śharīra*, *indriya*, *manas* and *ātma*. These detailed definitions provide a foundation and framework for professionals to apply the concept of *svastha* and reliably recognize its presence in highly individualized, unique presentations.

The line between *svastha* and *asvastha* is not demarcated by a single boundary.

Instead, various states of *svastha* to *asvastha* should be considered as ranges on a scale. These include:

1. Svastha
2. Fluctuation
3. Asvastha

Svastha indicates that all components which support the body are within their normal operating parameters, or *prākṛta* states. At a minimum, these components include the *doṣhas*, *dhātus* and *malas*.

Fluctuation from *svastha* is most commonly seen when any of these primary components are influenced by the major factors of *rasa*, *āhāra* or *ṛtu*. Their regular, repeated influence can cause one or more specific *guṇas* to increase or decrease into a state of *chaya* or *kṣhaya*. This state of deviation is heading toward presentations of *vaikṛta* but is not yet in a complete state of *vikṛti*.

If the *rasa*, *āhāra*, *ṛtu* or any other source of causative factors continue to manipulate the specific *guṇas* to produce increase or decrease, the component's state will eventually shift into *asvastha*. This is generally identified by the presence of a clear, recognizable pathology and often requires therapeutic intervention, in addition to the removal of the causative factors, to restore the individual to a state of *svastha*.

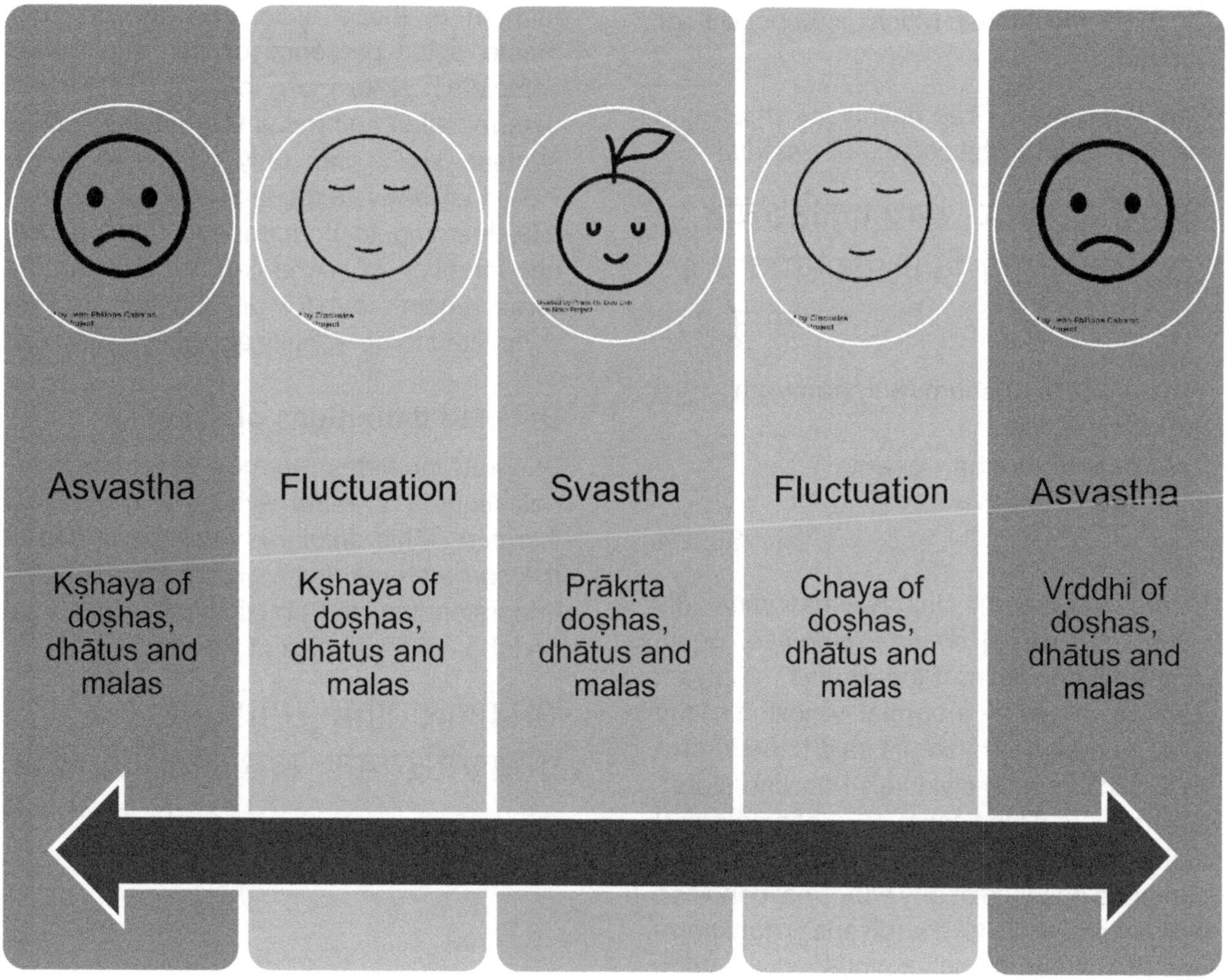

Within these ranges, the three main states can be further divided based on the *doṣha(s)*, their quantity, qualities, locations, duration and additional factors. Here, the focus is on understanding these factors and assessing them within the context of *svastha* and many possible presentations of fluctuation. Review the following definitions of *svastha* in detail to understand the classical approaches to assessing and measuring states of health.

General definitions of svastha

The classics provide direct and simple means for understanding *svastha* from a general perspective. These definitions explain the state of *svastha* in slightly more detail and also provide basic indicators for guiding untrained individuals in determining for themselves that which is beneficial or harmful.

Charaka provides two definitions which can be interpreted in the context of *svastha*:

विकारो धातुवैषम्यं, साम्यं प्रकृतिरुच्यते ।
सुखसंज्ञकमारोग्यं, विकारो दुःखमेव च ॥
च. सू. ९।४

Vikāro dhātuvaiṣhamyaṁ, sāmyaṁ prakṛtiruchyate |
Sukhasaṁjñakamārogyaṁ, vikāroduḥkhameva cha ||
Cha. Sū. 9/4

Vikāro (Disease) dhātuvaiṣhamyaṁ ([is considered to be] *dhātu vaiṣhamya*, or an abnormal condition of the *dhātus*), sāmyaṁ ([*dhātu*] *sāmya*, or a normal condition of the *dhātus*) prakṛtiruchyate (is said to be known as prakṛti. or an individual's baseline state). Sukha (Happiness, contentment) saṁjñakam (is known to be) ārogyaṁ (the complete absence of any abnormal condition or disease), while vikāra (disease) duḥkham-eva (is marked by unhappiness, discontent, sadness, etc).

कार्यफलं सुखावाप्तिः, तस्य लक्षणं - मनोबुद्धीन्द्रियशरीरतुष्टिः ॥
च. वि. ८।९०

Kāryaphalaṁ sukhāvāptiḥ, tasya lakṣhaṇaṁ - manobuddhīndriyaśharīratuṣhṭiḥ ||
Cha. Vi. 8/90

Kārya-phala (The goal of the practice of this science is) sukhāvāptiḥ (the achievement of a state of happiness, content, satisfaction, etc). Tasya lakṣhaṇaṁ (This can be recognized by the features of) mano, buddhi, indriya, śharīra tuṣhṭiḥ (satisfaction, pleasantness, contentment of the mental faculties, power of intelligence, senses and the physical body).

In both of these definitions, the common theme is the presence of *sukha* in a true, complete state of health. Ultimately, determination and recognition of this state of genuine *sukha* can only be made by the individual who is experiencing it. Because of this, learning to comprehend the meaning and intention of *sukha* can be considered a basic requirement for anyone who is truly committed to personally applying Āyurveda.

Detailed definitions of svastha

Suśhruta provides the most comprehensive definition of *svastha* available in classical literature. This *śhloka* is considered one of the cornerstones for a proper foundation in understanding and practicing Svastha Vṛtta and the entire science of Āyurveda.

समदोषः समाग्निश्च समधातुमलक्रियः ।
प्रसन्नात्मेन्द्रियमनाः स्वस्थ इत्यभिधीयते ॥
स. सू. १५।४१

Samadoṣhaḥ samāgniśhcha samadhātumalakriyaḥ |
Prasannātmendriyamanāḥ svastha ityabhidhīyate ||

Su. Sū. 15/41

Iti (And so,) svastha (a complete state of health) abhidhīyate (is known by the following):

Sama doṣhaḥ	*Doṣhas* in a state of *sama* (normal, healthy equilibrium)
Sama agni	*Agni* in a state of *sama*
Sama dhātu	*Dhātus* in a state of *sama*
Mala kriyaḥ	Proper function, action and elimination of *malas*
Prasanna	Happy, content state of:
ātma	the soul
indriya	the senses
manāḥ	the mind

This definition provides the framework to assess and measure an individual's current state of health, their levels of fluctuation and any health disorders. It allows the Āyurvedic professional to gauge where the individual currently stands on the scale of *svastha* to *asvastha* by properly assessing *lakṣhaṇas.*

For the detailed lists of *lakṣhaṇas* under each component, refer to Vol. 2, Siddhānta and Śhārīra.

Assessment component	Includes	Lakṣhaṇas to assess
Sama doṣha	Vāta Pitta Kapha	Prākṛta doṣha Vṛddha doṣha Kṣhīṇa doṣha
Sama agni	Samāgni Mandāgni Tīkṣhṇāgni Viṣhamāgni	Prākṛta agni Vaikṛta agni
Sama dhātu	Rasa Asthi Rakta Majja Māṁsa Śhukra Medas	Prākṛta dhātu Vṛddha dhātu Kṣhīṇa dhātu
Mala kriya	Mūtra Purīṣha Sveda	Prākṛta mala Vṛddha mala Kṣhīṇa mala
Prasanna ātma	Ātma	Jīva (ātma) lakṣhaṇas
Prasanna indriya	Indriya	Indriya lakṣhaṇas
Prasanna manas	Manas	Mano guṇa and karma Tri-guṇa lakṣhaṇas

Additionally, Charaka provides several key parameters to assess when measuring an individual's state of *svastha*. These are listed as the key *lakṣhaṇas* for clinical assessment of *dhātu sāmya* (Cha. Vi. 8/89).

Dhātu sāmya lakṣhaṇas	Split Devanāgarī and nearest English explanation
रुगुपशमनं Rugupaśhamanaṁ	*Ruk upaśhamana* Proper alleviation (correct management) of pain or suffering
स्वरवर्णयोगः Svaravarṇayogaḥ	*Svara varṇa yoga* Normal, healthy speech (ability to speak) and complexion
शरीरोपचयः Śharīropachayaḥ	*Śharīra upachaya* Proper, normal growth (healing, recovery) of the body
बलवृद्धिः Balavṛddhiḥ	*Bala vṛddhi* Proper, normal increase in strength (physical capacity to perform activities); ojas may also be considered here
अभ्यवहार्याभिलाषः Abhyavahāryābhilāṣhaḥ	*Abhyavahāri-ābhilāṣhaḥ* Desire to eat
रुचिराहारकाले Ruchirāhārakāle	*Ruchi āhāra kāle* Proper, normal presence of appetite at regular mealtimes
अभ्यवहृतस्य चाहारस्य काले सम्यग्जरणं Abhyavahṛtasya chāhārasya kāle samyagjaraṇaṁ	*Abhyavahṛtasya chāhārasya kāle samyak-jaraṇaṁ* Proper digestion of food which has been consumed in the right time
निद्रालाभो यथाकालं Nidrālābho yathākālaṁ	*Nidrā lābho yathā kālaṁ* The beneficial results of sleeping on a regular schedule
वैकारिणां च स्वप्नानामदर्शनं Vaikāriṇāṁ cha svapānāmadarśhaṁ	*Vaikāriṇāṁ cha svapānām adarśhaṁ* Non-appearance of abnormal dreams
सुखेन च प्रतिबोधनं Sukhena cha pratibodhanaṁ	*Sukhena cha pratibodhanaṁ* Contentment, satisfaction upon waking in the morning
वातमूत्रपुरीषरेतसां मुक्तिः Vātamūtrapurīṣharetasāṁ muktiḥ	*Vāta, mūtra, purīṣha, retasā mukti* Proper, normal, unimpaired release of flatus, urine, stools and ejaculation (orgasm)
सर्वाकारैर्मनोबुद्धिन्द्रियाणां चाव्यापत्तिरिति Sarvākārairmanobuddhindriyāṇāṁ chāvyāpattiriti	*Sarvākārair mano, buddhi, indriyāṇāṁ cha avyāpattir-iti* All activities of the mind, intellect and senses are free from disorder and disease (ie, free from unhealthy functioning)

It is clear from the detailed definitions, parameters, and measurable outcomes of *svastha* that the true meaning of the term cannot currently be conveyed through the simple translation of health. The classical Āyurvedic references provide a deeper, holistic picture beyond the absence of disease or disparate physical, mental and social health. When utilizing these terms in professional communications, always be aware of the intention and utilize the appropriate terminology.

TEST YOURSELF

Learn, review and memorize key terms from this section.

svastha

---

asvastha

---

sama doṣha

---

sama agni

---

sama dhātu

---

mala kriya

---

prasanna ātma

---

prasanna indriya

---

prasanna manas

---

dhātu sāmya

DIFFERENTIATING SVASTHA AND ASVASTHA

Identifying and measuring *svastha* and *asvastha*, and all the possibilities within their ranges, requires analyzing each component and assessing each of the *lakṣhaṇas*. In Suśhruta's detailed definition of *svastha* described above, these *lakṣhaṇas* are grouped into categories creating a methodical framework for assessment. The components of that definition refer to assessing and measuring the related *lakṣhaṇas* as described in the classics including *prākṛta* and *vaikṛta doṣha*, *agni*, *dhātu* and *mala*.

When assessing *svastha*, it is realistic to expect some type of deviation from complete health in virtually all individuals at all times. While the notion of "perfect health" may seem like an ambitious but realistic goal, it is extremely difficult to achieve in regular life when considering all the possible factors that can contribute to fluctuations. Several of these factors are typically out of the control of individuals, like seasonal influence, time and external stressors.

The goal in assessing *svastha* and striving towards it is not necessarily one of perfection, but rather learning to continuously work towards an optimal point of homeostasis, and accept the present reality with genuine satisfaction.

Measuring svastha

Classical Āyurvedic literature presents frameworks for assessing *svastha* along with the appropriate parameters to measure current states. Several variations of assessment methods are presented by different authors throughout their respective texts. These methodologies are intended to be used for assessing the range of *svastha* through *asvastha*, specific *vikāra*, and understanding their contributing factors.

Assessment methodologies are explained throughout the texts and often appear in the context of that which is being assessed. Associated *lakṣhaṇas* for each measured component may or may not be cited with the assessment methodology. These *lakṣhaṇas* indicate a specific sign or symptom, a quantity or level, or other boundary limits to measure the state of the assessment criteria.

Forming the complete assessment methodology requires combining many references from various chapters of entire treatises.

Fundamental assessment models

Charaka, Suśhruta and Vāgbhaṭa each present comprehensive assessment models in their works. While each model is unique based on minor variations in the number of components to assess, they each cover a complete review of an individual's state of health. The three major models include:

Assessment model	Reference	Number of components
Daśha-vidha parikṣha	Cha. Vi. 8/94	10
Ekādaśha-vidha parikṣha	AH Sū. 12/67	11
Dvādaśha-vidha parikṣha	Su. Sū. 35/	12

Although each model can be used independently, the approach in this textbook combines these frameworks, restructures them and organizes specific assessment criteria within the main categories. Review the structure of this assessment model next.

Clinical Svastha Assessment

Parikṣha	Measurements	Assessment category	CA	SU	AH
Deśha		Environment		✓	
Ṛtu / Kāla		Season, time period		✓	✓
Sātmya		Wholesome	✓	✓	✓
	Charyā (dina, rātri, ṛtu)	Schedules			
	(A)Brahmacharyā	Lifestyles			
	Nidrā	Sleep routines			
	Adhāranīya vegas	Natural release routines			

Parikṣha	Measurements	Assessment category	CA	SU	AH
Prakṛti		Baseline	√	√	√
	Sāra	Excellent dhatu	√		
	Pramāṇa	Measurements	√		
Vikṛti		Deviation	√		
	Vyādhi	Disorder		√	
	Duṣhya	Deranged dhātu(s)		√	
	Avastha	Stage			√
	Bheṣhaja	Treatment methodology		√	
	Guru-laghu vyādhitā	Stress tolerance			
Āhāra Śhakti / Agni / Āhāra		Digestive power	√	√	√
	Abhyavaharaṇa śhakti	Intake power	√		
	Jaraṇa śhakti	Processing power	√		
	Āhāra	Food, diet			√
Bala		Strength		√	
	Deha	Physical structure		√	
	Saṁhanana	Compactness	√		
	Vyāyāma Śhakti	Physical capacity	√		
	Ojas	Resistance to disease			
Sattva		Mental state	√	√	√
	Puruṣhārthas	Life goals			
	Dhāraṇīya vegas	Self-control			
Vayas and āyu		Age	√	√	√
	Āyu	Lifespan		√	

Each of the assessment categories in this framework will be reviewed in detail in this textbook and subsequent volumes. This volume focuses on the categories that can be more readily applied within the context of *svastha* and divides them into external and internal factors.

External factors that influence health include *deśha* and *kāla* (including *ṛtu*) which are reviewed in detail in Unit 1. Internal factors that influence health include *sātmya*, *prakṛti*, *ahāra śhakti* (including *agni* and *āhāra*), *bala*, *vyāyāma śhakti*, *sattva* and *vaya* which are reviewed in detail in Unit 2.

Assessment components are explained in each chapter starting with a review of classical knowledge. Each is then analyzed through its underlying laws and rules to determine the needs for its classical recommendations.

Then, each component is considered within the context of the current, modern local environment, time and people. Classical laws and rules can be applied in these new contexts; however, recommendations are not as easy to transpose.

It must be remembered that appropriate recommendations should be made based on a combination of theoretical guidance and sufficient practical application. This should include demonstrable evidence to provide a high level of confidence.

At the time of this writing, an insufficient amount of evidence is available to provide these types of recommendations from a viable, statistical perspective. Proper Āyurvedic research is required to create a solid foundation in the practice for long-term practical application and credibility of the science.

TEST YOURSELF

Learn, review and memorize key terms from this section.

daśha-vidha parikṣha

ekādaśha-vidha parikṣha

dvādaśha-vidha parikṣha

deśha

ṛtu

kāla

sātmya

prakṛti

vikṛti

āhāra śhakti

agni

āhāra

bala

sattva

āyu

PLANNING FOR SVASTHA OVER A LIFETIME

Planning for *svastha* over the course of a lifetime requires the correct combination of knowledge, practice and appropriate expectations. Classical guidance can provide a wealth of information, however, each classical recommendation should be reviewed and carefully analyzed to determine its applicability outside of the Indian subcontinent and in current global cultures.

One of the first aspects to consider is the expectation of *svastha* at various stages of life. The classics provide a detailed framework for the classification of *vayas* (see Vol 2, Chapter 13). The requirements for complete health vary greatly during each of these stages of life and they have a direct impact on how to apply Svastha Vṛtta appropriately. These requirements and appropriate expectations will be discussed in detail in Chapter 10.

From the broadest perspective, any factors that interact with an individual and create a change in the state of *āyu* (including *śharīra*, *indriya*, *manas* and *ātma*) can be considered to influence *svastha*. These factors fall under several categories in classical literature, including *nidāna* (causative factors for disease), *sātmya* (wholesome diets and regimens), *trayopastambha* (the three main supports of life), *āchāra rasāyana* (daily habits to promote vitality, mental health and regeneration) and many more. Each of these topics and their classical knowledge will be covered in detail in the related chapters throughout this volume.

Classical authors also considered the practice of proper Svastha Vṛtta as the personal responsibility of every individual. Traditional Āyurvedic practice provided a robust health care system complete with guidance that could empower each person in society to take control of their state of health, improve it and prevent disease to the best of their ability.

Charaka emphasizes the importance of personal responsibility many times throughout his text with references available at Cha. Sū. 5/103, Cha. Sū. 7/60, Cha. Sū. 17/119, Cha. Sū. 28/36-40, Cha. Sū. 30/84-85. Additional references include AH Sū. 2/47.

In Cha. Sū. 17/119, an important analogy is given:

नित्यं सन्निहितामित्रं समीक्ष्यात्मानमात्मवान्
। नित्यं युक्तः परिचरेदिच्छेन्नायुरनित्वरम् ॥
च. सू. १७।११९

Nityaṁ sannihitāmitraṁ samīkṣhyātmānamātmavān |
Nityaṁ yuktaḥ parícharedichchhennāyuranitvaram ||
Cha. Sū. 17/119

A person who seeks a long, complete life should continuously stay alert to do the right things as if surrounded by enemies (ie, that his life depends on it).

Classical Āyurvedic perspectives placed a significant amount of responsibility on each individual for proper health maintenance. Scholars were well aware of the fact that all disease and suffering could not be prevented. Accidents and untimely death were also considered unpreventable in certain situations (Cha. Vi. 3/29-36, Cha. Śhā. 1/). Today's concept of "good genes" (a strong, genetic resistance to disease) could be considered aligned with certain types of *prakṛti* having naturally higher vitality than others.

As a robust health care system, classical Āyurveda is also replete with its own unique methods for health planning, disease prevention, longevity and increasing quality of life. Many of these methods have extensive options for customization and can be applied in a wide variety of situations according to the requirements. Review several of these unique methods below.

Āyurveda's holistic and expansive perspective

Āyurveda's perspective towards life, health and happiness stands apart from Western scientific paradigms in many ways. Āyurveda has, since its earliest times, always considered life and health in a holistic manner. The entire science and all of its systematic approaches towards health are designed in this way. It also considers both expansionism and reductionism in its fundamental logical perspectives. This results in a non-limiting practice of health care on multiple, if not all levels.

Charaka demonstrates this by acknowledging the infinite possibilities of potential medicines and application of therapeutics that can be found in the world. He states:

अनेनोपदेशेन नानौषधिभूतं जगति किंचिद्द्रव्यमुपलभ्यते तां तां युक्तिमर्थे च तं तमभिप्रेत्य ॥

च. सू. २६।१२

Anenopadeśhena nānauṣhadhibhūtaṁ jagati kiṅchiddravyamupalabhyate tāṁ tāṁ yuktimarthe cha taṁ tamabhipretya ||

Cha. Sū. 26/12

Like it was just mentioned in the preceding verse, there is nothing which exists in this world that cannot be used for curative effects (as a medicine) when one's logical thought power is able to determine the correct application.

Sātmya

The concept of *sātmya* extends to almost every aspect of the application of Svastha Vṛtta within Āyurveda. It is based on the principle that foods and habits which are healthy for an individual are seen to provide positive benefits when used regularly and continuously.

While this may not be a completely foreign concept in Western paradigms, it appears to be one which is not regularly considered in the context of health. It can be compared to the methodology of physical or mental training to produce expected results of high quality.

Sātmya also highlights the importance of identifying appropriate diets, routines, behaviors and other habits that consistently produce healthy individuals within a subpopulation.

While many things can be considered as *sātmya* for individuals only, certain things which qualify as *sātmya* are seen to apply broadly to families, communities, geographical areas, ethnic populations, and even the entire human race.

Many of these concepts are considered new developments in the fields of Western medicine and health. Āyurveda has recognized and practiced these for centuries and provides a comprehensive language and framework to express them clearly.

Charaka summarizes the factors which promote and decrease *svastha* very succinctly. This statement is made by Punarvasu Ātreya to summarize his discussion with Agniveśha.

येषामेव हि भावानां संपत् संजनयेन्नरम् ।
तेषामेव विपद्व्याधीन्विविधान्समुदीरयेत् ॥

च. सू. २५।२९

Yeṣhāmeva hi bhāvānāṁ saṁpat saṁjanayennaram |
Teṣhāmeva vipadvyādhīnvividhānsamudīrayet ||
Cha. Sū. 25/29

The same factors can promote healthy growth of individuals or disease depending on their state of *sātmya*.

Pañchakarma (pañchaśhodhana)

The knowledge and practice of *pañchakarma* is perhaps one of the most intriguing areas of Āyurveda. Conceptually, it has taken on an almost infinite number of forms and explanations in commercialized, public spheres of Āyurveda. These misconceptions have lead to a great amount of confusion about what *pañchakarma* is and what it is not.

The classical definitions, however, are very clear in their explanations. *Pañchakarma* is a series of therapeutic interventions intended to remove the *doṣhas* from the body by way of their nearest route of exit.

The procedures themselves are often preceded and followed by preparatory and follow-up therapies that can include a wide variety of hands-on body-work comparable to massage, application of herbal pastes, heat, powder, oils, decoctions and many varieties of medicinal formulations.

Although supportive in the overall application of *pañchakarma*, these auxiliary treatments do not meet the classical definition of *pañchakarma* and are better referred to as *upakrama*.

Pañchakarma is cited throughout the classics as the main method for removing the root cause of a disorder and returning the body to its normal state. It can be likened to a reset button for a machine, and when done properly can eliminate many internal causative factors for disease and provide a clean foundation for health maintenance.

As a general rule, *pañchakarma* was intended to be done for individuals with a health disorder at the appropriate time indicated by the pathology.

As a preventive measure, it was recommended to be performed for all individuals on an annual basis during the period of middle age according to season. This annual practice provides the opportunity for regular bodily maintenance and improvement while giving the individual a few weeks of time to rest from the daily stressors of normal life.

Rasāyana

Rasāyana constitutes methods that lengthen the span of life and improve its quality. It is often translated as rejuvenation, longevity science or regenerative treatment. The practice of *rasāyana* in classical Āyurveda covers its approach and methodology in detail. This practice is well-developed beyond the superficial meanings of basic translations.

Rasāyana is best done following a proper *pañchakarma* to bring the body to a healthy, normal state. It also promotes the body to function in its best way to produce strong, healthy *dhātus*, *ojas* and other important characteristics.

Doṣha śhamana

Doṣha śhamana is a unique concept in Āyurveda because it is based on the *tri-doṣha siddhānta*. It refers to the process of returning the *doṣhas* to their normal states without expelling them from the body. This process may be induced therapeutically according to the individual's need through a wide range of methods that can include abstaining from causative factors to usage of specific *auṣhadhis* (medicinal formulations). *Doṣha śhamana* may also occur on its own based on changes in external factors like age, time and season.

Bṛmhana

Bṛmhana covers the processes of building up the strength of the individual's body in such a way that minimizes disturbance to normal, healthy *doṣhas*. When properly performed, *bṛmhana* acts as *doṣha śhamana* specifically for *vāta doṣha*, and as *rasāyana*.

These are just brief overviews of each of these methods. Effecting any of these methods appropriately requires a thorough understanding of all components of the applied science of Āyurveda. These will be introduced in this this textbook and the subsequent volume.

Extensive knowledge required for practice of complete *pañchakarma*, *rasāyana* and other advanced methods is within the scope of the Āyurveda Āchārya level. All methods discussed should be performed under supervision of a qualified Āyurvedic professional.

TEST YOURSELF

Learn, review and memorize key terms from this section.

nidāna

---

sātmya

---

trayopastambha

āchāra
rasayana

---

pañchakarma

---

rasāyana

---

doṣha śhamana

---

bṛmhana

Chapter 1: Review

ADDITIONAL READING

Read and review the references listed below to expand your understanding of the concepts in this chapter. Write down the date that you complete your reading for each. Remember that consistent repetition is the best way to learn. Plan to read each reference at least once now and expect to read it again as you continue your studies.

References marked with (skim) can be read quickly and do not require commentary review.

CLASSICS		1st read	2nd read
Charaka	Cha. Sū. 1/15 Cha. Sū. 5/103 Cha. Sū. 7/60 Cha. Sū. 9/4 Cha. Sū. 17/119 Cha. Sū. 25/29 Cha. Sū. 26/12 Cha. Sū. 28/36-40 Cha. Sū. 30/26 Cha. Sū. 30/84-85 Cha. Vi. 8/89-94		
Suśhruta	Su. Sū. 1/15 Su. Sū. 15/41 Su. Sū. 35/ Su. Sū. 41/5		
Aṣhṭāṅga Hṛdaya	AH Sū. 1/2 AH Sū. 12/67		
Bhāva Prakāśha			

JOURNALS & CURRENT RESOURCES

https://www.ncbi.nlm.nih.gov/pmc/articles/PMC3405450/

https://www.medscape.com/viewarticle/902769?src=WNL_topolexclsv_181013_MSCPEDIT&uac=145230DX&impID=1767494&faf=1

QUESTIONS & ANSWERS

Record your questions for this chapter here for further research and discussion.

Question:

Answer:

Question:

Answer:

Question:

Answer:

SELF-ASSESSMENT

1. What is the primary methodology in classical Āyurveda for prevention and maintenance of individual health?
   a. *Dharma*, *artha*, *kāma*, *mokṣha*
   b. Eating well
   c. Health
   d. *Svastha Vṛtta*
   e. All of the above

2. In order to provide guidance on basic recommendations for diet & lifestyle, what should be done?
   a. Consider the results
   b. Draw conclusions
   c. Propose recommendations
   d. Test and review recommendations
   e. All of the above

3. Why are Western definitions of health and wellness challenging to use in Āyurveda?
   a. They are complex terms for a layperson.
   b. They lack clear indicators.
   c. They lack measurable outcomes.
   d. Both B and C
   e. All of the above

4. How many components are included in *dvādaśha vidha parikṣha*?
   a. 9
   b. 10
   c. 11
   d. 12
   e. None of the above

5. Which two specific measurements are not mentioned in Charaka's or Vāgbhaṭa's parikṣhas?
   a. *Āhāra* and *avastha*
   b. *Deha* and *duṣhya*
   c. *Saṁhanana* and *deha*
   d. *Sāra* and *pramāṇa*
   e. *Vyadhi* and *jaraṇa śhakti*

6. Which assessment components does Suśhruta identify in the definition of *svastha*?
   a. *Mala kriya*
   b. *Prasanna indriya*
   c. *Sama agni*
   d. *Sama dhātu*
   e. All of the above

7. Āyurveda's approach to measuring health is most similar to
   a. Āyurveda doesn't measure health
   b. the scientific method
   c. the Western definition of wellness
   d. the WHO definition of health
   e. None of the above

8. Normal deviations from complete *svastha* are considered
   a. *asvastha*
   b. fluctuations
   c. *svastha*
   d. All of the above
   e. None of the above

9. In the practical application of Cha. Sū. 26/12, what is required?
   a. *Asātmya*
   b. Intuition
   c. Knowing all about *dravya*
   d. *Yukti*
   e. All of the above

10. Classical *pañchakarma* is meant to
    a. remove the *doṣhas* from the body via the nearest route or exit
    b. remove the root cause of disorders
    c. return the *doṣhas* to their normal states without expelling them
    d. Both A and B
    e. All of the above

CRITICAL THINKING

1. Consider Suśhruta's definition of svastha. How can each of the components mentioned be assessed individually?

2. In Suśhruta's definition of svastha, can the components be assessed inter-dependently? If so, how?

3. Choose any three popular English terms for health and explain how they meet at least one criteria from Suśhruta's definition of svastha.

4. Using any three *lakṣhaṇas* from Charaka's definition of svastha, explain their related siddhānta.

5. Based on what you learned so far, why is it challenging to simply transpose recommendations for Svastha Vṛtta from India to Western countries?

References

WHO Definitions of Health. http://www.who.int/suggestions/faq/en/

Chapter 2 : Key terms and concepts

KEY TERMS

agni	arogya	karma	√ ruj
Agrya Auṣhadha	asātmya	okasātmya	sama
āhāra	auṣhadha	pathya	sātmya
ahita	dravya	roga	viṣhama
apathya	hita	rogi	

The study and practice of Svastha Vṛtta utilizes specfic terms to denote an individual's state of health and the many factors which contribute to it. These terms are best understood as well-developed concepts. They do not have adequate English translations and will be used in their original Sanskrit forms.

These common terms may be used to elaborate an individual's health assessment based on any of the factors that contribute or detract from *svastha*. These terms will be used regularly throughout this volume and in clinical assessment.

SĀTMYA

Sātmya is a very broad concept that provides insight into an individual's habits and preferences over their lifetime. In cultures and communities where traditions are maintained generation over generation, it is easier to see how *sātmya* directly influences an individual's state of health.

Sātmya refers to any substance which is healthy for an individual when used regularly and continuously. Its opposite is *asātmya*, which contradicts the original definition in any manner.

Additionally, a substance may also be found to practically behave in a *sātmya* manner for an individual yet be known to cause harm. Anything which has become habituated to someone that falls in this category is termed *okasātmya.* Common examples of *okasātmya* can include regular consumption of small quantities of alcohol or tobacco for certain individuals.

The application of *sātmya*, *asātmya* and *okasātmya* is found in almost every aspect of clinical practice. *Sātmya* is considered as a primary, individual factor in svastha assessment. It can also be treated as a contributing, or secondary factor in every other assessment component.

Sātmya

The term *sātmya* is defined by the Monier-Williams dictionary through references from Charaka and Suśhruta.

sātmya	agreeable to one's nature or natural, innate constitution, wholesome
	suitableness, wholesomeness
	habit, habituation, diet (indeclinable "from habit"; at the end of a compound "used to")

The term is derived from *sātma* (*sa* + *ātman*) which indicates being with one's own nature, or natural state.

sātma(n)	together with one's own

source of being

That which is *sātmya* for an individual is aligned to produce *svastha* from the core state of the individual's basic nature.

Charaka defines *sātmya* at the beginning of *Vimāna-sthāna* to acknowledge its critical role in measuring health and all related factors. He states that *sātmya* is:

सात्म्यं नाम तद् यदात्मन्युपशेते; सात्म्यार्थो ह्युपशयार्थः ...

च. वि. १।२०

Sātmyaṁ nāma tad yadātmanyupaśhete; sātmyārtho hyupaśhayārthaḥ ...

Cha. Vi. 1/20

Sātmyaṁ nāma (Sātmya is known as) tad (that which) yadātmany-upaśhete (is suitable for an individual); sātmya artho (it includes those things which are used regularly) hi upaśhaya arthaḥ (and result in feeling better, or a positive state of health).

The two key requirements for *sātmya* are that it must be used regularly and produce a positive state of health.

The technical term mentioned by Charaka for producing this state of health is *upaśhaya*. This conveys the understanding that anything which is *sātmya* has a direct impact on making the individual feel a sense of relief or improvment in health and contentment.

Charaka reiterates the definition of *sātmya* at the end of *Vimāna-sthāna* in the context of explaining the *daśha-vidha parikṣha*.

सातत्येनोपसेव्यमानमुपशेते ।

च. वि. ८।११८

Sātatyenopasevyamānamupaśhete |

Cha. Vi. 8/118

Sātatyena (When continuously, regularly, habitually) upasevya (used or applied) mānam (in the correct amount) upaśhete (it is suitable [to the individual]).

Here, Charaka elaborates that *sātmya* is possible when the substance is utilized on a regular basis and in the correct amount for the individual.

Sātmya is often considered synonymous with *pathya*.

Asātmya

The opposite of *sātmya* is *asātmya*, which is anything that detracts from an individual's positive state of *svastha*. Charaka defines *asātmya* as:

असात्म्यमिति तद्विद्याद्यन्न याति सहात्मताम् ॥

च. शा. १।१२७

Asātmyamiti tadvidyādyanna yāti sahātmatām ||

Cha. Śhā. 1/127

Asātmyam iti (And so, *asātmya*) tad vidyādy-anna (is known as food) yāti sahātmatām (which is destructive to the individual).

Asātmya is that which is not conducive to the body. It diminishes an individual's state of *svastha* and produces a sense of *duḥkha*, discomfort or dissatisfaction, which may indicate that it is heading toward disease.

Asātmya is often considered synonymous with *apathya*.

Okasātmya

Okasātmya falls in between *sātmya* and *asātmya* because the individual has become accustomed to it through regular use even though it is generally detrimental to producing *svastha*.

यच्चेष्टाहारव्यपाश्रयम् । उपशेते
यदौचित्यादोकः सात्म्यं तदुच्यते ॥

च. सू. ६।४९

Yachcheṣhṭāhārvyapāśhrayam |
Upaśhete yadauchityādokaḥ sātmyaṁ
taduchyate ||

Cha. Sū. 6/49

Yat (Those) cheṣhṭa (activities) āhāra (and foods) vyapāśhrayam (which have become normal for the body) upaśhete yadauchityād (because of their regular use) okaḥ sātmyaṁ taducyate (are known as *okasātmya*).

Here, Charaka includes both foods and activities under the purview of *okasātmya*. Because of their long-term use, the individual develops a tolerance which can eventually lead to a dependency in the sense that they experience a sense of relief through their use. Since *okasātmya* foods and activities are generally not beneficial for a long-term state of *svastha*, Charaka later recommends that they be discontinued gradually and replaced with appropriate options.

सात्म्यमपि हि
क्रमेणोपनिवर्त्यमानमदोषमल्पदोषं वा
भवति ॥

च. वि. १।१९

Sātmyamapi hi
krameṇopanivartyamānamadoṣhamalpa
doṣhaṁ vā bhavati ||

Cha. Vi. 1/19

Sātmyamapi hi (Even if they [foods or activities] appear to be sātmya), krameṇa upanivartya mānam (they should be slowly and gradually removed [and replaced with more appropriate items if necessary]) adoṣham alpa-doṣhaṁ vā bhavati (as it will either produce no untoward effects on the *doṣhas* or very minimal effects).

Here, Chakrapāṇi comments that the use of the term *sātmya* in fact indicates *okasātmya*. Charaka provides a template schedule to follow for discontinuing *okasātmya* and replacing it with *sātmya* in Cha. Sū. 7/36-37.

उचितादहिताद्धीमान् क्रमशो विरमेन्नरः |
हितं क्रमेण सेवेत क्रमश्चात्रोपदिश्यते ||३६||

च. सू. ७।३६

Uchitādahitāddhīmān kramaśho
viramennaraḥ |
Hitaṁ krameṇa seveta
kramaśhchātropadiśhyate ||36||

Cha. Sū. 7/36

An individual should become aware of improper habits and gradually relinquish them in favor of wholesome ones. This should be done according to the correct sequence, as explained next.

प्रक्षेपापचये ताभ्यां क्रमः पादांशिको भवेत्
|
एकान्तरं ततश्चोर्ध्वं द्व्यन्तरं त्र्यन्तरं तथा
||३७||

च. सू. ७।३७

Prakṣhepāpachaye tābhyāṁ kramaḥ
pādāṁśhiko bhavet | Ekāntaraṁ
tataśhchordhvaṁ dvyantaraṁ
tryantaraṁ tathā ||37||

Cha. Sū. 7/37

Initially, one quarter of the improper habit should be relinquinshed and replaced by an equivalent amount of wholesomeness. Next, half of the original improper habit should be relinquised and continued for double the amount of initial time. Next, three quarters of the improper habit should be relinquised and continued for double the amount of time. Finally the entire improper habit is relinquised.

क्रमेणापचिता दोषाः क्रमेणोपचिता गुणाः |
सन्तो यान्त्यपुनर्भावमप्रकम्प्या भवन्ति च ||३८||

च. सू. ७।३७

Kramenāpachitā doṣāḥ kramenopachitā guṇāḥ |
Santo yāntyapunarbhāvamaprakampyā bhavanti cha ||38||

Cha. Sū. 7/37

Slowly and gradually relinquishing improper habits and replacing them with wholesome practices prevents reverting and encourages permanent adoption.

Sātmya bheda

Sātmya is classified by Charaka and Suśhruta into various types according to the context in which it is used. Charaka additionally provides a basic methodology for measuring an individual's application of *sātmya* within the context of *rasa*. This is a useful aid in understanding and determining additional factors which contribute to *svastha*.

Charaka's classification of *sātmya* includes:

सप्तविधं तु रसैकैकत्वेन सर्वरसोपयोगाच्च ।

च. वि. १।२०

Saptavidhaṁ tu rasaikaikatvena sarvarasopayogāchcha |

Cha. Vi. 1/20

Saptavidhaṁ tu (It can be classified as seven types) rasa-eka ekatvena (one for each individual rasa), sarva rasa upayogāt cha (and a seventh for all the rasas together).

Suśhruta's classification of *sātmya* includes:

सात्म्यानि तु देशकालजात्यृतुरोगव्यायामोदकदिवास्वप्न रसप्रभृतीनि प्रकृतिविरुद्धान्यपि यान्यबाधकराणि भवन्ति ॥ ३९
यो रसः कल्यते यस्य सुखायैव निषेवितः ।
व्यायामजातमन्यद्वा तत् सात्म्यमिति निर्दिशेत् ॥

सु. सू. ३५।४०

Sātmyāni tu deśha-kāla-jāti-ṛtu-roga-vyāyāma-udaka-divāsvapna-rasa-prabhṛtīni prakṛti-viruddhānyapi yānyabādhakarāṇi bhavanti || 38
Yo rasaḥ kalyate yasya sukhāyaiva niṣhevitaḥ | Vyāyāma-jātam-anyadvā tat sātmyamiti nirdiśhet ||

Su. Sū. 35/38-39

Sātmyāni tu (*Sātmya* can be considered within the context of) deśha (external environment), kāla (time), jāti (race, ethnicity), ṛtu (season), roga (disease), vyāyāma (exercise, physical training), udaka (water), divāsvapna (day-sleep), rasa (flavors), prabhṛtīni (and other things which are continuously used). Prakṛti-viruddhānyapi yānyabādhakarāṇi bhavanti (Even though these may be *prakṛti-viruddhā* [contrary, or antagonistic to the *prakṛti*], they are not harmful).

Yo rasaḥ (That *rasa* [is considered *sātmya*]) kalyate yasya (which produces) sukhāyaiva (happiness, satisfaction, contentment) niṣhevitaḥ (even when continuously used). Vyāyāma (Exercise, physical training), jātam (predisposition based on ethnicity) anyadvā (and other factors) tat sātmyamiti nirdiśhet (should all be considered in this way to understand an individual's *sātmya*).

Suśhruta's classification of *sātmya* can be summarized in the following table.

Sātmya	Nearest English equivalent	Practical application and examples
Deśha	External environment	Certain geographical locations are more conducive to promoting *svastha*, like *sādhārana deśha*. Also, a specific *deśha* may also be *sātmya* for an individual because they are born and raised there.
Kāla	Time	Certain times are more conducive to promoting *svastha*, including specific stages of life, seasons, times of day, etc.
Jāti	Race, ethnicity	Certain tendencies can be more conducive to promoting *svastha* in general among ethnic groups, genetic subpopulations, communities or large families.
Ṛtu	Season	Certain seasons are more conducive to promoting *svastha* in specific individuals.
Roga	Disease	Diseases which may be incurable from birth or developed over time become an inseparable part of the individual.
Vyāyāma	Exercise, physical training	Certain types, methods, schedules and durations of physical activity are more conducive to promoting *svastha* in specific individuals. Also, certain individuals have a preset capacity for specific types or amounts of *vyāyāma*.
Udaka	Water	Certain types, sources, quantities or amounts of water consumption are more conducive to promoting *svastha* in specific individuals.
Divāsvapna	Day-sleep	Certain sleep schedules which include daytime napping or reversed sleep schedules (staying awake at night and sleeping during the day) can be more conducive to promoting *svastha* in specific individuals.
Rasa	Flavors	When the use of all six rasas in their proper proportion promotes *svastha*, it is considered as the highest level of *sātmya*. When regular use of a single rasa promotes *svastha*, it is considered the lowest level of *sātmya*, and two to five *rasas* are moderate. That rasa which is always satisfying and healthy for an individual is *sātmya*.

TEST YOURSELF

Learn, review and memorize key terms from this section.

sātmya

---

asātmya

---

okasātmya

PATHYA, APATHYA

Pathya and *apathya* convey meanings similar to *sātmya* and *asātmya* except that they are only used in the context of dietary items in therapeutic interventions. *Pathya* and *apathya* specifically indicate that which produces a positive or negative result for an individual when applied as a supportive component in a larger management protocol for a specific disorder.

Charaka defines *pathya* as:

पथ्यं पथोऽनपेतं यद्यच्चोक्तं मनसः प्रियम्
।

च. सू. २५।४४.५

Pathyaṁ pathy ‘ napetaṁ
yadyachchoktaṁ manasaḥ priyam |

Cha. Sū. 25/44.5

Pathyaṁ (*Pathya* includes) pathya anapetaṁ (those *dravya*, ie, substances, foods, medicines) yadyachchoktaṁ (which produce) manasaḥ (a mental state which) priyam (likes the *dravya* and desires more).

Classically, a cornerstone of successful management is the ability of the individual to associate a positive health outcome in their own state of being with the treatment being applied.

Individual, subjective response is considered as a very strong indicator of appropriate outcomes in Āyurvedic management. It is assumed that an individual's capacity to correctly and accurately understand the benefits of any *dravya* required that they have a clean, clear state of mind first.

Charaka defines *apathya* as:

यच्चाप्रियमपथ्यं च नियतं तन्न लक्ष्येत् ॥

च. सू. २५।४५

Yachchāpriyamapathyaṁ cha niyataṁ
tanna lakṣhyet ||

Cha. Sū. 25/45

Yat-cha (And that which causes) apriyam (dislike, deterrence) apathyaṁ ([is] *apathya*) cha niyataṁ tanna lakṣhyet (and it is known by recurrent features, signs and symptoms [of the *dravya* producing a negative result]).

Measuring outcomes of *pathya* and *apathya* are major components of regular clinical monitoring and can be primarily understood through assessing *agni*.

In Cha. Sū. 25/, Charaka provides two lists of the best known *pathya* and *apathya drayvas* at the time. These lists are categorized by dietary food groups. They are intended for generally healthy individuals and may be used in management protocols as appropriate. For example, in advanced states of vitiated *doṣhas*, certain *apathya dravyas* may be temporarily beneficial.

Cha. Sū. 25/		
Dietary food group	Pathya dravya	Apathya dravya
Śhūkadhānya Paddy having bristles	*Lohita śhāli* Red rice (Oryza sativa)	*Yavaka* Small barley (Hordeum vulgare)
Śhāmīdhānya Pulses	*Mudga* Green gram (Phaseolus mungo)	*Māṣha* Black gram Phaseolus radiatus
Udaka Drinking water	*Āntarikṣha* Rain water	*Varṣhānādeya* River water during rainy season
Lavaṇa Salts	*Saindhava* Rock salt	*Ūṣhara* Salt collected from saline soil
Śhākā Leafy greens, herbs	*Jīvantī* Leptadenia reticulata	*Sarṣhapa śhākā* Mustard leaves (greens)
Mṛga-māṁsa Meat of large forest animals	*Eṇa* Antelope	*Go māṁsa* Beef (cow's meat)
Pakṣhi-māṁsa Meat of birds	*Lāva* Common quail	*Kāṇakapota* Young dove, or pigeon
Vileśha-māṁsa Meat of reptiles	*Godhā* Iguana	*Bheka* Frog
Mastya-māṁsa Meat of fish	*Rohita* An unknown type of fish	*Chilichima* An unknown type of fish
Sarpi Ghees	*Gavya sarpi* Cow's ghee	*Avika sarpi* Sheep's ghee
Kṣhīra Milks	*Go kṣhīra* Cow's milk	*Avi kṣhīra* Sheep's milk
Sthāvara-jāta sneha Vegetable oils	*Tila taila* Sesame oil (Sesamum indicum)	*Kusumbha sneha* Kusumbha oil (Canthamus tinctorius)
Ānūpa-mṛga vasā Muscle fat of marshy animals	*Varāha vasā* Muscle fat of boar	*Mahiṣha vasā* Muscle fat of buffalo
Matsya vasā Muscle fat of fish	*Chulukī vasā* Muscle fat of Gangetic dolphin	*Kumbhīra vasā* Muscle fat of crocodile

Jalacharavihaṅga vasā Muscle fat of aquatic birds	*Pākahaṁsa vasā* Muscle fat of white swan	*Kākamadgu vasā* Muscle fat of water fowl
Viṣhkiraśhakuni vasā Muscle fat of gallinaceous birds	*Kukkuṭa vasā* Muscle fat of hen	*Caṭaka vasā* Muscle fat of sparrow
Śhākhāda medas Fat of branch-eating animals	*Aja medas* Fat of goat	*Hasti medas* Fat of elephant
Kandā Tubers (rhizomes and roots)	*Śhṛṅgavera* Ginger	*Nikucha* Atrocarpus nikucha
Phala Fruits	*Mṛdvīka* Grapes	*Āluka or mūlaka* Potato or radish
Ikṣhuvikāra Preparations of sugarcane	*Śharkara* Rock sugar	*Phāṇita* Quarter-reduced sugar

Following this list of *pathya* and *apathya*, Charaka then goes on to describe an extensive list of *dravya*, *karma* and *auṣhadha* (foods, activities and medicines) which are most effective at producing specific results. This list is commonly referred to as the *Agrya Auṣhadha*. It is one of several methods provided in the classics to aid practical application of the science in both preventative and curative efforts

TEST YOURSELF

Learn, review and memorize key terms from this section.

pathya

---

apathya

---

dravya

---

karma

---

auṣhadha

Agrya Auṣhadha

HITA, AHITA

The concepts of *hita* and *ahita* are explained in Cha. Sū. 25/31 during a lesson between the student, Agniveśha, and the teacher, Punarvasu Ātreya. Because these concepts have great range of depth and breadth, they can be challenging to understand initially. The discussion between teacher and student provides an excellent opportunity to understand the train of thought in the learning process.

In response to Agniveśha's question about the cause of growth of health versus disease, Punarvasu Ātreya explains the role of *hita āhāra*:

हिताहारोपयोग एकएव पुरुषवृद्धिकरो भवति,

च. सू. २५।३१

Hitāhāropayoga ekaeva puruṣhavṛddhikaro bhavati,

Cha. Sū. 25/31

Hita āhāra upayoga (Wholesome food when regularly consumed) ekaeva bhavati (is the primary factor for) puruṣha vṛddhi karo (causing growth in human beings).

Ahita āhāra is stated to be:

अहिताहारोपयोगः पुनर्व्याधिनिमित्तमिति ॥

च. सू. २५।३१

Ahitāhāropayogaḥ punarvyādhinimittamiti ||

Cha. Sū. 25/31

Ahita āhāra upayogaḥ (Unwholesome food when regularly consumed) punar-vyādhi nimittam iti (as mentioned earlier, is the cause for disease).

Agniveśha immediately recognizes that this cannot be considered a rule on its own because many other factors influence the final result of food items being *hita* or *ahita* depending on their quantity, timing, method of preparation, and more. This is validated by Punarvasu Ātreya and explained by considering *hita* and *ahita* as synonyms with *sama* and *viṣhama*.

Chakrapāṇi's commentary on this section provides valuable insight into practical examples which demonstrate the principles explained by the teacher.

Additional definitions provide insight into the specifics of the concepts of *hita* and *ahita*:

यत् किञ्चिद्दोषमास्राव्य न निर्हरति कायतः । आहारजातं तत् सर्वमहितायोपपद्यते ॥

च. सू. २६।८५

Yat kiñchiddoṣhamāsrāvya na nirharati kāyataḥ | Āhārajātaṁ tat sarvamahitāyopapadyate ||

Cha. Sū. 26/85

Āhārajātaṁ (Any *āhāra*, *dravya* or *auṣhadha*) kiñchid-doṣham-āsrāvya (which completely loosens or dislodges the *doṣhas*) na nirharati kāyataḥ (yet does not expel or eliminate them from the body) sarvam-ahitā-yopapadyate (should be considered *ahita*).

This definition is much more specific about the recognizable and measurable actions of *ahita dravya*. It demonstrates appropriate clinical application of the concept of *ahita* by providing a general rule for expected outcomes. Any *doṣha lakṣhaṇas* or *karmas* which indicate the presence of dislodged but non-expelled *doṣhas* can be considered in this scope. This practical application of this definition is more common with *auṣhadha* than *āhāra*.

The role of *hita* and *ahita* in the development of disease is explained as:

हिताहितोपयोगविशेषास्त्वत्र शुभाशुभविशेषकरा भवन्तीति ।

च. सू. २८।५

Hitāhitopayogaviśheṣhāstvatra śhubhāśhubhaviśheṣhakarā bhavantīti |

Cha. Sū. 28/5

Hita ahita upayoga (Regular consumption of wholesome or unwholesome foods) viśheṣhāstu atra (is the specific cause for) śhubha aśhubha viśheṣha karā (the specific or particular healthy or unhealthy growth of the body, ie, health or disease).

This statement carries particular significance because it is included in the explanation of the normal processes of *agni*. This is to reiterate that the *hita* or *ahita* quality of consumed foods is a major factor in determining the individual's state of *svastha*.

Charaka elaborates this concept by stating:

एवभ्यश्चैवापथ्याहारदोषशरीरविशेषेभ्यो
व्याधयो मृदवो दारुणाः
क्षिप्रसमुत्थाश्चिरकारिणश्च भवन्ति ।

च. सू. २८।७

Evabhyaśhchaivāpathyāhāradoṣhaśharī raviśheṣhebhyo vyādhayo mṛdavo dāruṇāḥ
kṣhiprasamutthāśhchirakāriṇaśhcha bhavanti |

Cha. Sū. 28/7

Apathya āhāra, doṣha, śharīra viśheṣhebhyo (The significant factors including unwholesome food, the *doṣhas*, and the specific condition of the body) bhavanti (produce) vyādhayo mṛdavo dāruṇāḥ (diseases of mild and severe nature) kṣhipra-samutthāśh-chira-kāriṇa-śhcha (and diseases of acute and chronic nature, and many other types and variations).

It is significant to note here that the effects of *pathya* and *apathya āhāra* may express themselves quickly or slowly depending on the co-existing factors which contribute to an individual's current state of *svastha*. Even though the right food may appear to reduce or alleviate health issues in certain situations, food alone is never considered the equivalent of *auṣadha* (medicine) in classical therapeutics.

TEST YOURSELF

Learn, review and memorize key terms from this section.

hita

---

ahita

āhāra

---

agni

SAMA, VIṢHAMA

Sama and *viṣhama* are provided as synonyms for *hita* and *ahita* to help explain the specific effects that are produced by each. These are explained during the lesson between Punarvasu Ātreya and Agniveśha.

समांश्चैव शरीरधातून् प्रकृतौ स्थापयति
विषमांश्च समीकरोतीत्येतद्धितं विद्धि,
विपरीतं त्वहितमिति;

च. सू. २५।३३

Samāṁśhchaiva śharīradhātūn prakṛtau sthāpayati viṣhamāṁśhcha saīkarotītyetaddhitaṁ viddhi, viparītaṁ tvahitamiti;

Cha. Sū. 25/33

Samāṁ-śhchaiva (And so *sama* is that which) śharīra-dhātūn-prakṛtau sthāpayati (holds up, maintains the *śharīra*, *dhātus* and *prakṛti*), viṣhamāṁ-śhcha saīkarotītyetaddhitaṁ viddhi (and promotes their normal states and eliminates the causes or presence of abnormality); viparītaṁ tu-ahitam-iti (the opposite is *ahita*, or *viṣhama*).

TEST YOURSELF

Learn, review and memorize key terms from this section.

sama

viṣhama

AROGYA, ROGI, ROGA

Arogya, *rogi* and *roga* originate from the Sanskrit *dhātu*, √ *ruj*, meaning to cause pain, afflict, injure, or cause to break. Modifications of this root result in several terms which are frequently used in the classics in the context of *svastha*.

Roga	Disease
Rogi	(The person who is) diseased, the patient, or person suffering
Arogya	Free from disease, having returned to normal health

These terms are frequently used in clinical management and applied therapeutics. They are also commonly seen in the context of Svastha Vṛtta to denote states of *svastha* or *asvastha*, and the individual involved.

TEST YOURSELF

Learn, review and memorize key terms from this section.

roga

rogi

arogya

√ ruj

Chapter 2: Review

ADDITIONAL READING

Read and review the references listed below to expand your understanding of the concepts in this chapter. Write down the date that you complete your reading for each. Remember that consistent repetition is the best way to learn. Plan to read each reference at least once now and expect to read it again as you continue your studies.

References marked with (skim) can be read quickly and do not require commentary review.

CLASSICS		1st read	2nd read
Charaka	Cha. Sū. 6/49 Cha. Sū. 25/31-33 Cha. Sū. 25/44-45 Cha. Sū. 26/85 Cha. Sū. 28/5-7 Cha. Vi. 1/19-20 Cha. Vi. 8/118 Cha. Śhā. 1/127		
Suśhruta	Su. Sū. 35/38-39		
Aṣhṭāṅga Hṛdaya			
Bhāva Prakāśha			

JOURNALS & CURRENT RESOURCES

QUESTIONS & ANSWERS

Record your questions for this chapter here for further research and discussion.

Question:

Answer:

Question:

Answer:

Question:

Answer:

SELF-ASSESSMENT

1. The two requirements for *sātmya* are that it
    a. acts as its own individual factor and a contributing factor
    b. must be used regularly
    c. produces a positive state of health
    d. provides insight to individual habits and cultural traditions
    e. Both B and C

2. The Sanskrit *dhātu* √ *ruj* means
    a. to be rough
    b. to be dry
    c. to carry
    d. to cause pain
    e. All of the above

3. *Sama* and *viṣhama* are synonyms for
    a. *pathya* and *apathya*
    b. *sātmya* and *asātmya*
    c. *sāma* and *nirāma*
    d. *hita* and *ahita*
    e. None of the above

4. What does an individual need to accurately understand the benefits of a *dravya* they've taken?
    a. A clean, clear state of mind
    b. *Divāsvapna*
    c. Good digestion and metabolism
    d. *Saṁhanana*
    e. All of the above

5. Suśhruta's *sātmya bheda* includes
    a. *kāla*
    b. *rasa*
    c. *udaka*
    d. *vyāyāma*
    e. All of the above

6. According to Charaka, *sātmya* is
    a. consuming things which make one feel better
    b. that which is suitable for an individual
    c. things that are used regularly
    d. All of the above
    e. None of the above

7. The *Agrya Auṣhadha* is a list that includes the 3 categories of
    a. *auṣhadha*, *rasa*, *āhāra*
    b. *dravya*, *āhara*, *auṣhadha*
    c. *dravya*, *auṣhadha*, *karma*
    d. *kāla*, *rasa*, *āhāra*
    e. *karma*, *guṇa*, *lakṣhaṇa*

8. The term *ahita* is more common with
    a. *āhāra* than *auṣhadha*
    b. *apathya* than *dravya*
    c. *pathya* than *apathya*
    d. *sātmya* than *asātmya*
    e. All of the above

9. Based on Charaka's list in Cha. Sū. 25/, what are some examples of *pathya dravya*?
    a. *Aja medas*, *ūṣhara*, *gavya sarpi*
    b. *Avika sarpi*, *lāva*, *godhā*
    c. *Gavya sarpi*, *go kṣhīra*, *tila taila*
    d. *Māsa*, *ena*, *lāva*
    e. *Yavaka*, *saindhava*, *phāṇita*

10. If a certain dravya always promotes one's *svastha*, it is
    a. *ahita*
    b. *apathya*
    c. *dhātu sāmya*
    d. *pathya*
    e. *sātmya*

CRITICAL THINKING

1. List three or more things which are *sātmya*, *okasātmya* and *asātmya* for you.

2. Using your examples above, classify their types according to Suśhruta's *sātmya bheda*.

3. Review Charaka's *Agrya Auṣhadha*. Do you find any *dravya* surprising?

4. Pick any one of Charaka's *Agrya Auṣhadha*, and research it's *guṇa* and *karma* profile in Cha. Sū. 27/.

5. Consider the meaning of *pathya*. Are you familiar with any home-remedies that would meet the definition of *pathya*?

Chapter 3 : Deśha

KEY TERMS

āhāra	ātura	deśha sātmya	sādhārana
āmayā	cheṣhṭa	janapadoddhvaṁśha	sama doṣha
ānūpa	deśha	jāṅgala	svapna

Classical Āyurvedic *siddhānta* provide a comprehensive and robust framework for understanding the influence of *deśha* on *svastha* and reliably interpreting the effects.

This chapter covers these classical perspectives in a thorough review. This is followed by an analysis of the principles which underlie the mechanisms of action of *deśha*. The chapter concludes with a review of current practical applications of *deśha* in common, modern environments.

CLASSICAL REVIEW

The term *deśha* is used classically in Āyurveda to refer to two main concepts.

Deśha can indicate:

1. The external environment
2. A location on the physical body for applying therapeutic intervention

Paribhāṣhā

Definition #1

Charaka defines the term's usage in both contexts in Cha. Vi. 8/92.

देशस्तु भूमिरातुरश्च ॥

च. वि. ८।९२

Deśhastu bhūmirāturaśhcha ||

Cha. Vi. 8/92

Deśhastu (The term *deśha* is used in the context of) bhūmiḥ (the earth, land, external environment), cha (and) ātura (the individual suffering from disease, the patient).

Definition #2

In context of *ātura*, Charaka further clarifies that *deśha* indicates the location for therapeutic application.

देशस्त्वधिष्ठानम् ॥

च. वि. ८।७५

Deśhastvadhiṣhṭhānam ||

Cha. Vi. 8/75

Deśha-stu (The term *deśha* explains) adhiṣhṭhāna (the location, specifically for application of therapy).

This should be understood as the location which is indicated for therapeutic treatment. This definition is provided within the context of the *daśha-vidha parikṣha* which must be assessed before initiating any therapeutic protocols.

Tri-deśha bheda and lakṣhaṇas

All classical authors specify three types of *deśha* as environmental locations.

Deśha bheda:

Jāṅgala	Dry, arid, desert-like
Ānūpa	Damp, humid, marshy
Sādhārana	Moderate, neither too wet nor too dry

Each type is described in detail according to the author's geographical scope. Most of the classical descriptions are specific to the Indian-subcontinent and reflect predominant features found at the time of writing. These specific features highlight prevalent flora and fauna and climate patterns of the time.

Many of the species mentioned depend on characteristics of the geographical location and delicate climate conditions. Additionally, the *lakṣhaṇas* mentioned in each type of *deśha* may have limited application in other geographical regions. Still, a careful review and analysis of their qualities and features is worthwhile as it provides a more comprehensive understanding of how the science of Āyurveda was practically applied within the context of environmental conditions in the Indian subcontinent during its time.

Suśhruta provides a more general description of *deśha* while Charaka adds specific flora and fauna. Bhāvamiśhra documents information compiled from several sources.

Compare the references using the following charts.

Jāṅgala deśha lakṣhaṇas Characteristics of dry external environments	Cha. Ka. 1/8	Su. Sū. 35/42	BP. Pū. 4/85-86
Ākāśha sama The sky is level with the ground; wide, open plains	✓	✓	✓
Pravirala alpa kaṇṭika vṛkṣha prāyas Trees are usually sparse, few, and thorny		✓	✓
Alpa varṣha prasravaṇa udapāna udaka prāyas Rain, springs and wells usually have less water		✓	✓
Uṣhṇa dāruṇa vāta Winds are hot and harsh		✓	
Pravirala alpa śhaila Mountains are sparse and low		✓	
Sthira kṛśha śharīra manuṣhya prāyas Physical bodies of most people are usually firm and thin		✓	
Vāta pitta roga bhūyiṣhṭha Diseases of vāta and pitta are common	✓	✓	✓
Tarubhirapi cha - kadara, khadira, asana, aśhva-karṇa, dhava, tiniśha, śhallakī, sāla, soma-valka, badarī, tinduka, aśhvattha, vaṭa, āmalakī Deep forests of trees (as listed)	✓		
Aneka śhamī, kakubha, śhiṁśhapā prāya Large groups of common trees (as listed)	✓		

Jāṅgala deśha lakṣhaṇas Characteristics of dry external environments	Cha. Ka. 1/8	Su. Sū. 35/42	BP. Pū. 4/85-86
Sthira śhuṣhka pavana bala vidhūyamāna pranṛtyat taruṇa viṭapa Continuous, dry winds cause the tender branches of these trees to dance and sway	✓		
Pratata mṛga tṛṣhṇi kopa gūḍha tanu khara paruṣha sikatā śharkarā bahutna Abundant in thin, dry, rough sand and gravel creating mirages	✓		
Lāva tittiri cakora anucarita bhūmi bhāga Inhabited by birds like varieties of partridges	✓		
Sthira kaṭhina manuṣhya prāyas Physical bodies of most people are usually stable (sturdy) and hard	✓		
Hariṇa eṇa kṣhapṛṣhata gokarṇa khara saṅkula Many animals like antelope, deer, bucks, donkeys			✓
Susvādu phala Many pleasantly sweet fruits			✓
Vātala A natural disposition to aggravated *vāta* often encouraging disorders of *vāta*			✓

Ānūpa deśha lakṣhaṇas Characteristics of damp external environments	Cha. Ka. 1/8	Su. Sū. 35/42	BP. Pū. 4/81-84
Bahu udaka Abundant water		√	√
Nimna unnata The ground (land) is depressed (low, sunken) and raised (elevated)		√	
Nadī varṣha gahano Many rivers and abundant rainfall create dense, thick and impenetrable forests, thickets and woods		√	
Mṛdu śhīta anila Soft (mild) and cool breeze		√	
Bahu mahā parvata vṛkṣha Many mountains and big (great, old) trees		√	√
Mṛdu sukumāra upachita śharīra manuṣhya prāyas Physical bodies of most people are usually soft, tender and well-developed		√	
Kapha vāta roga bhūyiṣhṭha Diseases of kapha and vāta are common	√	√	√
Hintāla tamāla nārikela kadalī vana gahana Deep forests of trees (as listed), including Crataeva roxburghii, coconut and banana	√		
Sarit samudra paryanta prāyas Generally located along rivers, near the sea	√		
Śhiśhira pavana bahutna Often has a heavy cool, refreshing breeze	√		
Vañjula vānīra upaśhobhitatīrābhi saridbhirupagata bhūmi bhāga Nearby rivers are adorned with beautiful plants (as listed)	√		
Kṣhitidhara nikuñja upaśhobhita Mountains covered with beautiful creepers	√		
Manda pavana anuvījita kṣhitiruha gahana Gentle breeze blows through thick, swaying forests	√		
Aneka vana rājī puṣhpita vana gahana bhūmi bhāga Many varieties of beautiful, flowering trees in thick forests	√		√

Ānūpa deśha lakṣhaṇas Characteristics of damp external environments	Cha. Ka. 1/8	Su. Sū. 35/42	BP. Pū. 4/81-84
Snigdha taru pratāna upagūḍha Covered with trees having thick, spreading branches	√		
Haṁsa chakravāka balākā nandīmukha puṇḍarīka kādamba mudgu bhṛṅgarāja śhatapatra matta kokila anunādi taru viṭapa Sounds of birds like swans, a type of female bird, cranes, and others (as listed)	√		√
Sukumāra puruṣha People are gentle and of tender build	√		
Śhaśha vārāha mahiṣha ururohikulākula Animals like rabbits, boars, elephants, deer and duck			√

Sādhārana deśha lakṣhaṇas Characteristics of moderate external environments	Cha. Ka. 1/8	Su. Sū. 35/42-43	BP. Pū. 4/88
Ubhaya deśha lakṣhaṇa Features and characteristics of both environments		√	
Sama śhīta varṣha uṣhma māruta Cold, rain, heat and wind are generally moderate		√	√
Doṣhāṇā samatā Doṣhas are generally in a state of equilibrium		√	√
Dvayordeśhayorvīrud vanaspati vānaspatya śhakunimṛ gagaṇayuta Creepers, trees having fruits without flowers, trees having fruits and flowers, birds and animals as described in the other two environments	√		
Sthira sukumāra bala varṇa saṁhanana upapanna sādhāraṇa guṇa yukta puruṣha People from this environment are generally sturdy (stable), tender, strong, have good complexion, proper bodily structure	√		

Vaikṛta lakṣhaṇas and janapadoddhvaṁśha

In contrast to the normal *deśha lakṣhaṇas*, Charaka explains in Cha. Vi. 3/3-23 that a *deśha* may be subject to the effects of *vaikṛta lakṣhaṇas*. This occurs when there are irregularities and vitiation in four areas that indicate increasing danger and intensity of vitiation.

Vaikṛta deśha lakṣhaṇas are due to:

Vāyu	air
Udaka	water
Deśha	land, environment
Kāla	time, season

These four constitute the common factors which can affect all inhabitants of a specific area to negatively impact health. From a classical perspective, this is quite different from the more common, fundamental rules which state that health is largely individual and influenced primarily by one's diet and activities. Because the four factors of *vāyu*, *udaka*, *deśha* and *kāla* have the potential for large scale impact, they are grouped under a concept called *janapadoddhvaṁśha*, which can also be translated as epidemics.

In Cha. Vi. 3/19-20, Agniveśha enquires about the underlying reasons and causes for the manifestation of epidemics. Punarvasu Ātreya answers this by stating:

तस्य मूलमधर्मः, तन्मूलं वाऽसत्कर्म पूर्वकृतं; तयोर्योनिः प्रज्ञापराध एव ।

च. वि. ३।२०

Tasya mūlamadharmaḥ, tanmūlaṁ vā ' satkarma pūrvakṛtaṁ; tayoryoniḥ prajñāparādha eva |

Cha. Vi. 3/20

Adharma (Going or acting against *dharma*) is the mūla (root cause), vā (or), tanmūlaṁ (the root cause is) asatkarma pūrvakṛtaṁ (untruthful actions done previously); tayoryoniḥ (ultimately, the root cause of both is) prajñāparādha eva (acting against one's consciousness, or better judgement).

This explanation goes on to state that a sufficient momentum may be reached by rulers of states and countries continuously engaging in egregious behavior and actions resulting in the loss of any accumulation of benefits from previous positive actions. This has the potential to put the entire population at risk. Seasonal impairment is common at this point which negatively impacts all life forms. *Vaikṛta lakṣhaṇas* are then seen at all levels of *vāyu*, *udaka*, *deśha* and *kāla*.

Additionally, these four are explained to be more dangerous to the population in increasing order. Each of these four is progressively more difficult to prevent and correct. Chakrapāṇi explains this in detail in the commentary of Cha. Vi. 3/9-11. Review the *vaikṛta lakṣhaṇas* of each of the four in Cha. Vi. 3/7-8.

Suśhruta provides a similar perspective in Su. Sū. 6/15-20 where he explains that seasonal deviations, which may not always fall under the category of epidemics, can be responsible for a variety of problems through the food chain. When the seasons are not demonstrating their normal characteristics of *śhīta*, *uṣhṇa*, *vāta* and *vārṣha* (cold, heat, wind and rain), then the resulting abnormalities negatively affect the water and growth of plants and subsequently, herbal medicines. However, when the seasons remain normal, they produce water and plants which are beneficial for the people of the location. This directly results in an increase in *prāṇa*, *āyu*, *bala*, *vīrya* and *ojas*.

Understanding the effects of deśha

Charaka succinctly explains the characteristics and effects of *deśha* in Cha. Vi. 3/47-48. Although this appears to be an interpolated line, it still provides a valuable perspective to understand the relationship between environment and disease.

अल्पोदकद्रुमो यस्तु प्रवातः प्रचुरातपः ।
ज्ञेयः स जाङ्गलो देशः स्वल्परोगतमोऽपि च ॥ ४७
प्रचुरोदकवृक्षो यो निवातो दुर्लभातपः ।
अनूपो बहुदोषश्च समः साधारणो मतः ॥
च. वि. ३।४८

Alpodakadrumo yastu pravātaḥ prachurātapaḥ |
Jñeyaḥ sa jāṅgalo deśhaḥ svalparogatamo ' pi cha || 47
Prachurodakavṛkṣho yo nivāto durlabhātapaḥ |
Anūpo bahudoṣhaśhcha samaḥ sādhārаṇo mataḥ ||
Cha. Vi. 3/47-48

Alpa (Less) udaka (water) drumo ([and] trees), yastu pravātaḥ (and more air, wind) prachura ātapaḥ (and more sun) jñeyaḥ sa (is known to be found in) jāṅgalo deśhaḥ (*jāṅgala deśha*, or a dry external environment) svalpa (and fewer) rogatamo (diseases of strong nature) api cha (are seen here).

Prachura (More) udaka (water) vṛkṣho (and trees which produce fruit and other useful products) yo nivāto (along with less or little wind, breeze) durlabhātapaḥ (and less direct sunlight) anūpo ([is found in] *ānūpa deśha*, or a wet external environment) bahu doṣhaśhcha (and many diseases, as well as diseases of strong nature [are found here]).

Samaḥ (Moderate environments [are known as]) sādhārаṇo (*sādhārana deśha*) mataḥ (which promote a moderate, normal or healthy state of the *doṣhas*).

TEST YOURSELF

Learn, review and memorize key terms from this section.

deśha
____

ātura
____

jāṅgala
____

ānūpa
____

sādhārana
____

janapad-oddhvaṁśha
____

KEY PRINCIPLES

The main principles described classically include the general assessment of the *deśha* along with methodologies to manage its effects appropriately. Management may include general adjustments for the *deśha* and specific adjustments for the individual.

In order to effectively manage the effects of a *deśha*, a thorough assessment is required to identify its type. This can be accomplished through reviewing the characteristics of the environment in detail. Once the *deśha* is determined, appropriate techniques may be employed to negate its detrimental effects.

Principle #1: Deśha assessment

Deśha assessment can be performed following classical guidance as described in Cha. Ka. 1/8, Su. Su. 35/42-45 and BP Pū. 4/81-88. These *lakṣhaṇas* are tabulated in detail earlier in this chapter.

Deśha assessment is summarized in the following table.

General *lakṣhaṇas*	*Jāṅgala deśha* Dry environment	*Sādhārana deśha* Moderate environment	*Ānūpa deśha* Damp environment
Sun	More	Moderate	Less
Wind	Hot, harsh, dry, steady	Features of both	Soft, cool breezes
Water (rain)	Less	Moderate	More
Water (humidity)	Less	Moderate	More
Water (lakes, rivers, etc)	Less	Moderate	More
Topography	Sparse, low mountains; flat plains, open sky	Features of both	Many mountains; undulating plains
Vegetation	Sparse, few, thorny	Features of both	Deep forests; productive trees
General human build	Thin, stable, sturdy, hard	Features of both	Bulky, thick, delicate, gentle, well-developed
Effect on *doṣhas*	More *vāta*, *pitta*	Promotes *sama doṣha*	More *kapha*, *vāta*
Diseases	Less severe	Moderate	More severe

Deśha assessment intends to assess the environment that is the primary location for the individual. Classically, this was practically seen to involve the greater, external environment outside of the home or resident space. Today, many individuals spend larger portions of their time inside controlled environments where light, temperature, humidity and other external factors are regulated.

To accurately understand an individual's *deśha* in modern environments such as these, two assessments are often required. First, the external environment should be assessed, followed by the immediate environment where the invidual spends the majority of their time. Both of these contribute to the indivudal's *deśha sātmya* and their current state of *svastha*.

Principle #2: General management

Certain features of each *deśha* may present challenges to maintaining *sama doṣha* and promoting *svastha* for all inhabitants. In these situations, adjustments and modifications can be made to reduce the negative effects of the *deśha*. This is most often seen practically in the classics through recommendations found in *ṛtu chārya*, or seasonal management.

In the context of *hemanta ṛtu chārya* (regimens for the winter season), Vāgbhaṭa provides a relevant recommendation that describes modifying the immediate environment to stabilize and promote *svastha*. This reference demonstrates that an individual's immediate environment or resident space could be modified accordingly.

अङ्गारतापसन्तप्तगर्भभूवेश्मचारिणः ।
शीतपारुष्यजनितो न दोषो जातु जायते ॥ १६

अ. हृ. सू. ३।१६

Aṅgāratāpasantaptagarbhabhūveśhmachāriṇaḥ |
Śhītapāruṣhyajanito na doṣho jātu jāyate || 16

AH Sū. 3/16

Aṅgāra-tāpa (Heated by coal or charcoal) santapta ([which is] burned) garbha-bhūveśhma (inside the innermost chambers of the dwelling) chāriṇaḥ (on a regular, daily basis) jāyate (wins over, negates) śhīta (the cold) pāruṣhya (and dryness) janito (produced [during the winter season]) na doṣho jātu (to avoid generating any *doṣhas*).

Similarly, cooling measures and adaptations through application of water and fans ae recommended during the summer. It is important to note here that these types of modifications of the individual's immediate environment or resident space are intended to be adjusted throughout the course of the year in response to changing conditions of the greater external environment.

Ultimately, general management of the immediate environment can be made by applying any modifications required for light, temperature, humidity and other factors.

Principle #3: Individual management

At the most personalized level, an individual can modify their immediate environment to suit their specific needs based on any factor or requirement for their current state of *svastha*. Modifications that are prioritized based on these needs often outweigh the general management protocols intended for those in a normal state of *svastha*.

Suśhruta describes a simple, generic method for counteracting the negative effects of *deśha* in general based on an individual's disease. He states:

उचिते वर्तमानस्य नास्ति देशकृतं भयम् ।
आहारस्वप्नचेष्टादौ तद्देशस्य गुणे सति ॥

सु. सू. ३५।४५

Uchite vartamānasya nāsti deśhakṛtaṁ bhayam | Āhārasvapnacheṣhṭādau taddeśhasya guṇe sati ||

Su. Sū. 35/45

Uchite (The correct) vartamānasya (methods of living) nāsti (do not) bhayam (create fear or anxiety [of destabilizing health]) deśha-kṛtaṁ (when they are formulated inline with the external environment [by ensuring that]) āhāra (food and diet), svapna (sleep), cheṣhṭādau (and all habits, regimens and activities) guṇe sati (oppose or offset the characteristics) tad-deśhasya (of the external environment).

For an individual with a recognized pathology, a change in their *deśha* can promote and support the normalization and healing processes by offseting the *guṇas* involved. To further strengthen this therapeutic effect, the characteristics of *āhāra*, *svapna*, and *cheṣhṭa* can also be customized to reduce negative effects of the disorder and support reestablishment of *sama doṣha*.

Charaka provides a similar statement in Cha. Sū. 6/50.

देशानामामयानां च विपरीतगुणं गुणैः ।
सात्म्यमिच्छन्ति सात्म्यज्ञाश्चेष्टितं चाद्यमेव च ॥

च. सू. ६।५०

Deśhānāmāmayānāṁ cha
viparītaguṇaṁ guṇaiḥ |
Sātmyamichchhanti
sātmyajñāśhcheṣhṭitaṁ chādyameva
cha ||

Cha. Sū. 6/50

Deśha-ānāmāmayānāṁ cha (According to the external environment and the disease of the individual), viparīta-guṇaṁ (the opposite characteristics of these conditions) guṇaiḥ (should be employed as the characteristics for regular usage) sātmyam ichchhanti ([which the individual should learn to] desire on a regular, habitual basis) sātmya (to create stability and regularity) jñāśh (with these known) cheṣhṭitaṁ (activities, habits, routines) chādyameva cha (and all of the other components, including food and sleep).

Chakrapāṇi elaborates on this principle and provides examples demonstrating how the effects of the *deśha* should influence the choices of the individual in maintaining *svastha*. For example, if a person lives in a very cold place, they would have to offset the cold with heat.

An individual living in *ānupa deśha* and having disorders that are similar to the environment would need to adapt to regularly consuming food of opposite qualities like meat of animals from *jāṅgala deśha* for their dry and light *guṇas*.

This method of individual management based on *deśha* and *āmayā* (disease) demonstrates the application of an opposite approach compared to the standard recommendations for an individual in a state of *svastha*.

Recommendations for modifications of an individual's environment based on disease have been utilized throughout the history of medicine. Notably, during the 19th century, Western medical physicians often recommended that tuberculosis patients relocate to moderately high altitudes with drier climates. A recent epidemiological study found a statistically significant incidence of the disorder in specific geographical climates that correlates and supports these recommendations. Further research is required to demonstrate connections between environment and states of health.

TEST YOURSELF

Learn, review and memorize key terms from this section.

deśha sātmya

---

sama doṣha

āhāra

---

svapna

---

cheṣhṭa

āmayā

DEŚHA ASSESSMENT

Today, the classical knowledge of *deśha* can be applied successfully to determine the type of environment and its appropriate modifications for promoting *svastha*.

The general rules and descriptions found in the classics are sufficient to guide the creation of specific rules that are applicable in a variety of geographical locations outside of the Indian subcontinent.

Not only do the presentations of *deśha* vary considerably in different locations, but modern technology has also insulated many people from direct effects of their *deśha* by providing wider availability of climate control systems with complete heating and cooling available year-round.

The distinct effects of these systems must also be considered when analyzing the current effects of *deśha* on individuals especially when significant portions of time are spent in these types of controlled environments.

A thorough *deśha* assessment is a required component of each complete Clinical Svastha Assessment. *Deśha* assessment includes two areas to review.

External environment – the larger, outdoor environment that surrounds the individual

Dwelling environment – the immediate environment or resident space where the individual spends a significant portion of their time regularly

Assessing external environments

The three major classifications of *deśha* (*ānūpa*, *jāṅgala* and *sādhārana*) provide the basis for general external classification. These primarily analyze water content in the environment as ground saturation, precipitation (rainfall, snowfall, sleet, hail, etc.) and suspended moisture in the atmosphere, or humidity.

The classics do not clearly explain the implications of each of these forms of water presence in specific ways, however, that knowledge may be inferred based on the specific conditions of the location.

Today, research is required to fully understand these variations and determine how to measure their effects for reliable, predictable classification methods.

A basic assessment model for *deśha* in new locations can be created using the general classical rules. This model includes assessment parameters and measurable outcomes based on light, wind and three types of water presence - ground saturation, precipitation and humidity.

Additionally, the classical *deśha lakṣhaṇas* must be adjusted to incorporate local flora and fauna which accurately represents the type of *deśha*. Advanced assessment models for *deśha* can then incorporate parameters which require longer-term study, such as the prevalent *doṣhas* and predispositions to disease in the local region.

Deśha assessment may be performed in multiple ways depending on the resources available for assessment. In its simplest, most accessible format, *deśha* can be assessed according to the individual's responses to questions that approximate the influence of sun, wind and water in the area.

This method is often sufficient to provide the basic information needed for a basic classification of *ānūpa*, *jāṅgala* and *sādhārana*. At an advanced level, long-term climate data can be analyzed statistically to determine actual numbers of sunny days, cloudy days, precipitation days and other indicators that can more definitively demonstrate the scientific reasoning for the *deśha*'s classification.

For the Clinical Svastha Assessment, the *deśha* component can be determined for locations in the United States based on a general classification of the country. This can be supplemented by the individual's assessment of their specific location to account for microclimates and other special local conditions.

Use the table and questions on the following page to perform a *deśha* assessment.

Clinical Svastha Assessment: *Deśha*

Approximate the individual's location to estimate their predicted *deśha*. Answer these additional questions to further evaluate the specific location.

1. Choose the most appropriate answer for each assessment criteria.
2. Count the number of responses in each column to determine the total. The column with the highest count is the assessed *deśha* for the location.
3. Correlate this result with the expected results based on the actual location.

Question	Response			
Location (city, state, zip code)				
Latitude, longitude				
Altitude				
Zone	Subtropical	Temperate		
General topography	Coastal	Plains	Forest	Mountains
Located in a microclimate?	Yes	No	Unsure	
Local residential area	Urban	Suburban	Rural	
Predicted *deśha*	*Jāṅgala*	*Ānūpa*	*Sādhārana*	

Assessment criteria	*Jāṅgala*	*Ānūpa*	*Sādhārana*
Is it generally sunny?	More often	Less often	Moderately
What are the winds usually like?	Hot, harsh, dry, steady	Soft, cool breezes	Features of both
How often does it rain?	Infrequently	Frequently	Moderately
Is it generally humid?	Infrequently	Frequently	Moderately
Are there natural water bodies nearby?	Few	Many	Moderate
What is the topography like?	Sparse, low mountains; flat plains, open sky	Many mountains or hills; undulating plains	Features of both
What is the vegetation generally like?	Sparse, few, thorny	Deep forests; productive trees	Features of both
Total count			
Assessed *deśha*	*Jāṅgala*	*Ānūpa*	*Sādhārana*

Assessing dwelling environments

The widespread use of heating and cooling systems affects a large majority of the modern, urban world today, especially in Westernized countries. Climate control systems that regulate heating, cooling and humidity proliferate in homes, offices, shopping centers, indoor recreation areas and almost every enclosed building. This insulates inhabitants from fully experiencing the effects of the *deśha* and changes caused by the annual *ṛtu* cycles. This likely impacts the normal, expected cycles of *doṣhas* in *chaya*, *prakopa* and *praśhamana*. The changes that may result can be unexpected, varied and unpredictable.

A thorough understanding of how these heating and cooling systems work from a classical Āyurvedic perspective will help make their effects more recognizable.

Review the following tables and common methods of heating and cooling. Notice their typical results in terms of the *guṇas* affected. These general results can be altered and customized further, depending on the situation.

For example, in homes heated by steam radiators or wood stoves, a wide, shallow pan of water can be placed on top of the heating element to evaporate the water slowly. This increases the ambient humidity and offsets some of the dryness produced by the heat.

Humidifiers, plants, cooking and showers may also add small amounts of humidity to local areas within a home or dwelling. All of these should be reviewed during a thorough, Clinical Svastha Assessment to fully understand the immediate environment and living conditions of the individual.

Heating systems, methods, examples		Rūkṣha	Snigdha	Laghu	Guru	Cala	Sthira
Forced hot air Air is heated directly then circulated through ventilation ducts.							
	Gas furnace	++		++		++	
	Oil furnace	+++		++		++	
	Space heaters with blowers	+++		+++		+++	
Convection Air is heated and circulated slowly by air movement based on temperature differences. Heating elements that heat up quickly also cool quickly.							
	Electric baseboards	++		++		++	
	Space heaters (ceramic)	++		++		+	
	Portable oil-filled radiators	++		+	+	+	+
	Non-steam radiators	++		+	+	+	+
	Steam radiators		+		+	+	
Radiant Heats cooler objects directly							
	Radiant floor heating with hot water tubes	+		+	+	+	+
	Hydronic baseboards	+		+	+	+	+
	Wood and pellet stoves	+	+	+	+	++	
	Infrared heaters		++		++		++

Cooling systems, methods, examples		Rūkṣha	Snigdha	Laghu	Guru	Cala	Sthira
Air conditioning Air is cooled and dehumidified directly then circulated through ventilation ducts.							
	Evaporative water cooler		++		++	+	
	Single room a/c	++		+	+	++	
	Central a/c	++		+	+	+	

Key: + = Mild increase ++ = Moderate increase +++ = Large increase

The effects described above apply to the area that these heating and cooling methods are able to control. These effects should then transfer to the individuals present in those controlled environments. This does not mean, however, that each person in the controlled environment will realize and experience these effects in the same way. Each individual's unique state of *svastha* will have a direct impact on their experience.

When applying the rules and logic of the classical Āyurvedic principles, it must be remembered that each factor can influence the outcome of other factors, and vice versa. Performing an assessment of an individual's *deśha* and its effects on their overall level of *svastha* requires understanding the complete presentation from the following aspects:

1. Independent assessment of the *deśha*
2. Known, expected effects of the *deśha* on specific types of individuals (largely based on *prakṛti*)
3. Complete assessment of the individual with outcomes for all factors
4. Logical deduction of the influence of the *deśha* on the individual's state of *svastha*

This application of *yukti* applies to each of the factors being assessed. In the remaining chapters throughout this textbook, look for ways to use all of the types of *pramāṇa* within each component of the assessment.

Chapter 3: Review

ADDITIONAL READING

Read and review the references listed below to expand your understanding of the concepts in this chapter. Write down the date that you complete your reading for each. Remember that consistent repetition is the best way to learn. Plan to read each reference at least once now and expect to read it again as you continue your studies.

References marked with (skim) can be read quickly and do not require commentary review.

CLASSICS		1st read	2nd read
Charaka	Cha. Sū. 6/50 Cha. Vi. 3/ Cha. Vi. 8/75 Cha. Vi. 8/92 Cha. Ka. 1/8		
Suśhruta	Su. Sū. 35/42-45		
Aṣhṭāṅga Hṛdaya	AH Sū. 3/16		
Bhāva Prakāśha	BP. Pū. 4/81-88		

JOURNALS & CURRENT RESOURCES

https://www.saveonenergy.com/climate-equivalences/

https://www.atsjournals.org/doi/full/10.1164/rccm.201311-2043OE

https://www.ncbi.nlm.nih.gov/pmc/articles/PMC4822399/

QUESTIONS & ANSWERS

Record your questions for this chapter here for further research and discussion.

Question:

Answer:

Question:

Answer:

Question:

Answer:

SELF-ASSESSMENT

1. Why are the classical explanations of *deśha* limited in application?
    a. Many species are specific to certain locations.
    b. Most descriptions are specific to the Indian subcontinent.
    c. The *deśha lakṣhaṇas* are limited for other geographic regions.
    d. They highlight the prevalent flora and fauna of the time.
    e. All of the above

2. How is classical information on *deśha* relevant today?
    a. It explains how the science of Āyurveda was applied.
    b. It provides such specific details.
    c. The present-day geography is the same.
    d. All of the above
    e. None of the above

3. What are the two *jāṅgala lakṣhaṇas* shared by Charaka, Suśhruta and Bhāva Prakāśha?
    a. *Sthira kaṭhina manuṣhya prāyas* and *susvādu phala*
    b. *Susvādu phala* and *pravirala alpa śhaila*
    c. *Uṣhṇa*, *dāruṇa vāta* and *ākāśha sama*
    d. *Vāta*, *pitta roga bhūyiṣhṭha* and *ākāśha sama*
    e. *Vātala* and *aneka*, *śhamī kakubha*, *śhiṁśhapā prāya*

4. If a *deśha* has *bahu udaka*, *bahu mahā parvata vṛkṣha* and *snigdha taru pratāna upagūḍha*, it would be called
    a. *ānupa deśha*
    b. *jāṅgala deśha*
    c. *sādhārana deśha*
    d. *sātmya deśha*
    e. None of the above

5. Which classical factors indicate that health is not just about diet and activity?
    a. *Kāla lakṣhaṇas*
    b. *Udaka lakṣhaṇas*
    c. *Vaikṛta deśha lakṣhaṇas*
    d. *Vāyu lakṣhaṇas*
    e. None of the above

6. According to Punarvasu Ātreya, the root cause for *janapadoddhvaṁśha* is
    a. Acting against *dharma*
    b. Acting against one's consciousness
    c. Epidemics
    d. Previous, untruthful actions
    e. All of the above

7. Suśhruta mentions seasonal deviations that can result in abnormalities. What are these deviations?
    a. *Śhīta*
    b. *Uṣhṇa*
    c. *Vārṣha*
    d. *Vāta*
    e. All of the above

8. What is the best way to address the challenges of *deśha* in order to maintain *sama doṣha*?
    a. *Agni*
    b. Relocate to a different *deśha* during the year
    c. *Ṛtu carya*
    d. *Svastha*
    e. All of the above

9. According to this chapter, which heating system does not increase *rūkṣha*?
    a. Ceramic space heaters
    b. Electric baseboards
    c. Gas furnace
    d. Infrared heaters
    e. None of the above

10. Which *siddhānta* most thoroughly explains Chakrapani's reasoning and examples for maintaining *svastha* in a particular *deśha*?
    a. *Kārya-kāraṇa bhāva*
    b. *Loka-puruśha sāmya*
    c. *Samavāya-samavāyi*
    d. *Saṁyoga-vibhāga*
    e. *Samanya-viśheṣha*

CRITICAL THINKING

1. Think about your immedate local geographical region (within a radius of 5 miles). How would you classify this and why?
2. Think about your larger geographical region (within a radius of 100 miles). How would you classify this and why?
3. Using the map of the United Sates, shade the areas of *ānupa*, *jāṅgala* and *sādhārana deśhas*.
4. Explain what is practically observed in geographical areas that transition from one *deśha* to another.
5. Consider the types of ventilation and air conditioning systems that you commonly use. How do these affect your living environment?

Chapter 4 : Kāla and ṛtu

KEY TERMS

ādāna kāla	grīṣhma	ṛtu	uṣhṇa
agneya	hemanta	ṛtu sandhi	uttarāyana
agni	kāla	śhamā	vamana
ahorātri	kāla chakra	śharad	varṣha
ayana	kopa	saumya	varṣhā
ayana sandhi	māsa	śhiśhira	vasanta
basti	muhūrta	śhīta	vāyu
chaya	pariṇāma	śhodhana	virechana
dakṣhiṇāyana	prāvṛt	soma	visarga kāla
dina	rātri		

The concept of *kāla* in Āyurveda is wide and pervasive. It influences all aspects of life, health and treatment. It is a common factor which exerts its control over everything in the world and it has been recognized in many streams of Vedic sciences throughout history.

Within the context of Āyurveda, *kāla* is considered using specific divisions which are applicable to the practice of the science. These measurements are often found throughout classical references with instructions for preparing medicinal formulations and applying clinical treatments.

The effects of *kāla* connect every aspect of life and ultimately health. Due to the influences of time on the environment and all living things, specific guidelines and recommendations were detailed in the classics to help prevent disease and promote health. These guidelines highlight the importance of doing certain activities at specific times to support the body and mind to be synchronized with the natural cycles and rhythms of time.

This chapter covers the fundamental knowledge of *kāla*, its classifications, functions and classical descriptions in the context of the year, seasons, days and nights. It includes recommendations for health-promoting regimens and routines from classical perspectives to provide a basis for understanding the application of the science in a known environment. Key principles derived from this knowledge are reviewed at the end of the chapter followed by a discussion of their practical application today.

CLASSICAL REVIEW

In classical Āyurvedic literature, time is generally known by two terms, *kāla* and *pariṇāma*. Although these can both be translated as time, they convey distinct meanings. *Kāla* has a wider scope to indicate time in any measurable form. *Pariṇāma* refers to the transformation caused by the passage of time. In this respect, *pariṇāma* often refers to the conversion of one thing into another form.

Paribhāṣhā

Definition #1:

In the context of explaining *rasa* and its appropriate usage in food consumption, Charaka defines *kāla* as *nityaga* and *avasthika*.

कालो हि नित्यगश्चावस्थिकश्च; तत्रावस्थिको विकारमपेक्षते, नित्यगस्तु ऋतुसात्म्यापेक्षः ॥

च. वि. १।२२(४)

Kālo hi nityagaśhchāvasthikaśhcha; tatrāvasthiko vikāramapekṣhate, nityagastu ṛtusātmyāpekṣhaḥ ||

Cha. Vi. 1/22(4)

Kālo hi (Kāla refers to) nityagaśhcha (that which is constantly going little by little, ie, time in the form of day and night) avasthikaśhcha (and stages [of life, states of health, stages of disease, etc]); tatra (and generally) avasthiko (avasthika, ie, considering time in the course of stages or phases) vikāram apekṣhate (is used in the context of diseases), nityagastu (while nityaga, ie, considering time in the course of a continous wheel) ṛtu-sātmya apekṣhaḥ (is used in the context of *ṛtu-sātmya*, or accustomization of proper food and routines on a seasonal basis).

Definition #2

In the context of assessing an individual, Charaka provides succinct definitions in two contexts in *Vimāna-sthāna* chapter 8. He first explains *kāla* within one of the assessment frameworks required by the Vaidya, and then within the context of *daśha-vidha parīkṣha.*

कालः पुनः परिणामः ॥

च. वि. ८।७६

Kālaḥ punaḥ pariṇāmaḥ ||

Cha. Vi. 8/76

Kāla (Time) punaḥ (again, as stated earlier) pariṇāma (is the process of transformation).

Here, Charaka clarifies the important point that *kāla* and *pariṇāma* may be considered equivalent in certain circumstances.

Definition #3

Charaka also explains *kāla* as *saṁvatsara* and *ātura*. *Kāla* measures the passage of time in intervals such as *saṁvatsara*, or the passage of one year and its subdivisions. *Kāla* also tracks the distinct stages of progression of a disease as seen in the *ātura*, or patient.

कालः पुनः संवत्सरश्चातुरावस्था च ।

च. वि. ८।१२५

Kālaḥ punaḥ saṁvatsaraśhchāturāvasthā cha |

Cha. Vi. 8/125

Kāla (Time) punaḥ (again, as stated earlier) saṁvatsaraśhcha (is used in the context of *saṁvatsara*, ie, a year, divided into seasons, and) ātura avasthā cha (the states, or stages seen in a patient or one suffering from disease).

Definition #4

Charaka also provides a definition for *kāla* as a synonym of *saṁvatsara*.

शीतोष्णवर्षलक्षणाः पुनर्हेमन्तग्रीष्मवर्षाः संवत्सरः, स कालः ।

च. सू. ११।४२

Śhītoṣhṇavarṣhalakṣhaṇāḥ punarhemantagrīṣhmavarṣhāḥ saṁvatsaraḥ, sa kālaḥ |

Cha. Sū 11/42

Sa kālaḥ (And so, time [in the context of]) saṁvatsaraḥ (a year), śhīta-uṣhṇa-varṣha lakṣhaṇāḥ (is known by the characteristics of cold, hot, and rainy) punar hemanta-grīṣhma-varṣhāḥ (respectively, in the seasons of winter, summer and monsoon).

The seasons of winter, summer and monsoon that are referenced here are specific to the Indian subcontinent. The months when they occur vary from most other geographical locations around the world due to unique climatological characteristics found only in this region.

Definition #5

Suśhruta provides a very comprehensive definition of *kāla* as he introduces Chapter six of *Sūtra-sthāna*. This chapter covers a full review of *kāla*, its divisions and practical application of annual seasons.

कालो हि नाम (भगवान्)
स्वयम्भुरनादिमध्यनिधनः । अत्र
रसव्यापत्सम्पत्ति जीवितमरणे च
मनुष्याणामायत्ते । स सूक्ष्मामपि कलां न
लीयते इति कालः, सङ्कलयति कालयति वा
भूतानीति कालः ॥

सु. सू. ६।३

Kālo hi nāma (bhagavān)
svayambhuranādimadhyanidhanaḥ |
Atra rasavyāpatsampatti jīvitamaraṇe
cha manuṣhyāṇāmāyate | Sa
sūkṣhmāmapi kalāṁ na līyate iti kālaḥ,
saṅkalayati kālayati vā bhūtānīti kālaḥ ||

Su. Sū. 6/3

Kālo hi nāma bhagavān (Kāla is known as Bhagavān, ie, comparable to god) svayambhur (it, itself is) anādi (having no beginning), madhya (having no middle, and) nidhanaḥ (having no end). Atra (In this manner), rasa-vyāpat (disorders or abnormal flavors and their qualities) sampatti (are born, created, come into existence), jīvita (life) maraṇe cha (and death) manuṣhyāṇām (of all human beings) āyate (is dependent upon it). Sa sūkṣhmāmapi kalāṁ (Since even for the smallest moment of time) na līyate (it does not disappear), iti kālaḥ (it is called time). Saṅkalayati (It kills) kālayati vā (or takes over, urges on) bhūtāni (all beings) iti kālaḥ (and is called time).

Kāla bheda

The general divisions of time are discussed in the classics by some authors. The primary reference is Su. Sū. 6/4-10, while Charaka's brief explanations in Cha. Sū. 6/3-4, Cha. Vi. 8/125 cover the divisions of time primarily for seasonal therapeutic use. These classical Āyurvedic divisions of time may vary from other streams of Vedic sciences.

Unit of time Su. Sū. 6/4-10	Definition Nearest English translation	Approximate duration
Akṣhi nimeṣha	*Laghu-akṣhara uchchhāraṇa mātra* The duration (time) required to speak a short syllable Literally, the time required to close the eyelids	0.32 seconds
Kāṣhṭhā	*Pañchadaśha akṣhi nimeṣhāḥ* 1 *kāṣhṭhā* = 15 *akṣhi nimeṣhas*	4.78 seconds
Kalā	*Triṁśhatkāṣhṭhāḥ* 1 *kalā* = 30 *kāṣhṭhās*	2 min 23.3 secs (143.3 secs)
Muhūrta	*Viṁśhatikalo muhūrtaḥ kalā daśhabhāgaśhcha* 1 *muhūrta* = 20 + 1/10th of a *kalā*	48 minutes
Ahorātra	*Triṁśhanmuhūrtaṁ ahorātraṁ* 1 *ahorātra* = 30 *muhūrta*	1440 minutes 24 hours
Pakṣha	*Pañchadaśha ahorātrāṇi pakṣhaḥ, sa cha dvividhaḥ - śhuklaḥ kṛṣhṇaśhcha* 1 *pakṣha* = 15 *ahorātra*	15 days
Māsa	*Tau māsaḥ* 1 *māsa* = 2 *pakṣhas* *Tatra dvāśha māsāḥ* And then there are 12 months	30 days, or 1 month 12 months total
Ṛtu	*Dvimāsikamṛtuṁ kṛtvā ṣhaḍṛtavo bhavanti* Two months constitute a season, of which there are six	2 months 6 seasons total
Ayana	*Kāla-vibhāga-karatvādyane dve bhavato dakṣhiṇamuttaraṁ cha* Subdivided into two based on *dakṣhiṇa* (southern) and *uttara* (northern) inclinations	6 months 2 *ayanas* total
Saṁvatsara	*Atha khalvayane dve yugapat saṁvatsaro bhavati* Two such *ayana* together are a *saṁvatsara* (year)	12 months 1 *saṁvatsara* total
Yuga	*Te tu pañcha yugamiti saṁjñā labhante* Five of these are known as a *yuga*	5 years 1 *yuga* total

Here, Suśhruta's usage of the term *yuga* differs greatly from Charaka's in Cha. Vi. 3/24-27 which refers to very large periods of time.

The cycle from *akṣhi nimeṣha* through *yuga* is defined by Suśhruta as a calendar system known as the *kāla chakra*. This indicates the continuous, cyclical and revolving nature of the periods of time. Within this system, the six seasons and twelve months are slightly different from the currently popular Hindu calendar, which is called the Āyurvedic calendar.

Notice that the *kāla chakra* calendar aligns with the seasonal divisions mentioned by Charaka in Cha. Sū. 6/4. From a practical standpoint, both of these seasonal presentations can be seen within the Indian subcontinent depending on the geographical location. In Southern India, there tends to be a much longer rainy season which warrants two periods covering early rains and late rains. While in Northern India there is a longer period of winter, warranting an early and late period. This is a significant demonstration of customization of the classical science and must be understood well. It provides insight into recognizing the factors for seasonal change and will provide support for creating seasonal divisions in new regions when the underlying laws are applied properly.

These different monthly and seasonal calendar systems are classically detailed in the following table.

Kāla chakra Su. Sū. 6/6 and Cha. Sū. 6/4		Āyurvedic calendar Su. Sū. 6/10 and Cha. Vi. 8/125	
Ṛtu Season	*Māsa* Months	*Ṛtu* Season	*Māsa* Months
Uttarāyana			
Śhiśhira Late winter	*Māgha, Phālguna*	*Vasanta* Spring	*Phālguna, Chaitra*
Vasanta Spring	*Chaitra, Vaiśhākha*	*Grīṣhma* Summer	*Vaiśhākha, Jyeṣhṭha*
Grīṣhma Summer	*Jyeṣhṭha, Āṣhāḍha*	*Prāvṛt* Early rains	*Āṣhāḍha, Śhrāvaṇa*
Dakṣhiṇāyana			
Varṣhā Rainy	*Śhrāvaṇa, Bhādrapada*	*Varṣhā* Late rains	*Bhādrapada, Āśhvina*
Śharad Autumn	*Āśhvina, Kārttika*	*Śharad* Autumn	*Kārttika, Mārgaśhīrṣha*
Hemanta Winter	*Mārgaśhīrṣha, Pauṣha*	*Hemanta* Winter	*Pauṣha, Māgha*

In Su. Sū. 6/10 and Cha. Vi. 8/125, a slightly different classification is provided, commonly known as the Āyurvedic calendar. Chakrapāṇi explains the reasons for these differences in the commentary following the same line. He states that the *Kāla chakra*, the first seasonal classification, includes early and late winter seasons which are commonly seen in regions north of the Ganges. The Āyurvedic calendar, the second classification, includes early and late rainy seasons which are commonly seen in regions south of the Ganges. Similar statements are also found in Kāśhyapa Saṁhitā.

Chakrapāṇi further elaborates that the Āyurvedic calendar, with early and late rains, allows for proper application of therapeutics, particularly *pañchakarma*. Charaka confirms this with the following statement.

एवमेते संशोधनमधिकृत्य षट् विभज्यन्ते ऋतवः ॥

च. वि. ८।१२५

Evamete saṁśhodhanamadhikṛtya ṣhaṭ vibhajyante ṛtavaḥ ||

Cha. Vi. 8/125

Evam-ete (And so, with this being the main purpose), saṁśhodhanam-adhikṛtya (the application of elimination therapies) vibhajyante (divides) ṛtavaḥ (the seasons into) ṣhaṭ (six).

He states that the *Kāla chakra* classification with early and late winter is to allow the *ṣhad-rasa* to manifest completely throughout the course of the year.

It is important to note that multiple formats of seasonal classifications were accepted and regularly applied in classical literature and practice. Each method has its specific purpose and was intended to be utilized in the appropriate context. Charaka validates this in Cha. Vi. 8/125 by stating the following.

तत्र संवत्सरो द्विधा त्रिधा षोढा द्वादशधा भूयश्चाप्यतः प्रविभज्यते तत्तत्कार्यमभिसमीक्ष्य ।

च. वि. ८।१२५

Tatra saṁvatsaro dvidhā tridhā ṣhoḍhā dvādaśhadhā bhūyaśhchāpyataḥ pravibhajyate tattatkāryamabhisamīkṣhya |

Cha. Vi. 8/125

Tatra (And so), saṁvatsaro (a year) dvidhā (in two), tridhā (or three), ṣhoḍhā (or six), dvādaśhadhā (or twelve) bhūyaśhchāpyataḥ (or even more) pravibhajyate (may be accepted as having appropriate divisions) tattat-kāryamabhisamīkṣhya (based on the need or requirement).

This statement provides a key reference which allows calendar systems to be modified and applied as appropriate in any location. Time may be divided to create the number of seasons which are practically experienced in any area.

In the commentary of Cha. Sū. 6/4, Chakrapāṇi also states that the number of seasons may vary according to the purpose. He notes that the classification of six seasons provided in both references may also be reduced to three for the purposes of therapeutic management. He also reconfirms that the importance of knowing the seasons is to be able to provide appropriate recommendations for diet and activities according to each season. When properly applied, this knowledge could allow an individual to potentially avoid or reduce the negative effects of natural cycles of *doṣhas* occurring in the external environment.

Vāgbhaṭa follows a similar approach by classifying the seasons for therapeutic action. He summarizes the entire concept in a very simple way by classifying them based on their primary characteristics.

कालस्तु शीतोष्णवर्षामेदात्रिधा मतः ॥

अ. हृ. सू. १२।३८

Kālastu śhītoṣhṇavarṣhāmedātridhā mataḥ ||

AH Sū. 12/38

Kālastu (Kāla, or time, is known as) śhīta (cold), uṣhṇa (hot) varṣhāmedā (and rainy) tridhā mataḥ (in its three main divisions).

Vāgbhaṭa further explains that these three primary seasons of cold, heat and rain are separated by seasons of moderate nature. It is during this intermediate time that any accumulated *doṣhas* should be expelled from the body.

अत्युष्णवर्षशीता हि ग्रीष्मवर्षाहिमगमाः ॥
सन्धौ साधारणे तेषां दुष्टान् दोषान्
विशोधयेत् ।

अ. हृ. सू. १३।३४

Atyuṣhṇavarṣhaśhītā hi grīṣhmavarṣhāhimagamāḥ ||
Sandau sādhāraṇe teṣhaṁ duṣhṭān viśhodhayet |

AH Sū. 13/34

Ati-uṣhṇa-varṣha-śhītā (Too much heat, rain, and cold) hi grīṣhma-varṣhā-hima gamāḥ (are seen in summer, rains, and winter). Sandau (Between each of these) sādhāraṇe (is *sādhāraṇa*, a moderate season), teṣhaṁ (which is the appropriate time) duṣhṭān viśhodhayet (to expel that which has become *duṣhṭa*, ie, vitiated or impure).

Comparing calendar systems

The currently popular Gregorian calendar tracks the passage of time based on the earth's movement around the sun. This is known as a solar calendar which constitutes 365.25 days annually. Every four years, an additional day is added to account for the extra quarter days to keep the calendar in synch with the movements of celestial bodies, seasonal manifestations, equinoxes and solstices.

Like many Old-World calendars, the classical Vedic calendar system is based on a luni-solar system. Each month consists of the waxing and waning periods of the moon, called *śhuklaḥ pakṣha* (the white or bright half, the waxing period) and *kṛṣhṇa pakṣha* (the black or dark half, the waning period). Based on these cycles, each month contains 29.5 days.

The lunar month system generates a total of 354 days per year, having 11.25 days less than a solar calendar calculation. To accommodate this and maintain alignment of the calendar system, a 13th month is added almost every three years, or after 32.5 months.

Today, the luni-solar calendar system is still used in India and many other traditional cultures to calculate holidays and festivals. Because of the fluctuations in aligning dates between these systems and the Gregorian calendar, it appears as though traditional holidays and festivals move back by approximately ten days for several years in a row. Then they jump forward by a month approximately every three years.

Influence of vāyu, agni and soma

Understanding the intricacies of the seasons and the overall effects of annual cycles on the environment and human health requires a strong foundation in knowing the underlying causative factors. Classically, these are considered to be *vāyu*, *agni* and *soma*, or the wind, the sun and moon in the external world.

Charaka identifies these three specifically by stating that they form the basis for all seasonal changes.

तावेतावर्कवायू सोमश्च कालस्वभावमार्गपरिगृहीताः कालर्तुरसदोषदेहबलनिर्वृत्तिप्रत्ययभूताः समुपदिश्यन्ते ।

च. सू. ६।५

Tāvetāvarkavāyū somaśhcha kālasvabhāvamārgaparigṛhītāḥ kālarturasadoṣhadehabalanirvṛttipratyay abhūtāḥ samupadiśhyante |

Cha. Sū. 6/5

Tāvetāv-arka-vāyū (These two, the sun and wind, taken together), somaśhcha (and the moon), kāla-svabhāva-mārga-parigṛhītāḥ (restricted by time, their own nature, and path of motion), kāla-rtu-rasa-doṣha-deha-bala-nirvṛtti-pratyaya-bhūtāḥ (constitute the basis for expression of time, seasons, flavors, *doṣhas*, growth of bodies, and strength), samupadiśhyante (and they are being described as follows).

The sun and wind are considered together within the context of *ādāna kāla*, while the moon is primarily responsible for *visarga kāla*. The explanation which follows in Cha. Sū. 6/ explains how these factors exert their effects. Later, in Cha. Sū. 12/, Charaka provides a more extensive overview with a broader and deeper understanding of how these three forces can be understood in both external and internal contexts.

Suśhruta provides a slightly different perspective by stating:

शीतांशुः क्लेदयत्युर्वीं विवस्वान् शोषयत्यपि । तावुभावपि संश्रित्य वायुः पालयति प्रजाः ॥

सु. सू. ६।८

Śhītāṁśhuḥ kledayatyurvīṁ vivasvān śhoṣhayatyapi | Tāvubhāvapi saṁśhritya vāyuḥ pālayati prajāḥ ||

Su. Sū. 6/8

Urvīṁ vivasvān (By these two celestial bodies, ie, the moon and the sun) śhītāṁśhuḥ kledayati (coolness and moisture are maintained), api (and also) śhoṣhayati (dried up). Tāvubhāvapi saṁśhritya (And both of these two) vāyuḥ (along with *vāyu*) pālayati (help to maintain) prajāḥ (mankind).

Recall that the *tri-doṣha siddhānta* originated from the base principles of *vāyu*, *agni* and *soma* representing the functions of *vikṣhepa*, *ādāna* and *visarga* (Su. Sū. 21/8, 42/5). Charaka elaborates the reasons for the similarities based on *loka-puruṣha sāmya* in Cha. Sū. 12/.

The name of this chapter is "*Vāta kala-akalīya adhyāya*," and it refers to the good and bad effects of *vāta*. The remaining two *doṣhas* are discussed in the chapter after the explanation of *vāta* which takes primary importance because it is the most powerful among the three.

Review the following references to compare the functions of *vāyu*, *agni* and *soma* in their normal and abnormal presentations both externally and internally. Notice that the external effects of *agni* and *soma* have not been described directly by Charaka. These two should be understood through the lens of the *ayana lakṣhaṇas*, which are discussed in the following section.

	External manifestation		Internal manifestation	
	Normal	Abnormal	Normal	Abnormal
Vāyu	Cha. Sū. 12/8(4)	Cha. Sū. 12/8(5)	Cha. Sū. 12/8(2)	Cha. Sū. 12/8(3)
Agni	*Ādāna kāla*		Cha. Sū. 12/11	Cha. Sū. 12/11
Soma	*Visarga kāla*		Cha. Sū. 12/12	Cha. Sū. 12/12

Suśhruta and Bhāvamiśhra also provide interesting perspectives on the effects of climate patterns and common weather phenomena on regular states of health. They explain how each one can promote health with moderate exposure or become detrimental with excessive use. These boundaries are unique to each individual depending on their tolerance levels.

Effects of vāyu

प्रवातं रौक्ष्यवैवर्ण्यस्तम्भकृद्दाहपक्तिनुत् ।
स्वेदमूर्च्छपिपासाघ्नमप्रवातमतोऽन्यथा ॥
८४
सुखं वातं प्रसेवेत ग्रीष्मे शरदि मानवः ।
निवातं ह्यायुषे सेव्यमारोग्याय च सर्वदा ॥
८५

सु. चि. २४।८४-८५

Pravātaṁ raukṣhyavaivarṇyastambhakṛddāhapaktinut |
Svedamūrchchhapipāsāghnampravātamato ' nyathā || 84
Sukhaṁ vātaṁ praseveta grīṣhme śharadi mānavaḥ | Nivātaṁ hyāyuṣhe sevyamārogyāya cha sarvadā || 85

Su. Ci. 24/84-85

Pravātaṁ (Strong wind, especially blowing directly in one's face, causes) raukṣhya (dryness), vaivarṇya (discoloration), stambha kṛd (and creates obstruction). Dāha (It prevents burning sensation internally), paktinut (impedes the functions of agni), sveda (and reduces sweating), mūrchchha (fainting or loss of consciousness), pipāsāghnam (and thirst) pravātamato anyathā (and so these are the effects of strong wind).

Sukhaṁ (Comfortable, pleasant) vātaṁ (wind or breeze) praseveta (can be regularly enjoyed) grīṣhme (in the summertime) śharadi (and second summer) mānavaḥ (by people). Nivātaṁ (Places free from wind or breezes) hyāyuṣhe (are life-promoting, or healthy for a long life) sevyam (and should be standard) ārogyāya (to promote health and prevent disease) cha sarvadā (for all people).

Here it can be seen that wind and breeze during hot seasons is helpful to promote a state of health for everyone. However, in cold environments, excessively strong winds can be detrimental to health. These phenomena are commonly experienced by people who live in cold regions and are regularly exposed to them. Even though people of these geographical areas usually build up a tolerance to the extreme effects of weather, they still notice their results.

Bhāvamiśhra elaborates on this topic in BP Pū. 5/190-201 with detailed descriptions of the effects of wind and breeze from specific directions. He also explains how the breeze produced by different types of leaves has distinct effects in temperature and on the *doṣhas*. While these effects are likely highly customized to the Indian subcontinent, they do provide excellent examples of how the science can be applied practically.

Effects of ātapa

आतपः पित्ततृष्णाग्निस्वेदमूर्च्छाभ्रमास्त्रकृत् । दाहवैवर्ण्यकारी च छाया चैतानपोहति ॥ ८६

सु. चि. २४।८६

Ātapaḥ pittatṛṣhṇāgnisvedamūrchchhābhramāst rakṛt | Dāhavaivarṇyakārī cha chhāyā chaitānapohati || 86

Su. Ci. 24/86

Ātapaḥ (The hot sun) strakṛt (causes increase of) pitta (pitta [*doṣha*]), tṛṣhṇa (thirst), agni (the power of *agni*, or digestion and metabolism), sveda (sweat), mūrchchhā (fainting or loss of consciousness) bhramā (and dizziness). Dāha (Internal burning sensation) vaivarṇya (and discoloration of normal complexion) kārī (increase) cha (and) chhāyā (staying in the shade) chaitānapohati (reduces these problems).

The strength of the sun in the Indian subcontinent can easily be considered extreme, especially during the Indian seasons of summer and post-monsoon. The sun can quickly take away one's strength and stability causing delerium, fainting and loss of consciousness. Shade alone can provide significant relief from the overpowering effects of direct sun. It is common to see people living in equatorial regions use umbrellas throughout the year to provide shade and protect themselves from the sun.

Bhāvamiśhra provides a similar description in BP Pū. 5/231.

Effects of agni

अग्निर्वातकफस्तम्भशीतवेपथुनाशनः । आमाभिष्यन्दजरणो रक्तपित्तप्रदूषणः ॥ ८७

सु. चि. २४।८७

Agnirvātakaphastambhaśhītavepathunā śhanaḥ | Āmābhiṣhyandajaraṇo raktapittapradūṣhaṇaḥ || 87

Su. Ci. 24/87

Agnir (Exposure to [the heat of] fire) nāśhanaḥ (eradicates) vāta (vāta [*doṣha*]), kapha (kapha [*doṣha*]), stambha (stiffness), śhīta (cold) vepathu (shivers), āmābhiṣhyanda (and obstruction due to *āma*). Pradūṣhaṇaḥ ([However] it can aggravate) jaraṇo (the onset of old age) raktapitta (and the disorder of *raktapitta*).

Suśhruta's explanation of exposure to fire is intriguing. With the correct amount of exposure, fire can help maintain proper functioning of the digestive and metabolic physiology to keep the channels clear and free from obstruction due to *āma*. Its effects are often found to be practically beneficial for the elderly who tend to suffer from cold, stiffness, shivers and other disorders due to vāta and kapha. Yet too much exposure to fire can accelerate the ageing process and disorders prevalant in pitta and rakta *doṣhas*, such as *raktapitta*.

Bhāvamiśhra reiterates this statement in BP Pū. 5/233.

Effects of varṣha

Bhāvamiśhra adds to Suśhruta's original explanations and includes descriptions of the effects of rain and fog in BP Pū. 5/232.

वृष्टिर्वृष्या हिमा बल्या निद्राऽऽलस्यविधायिनी । भयावहा मोहकरी कुहेलिः कफवातला ॥ २३२

भा. प्र. पू. ५।२३२

Vṛshṭirvṛṣhyā himā balyā nidrā ' ' lasyavidhāyinī | Bhayāvahā mohakarī kuheliḥ kaphavātalā || 232

BP Pū. 5/232

Vṛṣhṭir (Rain) vṛṣhyā (acts as an aphrodisiac), himā (is cool), balyā (strengthening), nidrā (promotes sleep), ālasyavidhāyinī (and encourages laziness). Bhayāvahā (Fear is increased) mohakarī (and delusion, confusion is increased) kuheliḥ (by fod) kaphavātalā (which also causes an increase in kapha and vāta).

The effects of natural weather patterns are strongly evident in the Indian subcontinent when residing in the environment for extended periods of time. The accumulation of the specific *guṇas* of the weather pattern become easily recognizable because they can persist for several months in a row.

Effects of dhūma

Bhāvamiśhra also includes a description of the effects of smoke in BP Pū. 5/234.

सद्यः श्लेष्मकरो धूमो नेत्रयोरहितो भृशम् ।
शिरोगौरवकृच्चापि वातपित्तं च कोपयेत् ॥
२३४

भा. प्र. पू. ५।२३४

Sadyaḥ śhleṣhmakaro dhūmo netrayorahito bhṛśham |
Śhirogauravakṛchchāpi vātapittaṁ cha kopayet || 234

BP Pū. 5/234

Sadyaḥ (An immediate) śhleṣhma-karo (increase in kapha) dhūmo ([is caused by] smoke) netrayor (which for the eyes) ahito bhṛśham (is extremely unhealthy). Śhiro-gaurava (Heaviness of the head) kṛchchāpi (is also produced) vātapittaṁ cha (and vāta and pitta) kopayet (become greatly aggravated).

Effects of jyotsnā

Bhāvamiśhra adds a unique description of the effects of moonlight in BP Pū. 5/263.

ज्योत्स्ना शीता स्मरानन्दप्रदा
तृट्पित्तदाहहृत् । ततो हीनगुणः
कुर्यादवश्यायोऽनिलं कफम् ॥ २६३

भा. प्र. पू. ५।२६३

Jyotsnā śhītā smarānandapradā
tṛṭpittadāhahṛt | Tato hīnaguṇaḥ
kuryādavaśhyāyo ' nilaṁ kapham || 263

BP Pū. 5/263

Jyotsnā (Moonlight) śhītā (is cold, cooling), smarānandapradā (produces desire for sexual intercourse), tṛṭ-pitta-dāha hṛt (and reduces thirst, pitta and internal burning sensation). Tato (And even) hīnaguṇaḥ (imparting slighly less effect [than moonlight]) kuryād-avaśhyāyo (is the dew or mist at nighttime) anilaṁ (which increases vāta) kapham (and kapha).

Bhāvamiśhra discusses both the direct effects of moonlight and the general atmosphere of the night as dewy or misty. Both impart certain effects through their *guṇas* with moonlight having the stronger effect.

Effects of tamas

Bhāvamiśhra also describes the effects of tamas as the effects of nighttime in BP Pū. 5/264.

तमो भयावहं मोहदिङ्मोहजनकं भवेत् ।
पित्तहृत्कफहृत्कामवर्धनं क्लमकृच्च तत् ॥
२६४

भा. प्र. पू. ५।२६४

Tamo bhayāvahaṁ
mohadiṅmohajanakaṁ bhavet |
Pittahṛtkaphahṛtkāmavardhanaṁ
klamakṛchcha tat || 264

BP Pū. 5/264

Tamo (Tamas, or the darkness of the night) bhayā-vahaṁ (increases fear), moha-diṅmoha-janakaṁ bhavet (and creates a sense of delusion or confusion and disorients one from their direction). Pitta hṛt (It reduces pitta [*doṣha*]), kapha hṛt (it reduces kapha [*doṣha*]), kāma vardhanaṁ (it increases lust and desire) klama-kṛchcha tat (and causes a sense of exhaustion).

This explanation of the effect of tamas due to the night also provides significant insight into understanding the *tri-guṇas* through their regular, daily presentations.

Kāla lakṣhaṇas

Understanding and applying the divisions of time to any geographical area requires thorough, comprehensive knowledge of a broad range of classical *siddhānta*. These laws establish the reasons for seasonal change and provide the basis for appropriate diet and lifestyle recommendations. The classics utilize three major divisions of time and describe them through specific *lakṣhaṇas*. These include the *ayanas*, *ṛtus* and *ahorātri* (day and night).

Ayana lakṣhaṇas

The first major division of *kāla* in this context includes the two halves of the year known as *ayanas*. Each *ayana* is classically named based on the movement of the sun during its period. The half of the year when the sun heads towards its northernmost point is called *ādāna kāla*. And the half of the year when the sun moves towards its southernmost point is called *visarga kāla*. Both of these periods affect all life forms on earth.

Charaka defines the two *ayanas* based on their effects of depleting and nourishing.

तत्रादित्यस्योदगयनमादानं ... दक्षिणायनं विसर्गं च ॥

च. सू. ६।४

Tatrādityasyodagayanamādānaṁ ... dakṣhiṇāyānaṁ visargaṁ cha ||

Cha. Sū. 6/4

Tatra (And so), udagayanam (the half year period from winter to summer solstice) ādityasya (of the sun) ādānaṁ (is depleting) ... cha (and) dakṣhiṇāyānaṁ (the half year period from summer to winter solstice) visargaṁ (is strengthening).

Vāgbhaṭa provides similar basic definitions of the two *ayanas*.

Uttarāyana (Ādāna kāla):

तदादत्ते नृणां प्रतिदिनं बलम् ॥

अ. हृ. सू. ३।२

Tadādatte nṛṇāṁ pratidinaṁ balam ||

AH Sū. 3/2

Tadādatte (It gradually takes away) balam (the strength) nṛṇāṁ (of the people) pratidinaṁ (every day).

Dakṣhiṇāyana (Visarga kāla):

यद्बलं विसृजत्ययम् ।

अ. हृ. सू. ३।४.५

Yadbalaṁ visṛjatyayam |

AH Sū. 3/4.5

Yad (This period) balaṁ visṛjatyayam (allows the strength of people to flow freely).

Ayana Biannual period	*Kāla* Effective period	Classical *ṛtus* (according to the *kāla chakra*) Approximate time (Gregorian)
Uttarāyana Northern-moving	*Ādāna kāla* Depleting period	*Śhiśhira*, *vasanta*, *grīṣhma* (from *Māgha* to *Āṣhāḍha*) Approx. mid-January through mid-July
Dakṣhiṇāyana Southern-moving	*Visarga kāla* Strengthening period	*Varṣhā*, *śharad*, *hemanta* (from *Śhrāvaṇa* to *Pauṣha*) Approx. mid-July through mid-January

Occassionally, *uttarāyana* and *dakṣhiṇāyana* may be translated as the northern solstice and southern solstice. This can be misleading because these two actually refer to the entire period of time, or half of the year where the sun moves towards its northern or southern maximum point. Presently, no English terms exist to refer to the entire bi-annual period of time denoted by the *ayanas*. These should be termed inter-ayana periods.

In older European and Viking times, two main periods of time between the spring and fall equinoxes were recognized as the major seasons of summer and winter. Today they are known as inter-equinoctial and by the Gregorian calendar they may appear to be three months later than the classical *ayanas*.

An additional discrepancy is found when comparing solstice dates on the Hindu calendar with the Gregorian solstices. In the Hindu calendar, the winter solstice is generally recognized around mid-January while the summer solstice falls somewhere in mid-July. These generally occur approximately three to four weeks later than the Gregorian solstices. From a practical perspective, the Hindu calendar dates generally fall closer to the appearance of the perceivable changes in *ayana lakṣhaṇas*.

The characteristics of each *ayana* have been described by both Charaka and Suśhruta prior to explaining the *ṛtu lakṣhaṇas*. Here they are covered in the same format.

Suśhruta provides the following description of the *ayana lakṣhaṇas*.

तेषु भगवानाप्यायते सोमः,
अम्ललवणमधुराश्च रसा बलवन्तो भवन्ति,
उत्तरोत्तरं च सर्वप्राणिनां बलमभिवर्धते ।
उत्तरं च शिशिरवसन्तग्रीष्माः, तेषु
भगवानाप्यायतेऽर्कः, तिक्तकषायकटुकाश्च
रसा बलवन्तो भवन्ति, उत्तरोत्तरं च
सर्वप्राणिनां बलमपहीयते ॥

सु. सू. ६।७

Teṣhu bhavānāpyāyate somaḥ, amla-lavaṇa-madhurā-śhcha rasā balavanto bhavanti, uttarottaraṁ cha sarvaprāṇināṁ balamabhi-vardhate | Uttaraṁ cha śhiśhira-vasanta-grīṣhmāḥ, teṣhu bhagavānāpyāyate ' rkaḥ, tikta-kaṣhāya-kaṭukā-śhcha rasā balavanto bhavanti, uttarottaraṁ cha sarvaprāṇināṁ balamapahīyate ||

Su. Sū. 6/7

Teṣhu bhavānāpyāyate somaḥ (During visarga kāla, soma predominates). Amla (Sour), lavaṇa (salty), madhurā-śhcha (and sweet) rasā (flavors) balavanto bhavanti (become stronger with each progressive season), uttara-uttaraṁ cha (and more and more) sarva-prāṇināṁ (all life forms) balamabhi-vardhate (are seen to grow progressively in strength during this time).

Uttaraṁ cha śhiśhira-vasanta-grīṣhmāḥ,

(Ādāna kāla includes late winter, spring and summer), teșhu bhagavānāpyāyate arkaḥ (and during this period the sun predominates). Tikta (Bitter), kaṣhāya (astringent), kaṭukā-śhcha (and pungent) rasā (flavors) balavanto bhavanti (become stronger with each progressive season), uttara-uttaraṁ cha (and more and more) sarva-prāṇināṁ (all life forms) balamapahīyate (gradually lose their strength).

Charaka describes the *ayana lakṣhaṇas* as follows.

विसर्गे पुनर्वायवो नातिरूक्षाः प्रवान्ति, इतरे पुनरादाने; सोमश्चाव्याहतबलः शिशिराभिर्भाभिरापूरयञ्जगदाप्याययति शश्वत्, अतो विसर्गः सौम्यः । आदानं पुनराग्नेयं; ।

च. सू. ६।५

Visarge punarvāyavo nāti rūkṣhaḥ pravānti, itare punarādāne; somaśhchāvyāhata-balaḥ śhiśhirābhirbhābhirāpūrayañjagadāpyāy ati śhaśhvat, atho visargaḥ saumyaḥ | Ādānaṁ punarāgneyaṁ; |

Cha. Sū. 6/5

Visarge (During visarga), punarvāyavo (as previously mentioned, the winds) nāti (are not too) rūkṣhaḥ (dry) pravānti (when they are blowing), itare punarādāne (as compared to *ādāna kāla*); somaśhchāvyāhata-balaḥ (and soma provides strength) śhiśhirābhirbhābhirāpūrayañjagadāpyāyati śhaśhvat (with its abundance of cooling rays continuously filling the world in the winter); atho (and so) visargaḥ (the period of *visarga kāla*) saumyaḥ (is *saumya*, or predominant in the characteristics of the moon).

Ādānaṁ (*Ādāna kāla*), punar-āgneyaṁ (as previously mentioned is predominant in the characteristics of *agni*).

तत्र रविर्भाभिराददानो जगतः स्नेहं वायवस्तिव्ररूक्षाश्चोपशोषयन्तः शिशिरवसन्तग्रीष्मेषु यथाक्रमं रौक्ष्यमुत्पादयन्तो रूक्षान् रसांस्तिक्तकषायकटुकांश्चाभिवर्धयन्तो नृणां दौर्बल्यमावहन्ति ॥

च. सू. ६।६

Tatra ravir-bhābhirād-adāno jagataḥ snehaṁ vāyavas-tīvra-rūkṣhā-śhcha-upaśhoṣhayantaḥ śhiśhira-vasanta-grīṣhmeṣhu yathākramaṁ raukṣhyam-utpādayanto rūkṣhān rasāṁs-tikta-kaṣhāya-kaṭukāṁ-śhchābhi-vardhayanto nṛṇāṁ daurbalyamāvahanti ||

Cha. Sū. 6/6

Tatra (And so), ravir-bhābhirād (the powerful sun) adāno (is *adāna*) jagataḥ (in the world). Upaśhoṣhayantaḥ (It dries up) snehaṁ (the unctuousness) vāyavas (by its winds) tīvra (that are strong, sharp, piercing) rūkṣhāśhcha (and dry) śhiśhira (in late winter), vasanta (spring and) grīṣhmeṣhu (in summer) yathākramaṁ (it continously increases) raukṣhyam (its dryness) utpādayanto rūkṣhān (and it also infuses the dryness) rasāṁs (into the fractional component of flavor by increasing) tikta (bitter), kaṣhāya (astringent), kaṭukāṁśhchābhi (and pungent) vardhayanto (which go on increasing) nṛṇāṁ (in human beings) daurbalyamāvahanti (resulting in a decrease in normal strength).

वर्षाशरद्हेमन्तेषु तु दक्षिणाभिमुखेऽर्के कालमार्गमेघवातवर्षाभिहतप्रतापे, शशिनि चाव्याहतबले, मादेन्त्रसलिलप्रशान्तसन्तापे जगति, अरूक्षा रसाः प्रवर्धन्तेऽम्ललवणमधुरा यथाक्रमं तत्र बलमुपचीयते नृणामिति ॥

च. सू. ६।७

Varṣha-śharad-hemanteṣhu tu dakṣhiṇābhimukhe ' rke kāla-mārga-megha-vāta-varṣhābhi-hata pratāpe śhaśhini chāvyāhatabale, māhendra-salila-praśhānta-santāpe jagati, arūkṣhā rasāḥ pravardhante ' amla-lavaṇa-madhurā yathākramaṁ tatra balam-upachīyate nṛṇām-iti ||

Cha. Sū. 6/

Varṣha (During the monsoon), śharad (second summer, and) hemanteṣhu (in early winter) tu dakṣhiṇābhimukhe arke (the sun moves to the south). Kāla (Time, and its transformative capabilities), mārga (the natural course of the earth), megha (the clouds, storms or cyclonic patterns), vāta (the winds), varṣhābhihata (the rains, etc) pratāpe śhaśhini chāvyāhatabale (gradually reduce the heat and the strength of the moon is not impeded). Māhendra-salila-praśhānta-santāpe jagati (The earth and human beings are relieved of their heat by the rain), arūkṣhā rasāḥ pravardhante (and a non-drying (moistening) effect is produced in people by the flavors of) amla (sour), lavaṇa (salty and), madhurā (sweet) yathākramaṁ (which grow progressively through these three seasons). Tatra (And so) balam (the strength) upachīyate nṛṇām-iti (of humans increases).

Because the *ayanas* have a direct effect on the *bala* of humans, Charaka and Vāgbhaṭa have both described the annual cycles of normal *bala* in this context.

आदावन्तो च दौर्बल्यं विसर्गादानयोर्नृणाम् । मध्ये मध्यबलं, त्वन्ते श्रेष्ठमग्रे च निर्दिशेत् ॥

च. सू. ६।८

Ādāna-vanto cha daurbalyaṁ visargādānayornṛṇām | Madhye madhyabalaṁ, tvante śhreṣhṭhamagre cha nirdiśhet ||

Cha. Sū. 6/8

Ādāna-vanto cha (And the period of *ādāna kāla* emits, ejects or throws out) daurbalyaṁ (the weakest strength [of human beings]) visargādānayornṛṇām (at the transition time between *ādāna* and *visarga kālas* [ie, approximately mid-July]). Madhye (At the midpoint of each period) madhya-balaṁ (bala is moderate), tvante (and at the transition time between *visarga* and *ādāna kālas*) śhreṣhṭhamagre cha nirdiśhet (*bala* is at its best, or highest level).

The correlations described here between *kāla* and *bala* are based on the assumption of normal seasons in the Indian subcontinent. These applications may operate differently in other geographical regions.

One of the unique climatic features found in the Indian subcontinent that likely contributes to the practical application seen in this location is the regularity of the annual monsoon. India is one of only a few locations in the world that experiences a true monsoon. This results in generally cool, wet conditions around the time of the summer solstice in the Gregorian calendar, with extreme periods of heat occurring before and afterwards.

Vāgbhaṭa explains the effects of extreme temperatures on *bala*.

शीतोऽग्र्यं वृष्टिधर्मेऽल्पं बलं मध्यं तु शोषयोः ।

अ. हृ. सू. ३।६.५

Śhīto ' gryaṁ vṛṣhṭidharme ' lpaṁ balaṁ madhyaṁ tu śhoṣhayoḥ |

AH Su. 3/6.5

Śhīto (Cold) agryaṁ (is best [to increase *bala*]); vṛṣhṭi-dharme (during monsoon) alpaṁ (it is at its lowest) balaṁ (strength) madhyaṁ tu śhoṣhayoḥ (and moderate in between).

Review the following table and summary.

	Ādāna kāla			*Visarga kāla*		
	Cha. Sū. 6/5-7	Su. Sū. 6/7	AH Sū. 3/2-6	Cha. Sū. 6/5-7	Su. Sū. 6/7	AH Sū. 3/2-6
Guṇa	Agni (agneya)			Soma (saumya)		
Ṛtus for śhodhana	Vasanta, grīṣhma, prāvṛṭ			Varṣhā, śharad, hemanta		
Ṛtus for rasa	Śhiśhira, vasanta, grīṣhma			Varṣhā, śharad, hemanta		
Rasas	Tikta, kaṣhāya, kaṭu			Amla, lavaṇa, madhura		
Bala	Uttama, madhyama, avara			Avara, madhyama, uttama		

Ṛtu lakṣhaṇas

Ṛtu lakṣhaṇas are the characteristics presented in the external environment during each season. These are well-documented in all major classical texts with detailed descriptions. Understanding the *ṛtus* in one's geographical region is a priority in traditional clinical practice.

Without the proper understanding of the seasons, Chakrapāṇi states that it is not possible to provide the appropriate recommendations for diet and routines (Cha. Sū. 6/4). Further, it should be understood that the knowledge of the seasons allows one to predict the cycles of the *doṣhas* and manage them more effectively.

The following table of references includes the classical descriptions of seasonal cycles in the Indian subcontinent. Note that Charaka, Vāgbhaṭa and Bhāvamiśhra explain *ṛtu lakṣhaṇas* and their related *ṛtu sātmya* in the same chapters. Suśhruta, however, separates these into theoretical and practical chapters. In this chapter, Suśhruta's format is followed with *ṛtu lakṣhaṇas* described in this chapter and *ṛtu sātmya* detailed in Chapter five.

Ṛtu	Charaka	Suśhruta	Aṣhṭāṅga Hṛdaya	Bhāva Prakāśha
Hemanta	Cha. Sū. 6/9-18	Su. Sū. 6/22-23	AH Sū. 3/7-16	BP. Pū. 5/316, 329
Śhiśhira	Cha. Sū. 6/19-21	Su. Sū. 6/24	AH Sū. 3/17	BP. Pū. 5/317, 330
Vasanta	Cha. Sū. 6/22-26	Su. Sū. 6/25-28	AH Sū. 3/18-25	BP. Pū. 5/317, 331-332
Grīṣhma	Cha. Sū. 6/27-32	Su. Sū. 6/29-30	AH Sū. 3/26-41	BP. Pū. 5/318, 333
Prāvṛṭ		Su. Sū. 6/31-32		
Varṣhā	Cha. Sū. 6/33-40	Su. Sū. 6/33-34	AH Sū. 3/42-44	BP. Pū. 5/318, 322-325
Śharad	Cha. Sū. 6/41-48	Su. Sū. 6/35-36	AH Sū. 3/49-54	BP. Pū. 5/316, 326-328

While each classical author covers a valid review of the *ṛtus*, there are slight variations and additional points in certain references. This may be a result of progression and advancement of the science over time. For example, Vāgbhaṭa adds key points about the prevalence of specific *rasas* during each *ṛtu* which Charaka and Suśhruta have not mentioned.

It is helpful to compile the significant statements from all authors and review these key points together to better comprehend the underlying principles. Use the following tables to reference the information from each author. The source references are color coded with the key at the top of the page.

Color-coded references			
Cha. Sū. 6/9-48	Su. Sū. 6/	AH Sū. 3/	BP. Pū. 5/

Consolidated review of classical *ṛtu lakşhaṇas* for the Indian subcontinent						
Kāla chakra	*Śhiśhira* Late winter	*Vasanta* Spring	*Grīşhma* Summer	*Varşhā* Monsoon	*Śharad* Second summer	*Hemanta* Early winter
Effect of the *ṛtu* on *doşhas* + chaya ++ prakopa - praśhamana						
Vāta	++		+	++	-	+
Pitta			+	+	++	-
Kapha	+	++	-			+
Effect of the *ṛtu* on *agni* and *bala* ++ uttama + madhyama - avara						
Agni	++	+ / -	-	- -	- / +	+
Bala	++	+ / -	-	- -	- / +	++
Ṛtu rasas and *pañchamahābhūtas*						
Rasa	Tikta	Kaşhaya	Kaṭu	Amla	Lavaṇa	Madhura
		M	T			
PMB based on rasa	Ākāśha + Vāyu	Vāyu + Pṛthvi	Tejas + Vāyu	Pṛthvi + Tejas	Tejas + Ap	Pṛthvi + Ap

Color-coded references			
Cha. Sū. 6/9-48	Su. Sū. 6/	AH Sū. 3/	BP. Pū. 5/

Ṛtu lakṣhaṇas (guṇas)						
Kāla chakra	*Śhiśhira* Late winter	*Vasanta* Spring	*Grīṣhma* Summer	*Varṣhā* Monsoon	*Śharad* Second summer	*Hemanta* Early winter
Śhīta	++			++		+
Uṣhṇa		+	++		++	
Snigdha		++		+	+	++
Rūkṣha	+		++			+
Guru	++			+	+	++
Laghu		+	++	+		
Manda	++			+		++
Tīkṣhṇa		+	++	+	++	
Pichchhila	++	+		++		+
Viśhada		++	++		+	

As discussed earlier, the classical seasons were divided in six for two main reasons:

1. To provide recommendations for proper seasonal usage of dietary items and lifestyle routines
2. To schedule *śhodhana* appropriately for eliminating the *doṣhas* at the safest time

Both of these reasons have significant implications in the states of all three *doṣhas* so that each can experience a full cycle of *chaya*, *prakopa* and *praśhamana* over the course of a year.

The need for six seasons for the manifestation of *rasas* and the elimination of *doṣhas* results in dividing the year into six, two-month periods. In the traditional Vedic or Hindu calendars, each month is identified by its *rāśhi*, or sun sign. This is explained in Bhāva Prakāśha.

चयकोपशमा यस्मिन्दोषाणां सम्भवन्ति हि । ऋतुषट्कं तदाख्यातं रवे राशिषु संक्रमात् ॥

भा. प्र. पू. ५।३०९

Chayakopaśhamā yasmindoṣhāṇāṁ sambhavanti hi |
Ṛtuṣhaṭkaṁ tadākhyātaṁ rave rāśhiṣhu saṁkramāt ||

BP. Pū. 5/309

Chaya kopa śhamā (The three stages of chaya, prakopa and praśhamana) yasmin doṣhāṇāṁ sambhavanti hi (occur in the doṣhas) ṛtu ṣhaṭkaṁ (throughout the six seasons) tadākhyātaṁ rave rāśhiṣhu saṁkramāt (which occur when the sun moves from one *rāśhi*, or sun sign, to the next).

Vāgbhaṭa recognizes a two-week period in between each of the six *ṛtus* as the seasonal transition time. He refers to the final week of the preceding *ṛtu* and the first week of the subsequent *ṛtu* as *ṛtu sandhi*. Literally, this means the joint between seasons, and it is the period where diet and habits are recommended to be gradually shifted to that which is appropriate for the coming season. By transitioning gradually, he states that one can avoid disorders caused by *asātmya*.

ऋत्वोरन्त्यादिसप्ताहावृतुसन्धिरिति स्मृतः ।
तत्र पूर्वो विधिस्त्याज्यः सेवनीयोऽपरः क्रमात् ॥
असात्म्यजा हि रोगाः स्युः सहसात्यागशीलनात् ।

अ. हृ. सू. ३।५८

Ṛtvorantyādisaptāhāvṛtusandhiriti smṛtaḥ |
Tatra pūrvo vidhistyājyaḥ sevanīyo ' paraḥ kramāt ||
Asātmyajā hi rogāḥ syuḥ sahasātyāgaśhīlanāt |

AH Sū. 3/58

Ṛtvorantyādi (The final seven days of the preceding *ṛtu*) saptāhāv (and the next seven days of the subsequent *ṛtu*) ṛtu-sandhir iti smṛtaḥ (are known as *ṛtu sandhi*). Tatra (And so), pūrvo vidhistyājyaḥ sevanīyo (those diets and routines which have been followed regularly during the previous [season]) aparaḥ kramāt (should be gradually reduced or removed [from the new routine for the coming season]). Asātmyajā hi rogāḥ syuḥ sahasātyāgaśhīlanāt (Following this schedule properly can help avoid disorders due to *asātmya*).

Ahorātri lakṣhaṇas

Just as the *doṣhas* experience more prominent, recognizable cycles annually through the *ṛtus*, they also undergo smaller, more mild fluctuations in each day and night cycle. Vāgbhaṭa describes the existence of this phenomenon very succinctly:

वयोहोरात्रिभुक्तानां तेऽन्तमध्याधिगाः
क्रमात् ।

अ. हृ. सू. १।७.५

Vayohorātribhuktānāṁ te ‘
ntamadhyādhigāḥ kramāt |

AH Sū. 1/7.5

Vaya ([In each stage of] lifespan), ahorātri (day and night), bhuktānāṁ (stages of digestion after eating a meal), te (they, ie, the *doṣhas*) anta madhya-adhigāḥ kramāt (undergo a cycle [of *chaya*, *prakopa* and *praśhamā*] in the end, the middle and the beginning of each).

Suśhruta provides more detail about how to recognize the *dina* and *rātri lakṣhaṇas* by comparing general periods of the day and night to the *ṛtus*. The more detailed understanding of the *ṛtus*, their *lakṣhaṇas* and their impact on the *doṣhas* can be applied to the shorter periods of typical days and nights.

तत्र पूर्वाह्णे वसन्तस्य लिङ्गं, मध्याह्ने
ग्रीष्मस्य, अपराह्णे प्रवावृषः, प्रदोषे वार्षिकं,
शारदमर्धरात्रे, प्रत्युषसि हैमन्तमुपलक्षयेत्;
एवमहोरात्रमपि वर्षमिव शीतोष्णवर्षलक्षणं
दोषोपचयप्रकोपोपशमैर्जानीयात् ॥ १४

सु. सू. ६।१४

Tatra pūrvāhṇe vasantasya liṅgaṁ,
madhyāhne grīṣhmasya, aparāhne
pravāvṛṣhaḥ, pradoṣhe vārṣhikaṁ,
śhāradamardharātre; pratyuṣhasi
haimantamupalakṣhayet;
evamahorātramapi varṣhamiva
śhītoṣhṇavarṣhalakṣhaṇaṁ
doṣhopachayaprakopopaśhamairjānīyāt
|| 14

Su. Sū. 6/14

Tatra (And so), pūrvāhṇe (the morning, or before noon) vasantasya liṅgaṁ (has characteristics like *vasanta*, or spring), madhyāhne (the midday, or around noon) grīṣhmasya (is like *grīṣhma*, or summer), aparāhne (the afternoon) pravāvṛṣhaḥ (is like *prāvṛt*, or the early part of rainy season) pradoṣhe vārṣhikaṁ (the evening is like *vārṣha*, or rainy season), śhāradam ardharātre (midnight is like *śhārat*, or second summer); pratyuṣhasi (and dawn) haimantam-upalakṣhayet (has characteristics of *hemanta*, or winter); evam (and so) ahorātram api (the day and night are like) varṣhamiva (the seasons of the year) śhīta-uṣhṇa-varṣha lakṣhaṇaṁ (having the characteristics of cold, hot and rain) doṣha (causing the *doṣhas*) jānīyāt (to undergo states of) upachaya (*chaya*, or accumulation), prakopa (*prakopa*, or great increase), upaśhamair (and *śhamana*, or restoration to normal equilibrium).

Ahorātri Day / night period	*Ṛtu* Similar season
Pūrvāhṇe Morning, before noon	*Vasanta* Spring
Madhyāhne Noon	*Grīṣhma* Summer
Aparāhne Afternoon	*Prāvṛt* Early rains
Pradoṣhe Evening	*Vārṣha* Monsoon
Ardharātre Midnight	*Śharad* Second summer
Pratyuṣhasi Dawn	*Hemanta* Winter

Additionally, identifying the distinctions in *dina* and *rātri lakṣhaṇas* could be known through the application of the *vimśhati guṇas*. This allows great flexibility in assessing new locations and time periods. The *lakṣhaṇas* are estimated using the *guṇas* for the known location of the Indian subcontinent.

Dina lakṣhaṇas Daytime characteristics		Kapha	Pitta	Vāta
First third (starts at sunrise)		++	+	-
Guru	Generally, the heaviest part of the day; highest humidity levels occur in the early morning			
Sthira	Feeling of stillness			
Snigdha, pichchhila	Dew, mist, fog			
Śhīta	Coolness			
Middle third (midday)		-	++	+
Uṣhṇa	Maximum period of direct sunlight increases heat retention			
Viśhada	As the sun rises, it tends to burn through the clouds to clear the sky			
Tīkṣhṇa	Generally, the time of day where sharpness and activity are at their peak			
Last third (ends at sunset)		+	-	++
Laghu	Generally, the lightest part of the day; lowest humidity levels occur in the afternoon and early evening			
Rūkṣha	The after-effects of midday heat cause moisture loss resulting in the driest period of the day			
Cala	Winds tend to increase especially as heat dissipates			
Rātri lakṣhaṇas (Su. Śha. 4/35) Nighttime characteristics		Kapha	Pitta	Vāta
First third (starts at sunset)		++	+	-
Tamas	Heaviness and tiredness due to the nature of the night			
Middle third (around midnight)		-	++	+
Rajas	Activity and awakening Some aspects of sattva may also be seen			
Last third (ends at sunrise)		+	-	++
Sattva	Clarity and vacuity Some characteristics of rajas may also be seen			

Although specific *dina* and *rātri lakṣhaṇas* may vary according to each *deśha* and *ṛtu*, the underlying cycles of *doṣhas* should remain the same over the course of day and night. The time durations of each period of predominant *doṣha* will change according to geographical location and season. Based on variations in *deśha* presentations and changes in duration of day and night in varying latitudes, the final effects on the *doṣhas* may be altered, extended or reduced according to the predominant *guṇas*.

TEST YOURSELF

Learn, review and memorize key terms from this section.

kāla

pariṇāma

śhīta

uṣhṇa

varṣha

muhūrta

kāla chakra

ayana

ṛtu

māsa

uttarāyana

ādāna kāla

agneya

dakṣhiṇāyana

visarga kāla

saumya

śhiśhira

vasanta

grīṣhma

prāvṛṭ

varṣhā

śharad

hemanta

vāyu

agni

soma

chaya

kopa

śhamā

ṛtu sandhi

ahorātri

dina

rātri

KEY PRINCIPLES

Understanding and applying the knowledge of *kāla* is possible in any geographic location using several key principles. These principles are derived from the practical application of the classics in the Indian subcontinent. They can be reverse-engineered, applied to new locations and tested within the scope of the classical Āyurvedic framework. This research and development will encourage advancement of the science.

Principle #1: Two ayanas

Each year is primarily divided into two *ayanas*, or periods of time that are predominant in producing effects of depletion and nourishment in human populations, the general environment and many life forms. These two periods include:

Uttarāyana Northern-moving	*Dakṣhiṇāyana* Southern-moving
Ādāna kāla Depleting period	*Visarga kāla* Strengthening period
Agneya guṇa *Agni* (sun) dominant	*Saumya guṇa* *Soma* (moon) dominant
Approximate timing (Gregorian calendar)	
Dec 20 – Jun 20	Jun 20 – Dec 20
Approximate timing (Hindu calendar)	
Jan 15 – Jul 15	Jul 15 – Jan 15

The approximate time periods of each *ayana* may be correlated to the solstices in the Gregorian calendar. In traditional Vedic or Hindu calendars, the approximate periods occur roughly one month following the Gregorian solstices. Note that the Vedic calendar dates can vary significantly depending on the year due to the addition of a 13th month during calendar correction years.

Determination of each *ayana* is made by assessing its *ayana lakṣhaṇas*. These *lakṣhaṇas* are extremely subtle to analyze on any given day. However, they can be more readily noticed as their cumulative effects build up over the course of the entire *ayana*.

Although an *ayana sandhi* has not been directly mentioned in the classics, it is plausible that it would exist at the junction of both *ayana* periods, or twice each year. Considerable research is required to assess, determine and confirm the timing of each *ayana* in any geographical region.

Principle #2: Ṛtu classifications

Seasonal divisions may be created for any geographical region as appropriate for the specific *lakṣhaṇas*. Charaka clearly states the flexibility of the science in this regard in Cha. Vi. 8/125 and in Cha. Sū. 6/4 in the Chakrapāṇi commentary.

The specific classifications of seasons mentioned by Charaka include:

1. Two
2. Three
3. Six
4. Twelve
5. More than twelve

It is interesting to note that a classification based on four seasons has not been mentioned here. The question that naturally arises is whether it was omitted as an example and still considered allowable, or if it is not intended to be used as a classification at all.

In many geographical regions today, popular Western culture considers four seasons of winter, spring, summer and fall. However, this can also be analyzed in context of the classical Āyurvedic perspective as two major seasons of winter and summer, or *śhīta* and *uṣhṇa*, separated by the transitional, moderate seasons of spring and fall. This may be appropriate in certain locations where rainfall occurs regularly throughout the year, rather than in a monsoon-like period. Extensive research is needed to determine the *ṛtu* classifications in any given location. A preliminary analysis has been attempted by the American Āyurvedic Journal of Health for six major geographical regions in the US by comparing their classical *lakṣhaṇas* with the National Oceanic and Atmospheric Administration's (NOAA's) 1981-2010 US Climate Normals data set. This includes thirty years of statistically normalized average climate data for major locations in the US.

Principle #3: Ṛtu cycles for rasa

The *Kāla chakra* calendar divides the seasons into six *ṛtus* to allow for the manifestation of the *ṣhad-rasa*. The manifestation of each one of the *ṣhad-rasa* is stated to occur during a specific *ṛtu* based on the *ṛtu's* predominance in specific *mahā-bhūtas*. These appear at certain times of the year due to the regular, cyclical events of heat, cold and precipitation in a unique presentation caused by the movement of the earth and the resulting seasons.

The *ṣhad-rasa* predominate in the *ṣhad-ṛtu* as follows.

Kāla chakra ṛtus	Predominant *rasa*	*Mahā-bhūtas*
Śhiśhira Late winter	*Tikta* Bitter	*Ākāśha* + *Vāyu*
Vasanta Spring	*Kaṣhaya* Astringent	*Vāyu* + *Pṛthvi*
Grīṣhma Summer	*Kaṭu* Pungent	*Tejas* + *Vāyu*
Varṣhā Monsoon	*Amla* Sour	*Pṛthvi* + *Tejas*
Śharat Second summer	*Lavaṇa* Salty	*Tejas + Ap*
Hemanta Early winter	*Madhura* Sweet	*Pṛthvi + Ap*

The primary application of the *Kāla chakra* calendar is for regions of the Indian subcontinent that experience a slightly longer winter period and slightly shorter monsoon period. For therapeutic applications, this calendar is also considered as the basis for practically understanding and utilizing the *ṣhad-rasa* for seasonal dietary and lifestyle routines.

Principle #4: Ṛtu cycles for śhodhana

The Āyurvedic calendar divides the seasons into six *ṛtus* to explain the annual cycles of the *doṣhas* and the appropriate time periods for expelling them to maintain normal health. The extensive processes required to safely remove *doṣhas* from the body in a controlled fashion using *śhodhana* are ideally advised during seasons that are not marked by significant cold, heat or precipitation.

The classical *ṛtus* and their appropriate type of *śhodhana* are listed below. Each type of *śhodhana* intends to target a specific *doṣha*.

Āyurvedic calendar *ṛtus*	*Ṛtu śhodhana* Seasonal therapy	Targeted *doṣha*
Hemanta Early winter	None	None
Vasanta Spring	*Vamana* Emesis	Kapha
Grīṣhma Summer	None	None

Prāvṛṭ Early rains	*Basti* Enema	Vāta
Varṣhā Late rains	None	None
Śharat Second summer	*Virechana* Purgation	Pitta

Charaka explains these recommendations in Cha. Vi. 8/125 and Suśhruta states them in Su. Sū. 6/12 and Su. Ci. 24/109.

Principle #5: Triggers for ṛtu changes

The change from one *ṛtu* to the next is always caused due to specific changes in the *guṇas* of the external environment. These are generally the result of the constant movement of the earth on its orbit around the sun which causes direct increases and decreases in heat, cold, wind and precipitation.

These external factors cause direct changes in the *guṇas* of the local region's environment which create its typical climate patterns. In the Indian subcontinent, climate patterns have for many centuries been very regular and predictable. Classical Āyurvedic principles for seasonal changes were created based on these predictable patterns using the *guṇa* framework.

Vāgbhaṭa provides the clearest explanations for seasonal triggers among all classical texts. He recognizes the three major periods of cold, heat and rains as the starting point. Each of these is predominated by a single *doṣha* which is also related to the prevalent *guṇas*. Between each of these primary seasons lies an intermediate, or moderate season.

Vāgbhaṭa further provides insight into the prevalence of each *doṣha* through its annual cycle of *chaya*, *prakopa* and *praśhamana*. He is able to identify the primary *guṇas* seen during each of these stages. Most importantly, he specifies the trigger *guṇas* that cause the *doṣha* to move from one stage to the next. These same principles can be applied to the changes of seasons that are seen throughout the year.

Review the explanations in the following table. Notice the pattern of *doṣhas*, their standard *guṇas* and their trigger *guṇas*.

Doṣhas	Guṇas	Chaya	Prakopa	Praśhamana
Vāta	Rūkṣha + others Laghu, cala, viśhada, khara	Uṣhṇa	Śhīta	Snigdha, etc + usna
Pitta	Tīkṣhṇa + others Rūkṣha, laghu, sara, drava	Śhīta	Uṣhṇa	Manda, etc + Sita
Kapha	Snigdha + others Guru, pichchhila, manda, etc	Śhīta	Uṣhṇa	Manda, etc + śhīta

Vāta and pitta are seen to enter their cycles of *chaya* and *prakopa* when their standard *guṇas* associate with their same and opposite *guṇas* based on temperature. However, kapha operates in the exact opposite manner. This special presentation of kapha is called *skannatva* and is explained in AH Sū. 12/19-28.

The reason for the opposite effects of kapha's cycle are due to its *svabhāva*. Consider the practical application of generating enough kapha to create a state of *chaya*. This involves the physical build-up of gross mass through its standard *guṇas*. It can be likened to filling an ice cube tray and placing it in the freezer. As the water gets colder, it expands slightly. When additional cold is applied to the water in the ice cube tray, it continues to expand until it freezes, reaching its maximum state of *chaya*.

Only through the application of *uṣhṇa* can the frozen ice, or accumulated kapha, be melted. This results in overflow and spreading. Taking a frozen ice cube and placing it on a plate during a hot summer day causes it to melt and spread quickly. Similarly, when *uṣhṇa* is applied to kapha in a state of *chaya*, it causes it to melt inside the body and spread out of its normal boundaries resulting in state of *prakopa*.

This same principle is seen in the seasons of winter and spring where kapha naturally experiences its states of *chaya* and *prakopa*.

Principle #6: Ahorātri classification

Day and night are classified as the daily time periods that occur between sunrise and sunset, and sunset and sunrise. These two approximate halves of a single day present with their own distinct *lakṣhaṇas* during three main phases. Each main phase is marked by specific *guṇas* which are practically seen to relate to a single *doṣha*.

The determination of day and night are straightforward. However, the three main phases that occur within each period of day and night are not always so obvious. Here, Vāgbhaṭa's principle must be applied. He states that the three *doṣhas*, vāta, pitta and kapha, appear at the end, middle and beginning of certain cycles, including the periods of day and night.

No additional details are provided on specific clock times or other demarcations. It should be understood that the involvement of each *doṣha* can be recognized based on the presentation of similar *lakṣhaṇas*. This provides a flexible framework that can be implemented in any geographical region where lengths of day and night periods vary greatly.

The duration of day and night, and the durations of the main phases marked by specific *doṣhas* may also have an impact on the factors which influence affected individuals. For example, in tropical zones, the day and night durations do not vary as much as they do in higher latitude temperate zones. Because of this change in the amount of time predominated by specific *guṇas*, the *doṣhas* are likely influenced accordingly.

Discerning the effects of the day and night for any geographical region may be done on a case-by-case basis until further research provides more conclusive recommendations.

TEST YOURSELF

Learn, review and memorize key terms from this section.

ayana sandhi

śhodhana

---

vamana

---

virechana

---

basti

KĀLA ASSESSMENT

The assessment of *kāla*, *ayana*, *ṛtu* and *ahorātri* in any geographical location outside of the Indian subcontinent is a practical application of the science of Āyurveda based on *yukti*. *Kāla* assessment is a key component of the application of the science for maintenance of health and management of disease because of its impacts on human health.

Classical *lakṣhaṇas* should be employed using their theoretical foundations to predict the expected, general outcome of the effects of *kāla* in any given location. With a known baseline for seasonal schedules and their anticipated effects, practitioners can then compare the presentations of specific individuals to determine whether their signs and symptoms are appropriate for the season or indicative of a deeper potential pathology.

The outcomes of annual and seasonal effects on human health can be considered in two major manifestations.

1. Acute, immediate effects
2. Chronic, cumulative effects

To distinguish these presentations clinically requires a thorough understanding of the individual's history, relevant causative factors and additional influential factors such as *deśha* and *kāla*. A carefully performed Clinical Svastha Assessment provides the framework for a complete review of all factors so that appropriate recommendations can be made.

For the *kāla* assessment, the individual's *ayana*, *ṛtu* and *ahorātri* must be analyzed and investigated. Significant information from the individual's main complaints and potential risk factors may be correlated in the process.

Determining ayana periods

The *ayana* periods are generally easier to approximate than the *ṛtu* periods. In the Northern and Southern Hemispheres, these larger, biannual cycles occur at opposite times of the year.

Hemisphere	*Uttarāyana* Period	*Dakṣhiṇ-āyana* Period
Northern Hemisphere	Jan 15 to Jul 15	Jul 15 to Jan 15
Southern Hemisphere	Jul 15 to Jan 15	Jan 15 to Jul 15

The potential *ayana sandhi* period should also be taken into account when determining the active *ayana* period. During the transitional time, the effects of the completed *ayana* period may be more pronounced. As the next *ayana* begins, it will not have accumulated its effects significantly yet.

To estimate the potential *ayana sandhi* period, note when the individual is within one month before or after the *ayana* transition date.

Use the following table and map to assess the *ayana* period.

Clinical Svastha Assessment: *Ayana*

Answer these questions to evaluate the current *ayana*.

Question	Response
Hemisphere	Northern Southern
Current date	
Expected current *ayana*	*Uttarāyana* *Dakṣhiṇāyana*
Within *ayana sandhi*?	One month prior One month after
Expected *ayana lakṣhaṇas*	
Current *ayana lakṣhaṇas*	

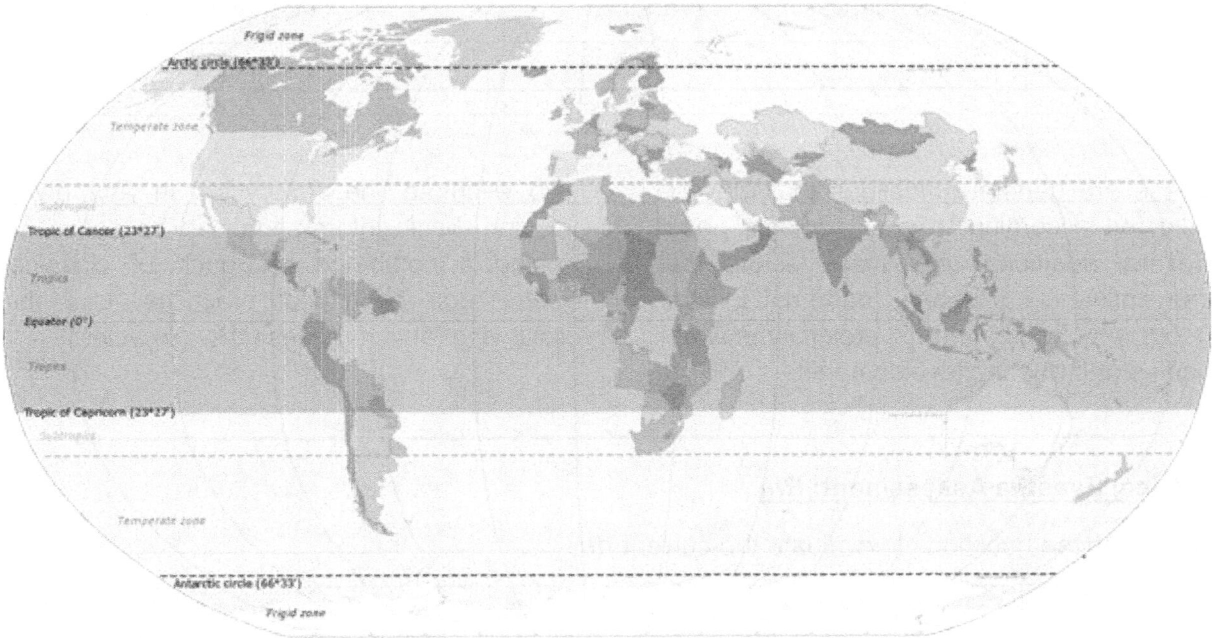

Determining ṛtu cycles

In new regions, the *deśha* and *ṛtu* are generally considered together in order to fully understand their implications on the *doṣhas* and *svastha*. The classics provide a flexible framework which can be utilized to describe and define seasonal cycles in any location.

Ultimately, the determination lies in accurately assessing the location's unique *lakṣhaṇas*. This allows the variances between seasons to be recognized so that the three predominant periods of cold, heat and possible rains can be established.

In different regions, these seasons may

occur independently or overlap each other, especially when considering precipitation. A few locations, which notably include the Indian subcontinent, do experience a true, annual monsoon period that spans for several months. However, many temperate locations do not experience clearly defined periods of wet and dry seasons. Precipitation in the form of rain, snow, sleet, hail, etc often occurs throughout the year and over the course of cold and hot seasons.

Using latitude and longitude and the major populated zones of tropical, subtropical and temperate, general seasonal patterns can be estimated for many locations. Review these general patterns with the approximate locations found on the map on the previous page.

Zones	Latitude range	Number of seasons	Common seasonal cycle
Temperate	40 – 66 degrees	2	Cold and hot, regular precipitation
Sub-tropical	23 – 40 degrees	Variable	Variable
Tropical	0 – 23 degrees	3	Cold, hot and wet

These are general guidelines that may be adjusted according to each region's need. Several additional, significant factors that can influence seasonal patterns include geography, wind patterns, proximity to water bodies and human developments.

To estimate the *ṛtu* cycles in any given region, basic information can be assessed using a combined approach of classical knowledge and local practices. Use the following table to assess the *ṛtu* cycles.

Clinical Svastha Assessment: *Rtu*

Answer these questions to evaluate the current *ṛtu*.

Question	Response
Current date	
Location	
Current local season	
Expected *ṛtu lakṣhaṇas*	
Current *ṛtu lakṣhaṇas*	
Estimated current *doṣha* cycles	V + / ++ / - P + / ++ / - K + / ++ / -

Determining ahorātri cycles

Determination of *ahorātri* cycles is most relevant to an individual's assessment of *svastha* when assessing the timing of the presentation of their primary *lakṣhaṇas*. This timing can be correlated to periods of the day or night which are known to be predominant in a specific *doṣha* and its related *guṇas*.

Use the following table to assess the local *ahorātri* cycles and correlate the primary *guṇas* with those found in the individual. If possible, estimate the *doṣha* states during the primary time period to determine whether the individual is in synch with the overall *ahorātri* cycle.

Clinical Svastha Assessment: *Ahorātri*

Answer these questions to evaluate the current *ahorātri*.

Question	Response
Local sunrise time	
Local sunset time	
Daytime duration (hours, mins)	
Nighttime duration (hours, mins)	
Primary times of *lakṣhaṇas*	
Primary manifested *lakṣhaṇas*	
Estimated *doṣha* states	V + / ++ / - P + / ++ / - K + / ++ / -

Chapter 4: Review

ADDITIONAL READING

Read and review the references listed below to expand your understanding of the concepts in this chapter. Write down the date that you complete your reading for each. Remember that consistent repetition is the best way to learn. Plan to read each reference at least once now and expect to read it again as you continue your studies.

References marked with (skim) can be read quickly and do not require commentary review.

CLASSICS		1st read	2nd read
Charaka	Cha. Sū. 6/ Cha. Sū. 12/ Cha. Sū. 17/114c Cha. Vi. 3/24-27 Cha. Vi. 8/76 Cha. Vi. 8/125-127		
Suśhruta	Su. Sū. 6/		
Aṣhṭāṅga Hṛdaya	AH Sū. 3/		
Bhāva Prakāśha	BP Pū. 5/309-338		

JOURNALS & CURRENT RESOURCES

http://aa.usno.navy.mil/faq/docs/rs_solstices.php

QUESTIONS & ANSWERS

Record your questions for this chapter here for further research and discussion.

Question:

Answer:

Question:

Answer:

Question:

Answer:

SELF-ASSESSMENT

1. In the context of Āyurveda, *kāla*
   a. has specific divisions that are applicable to the practice of the science.
   b. influences all aspects of life.
   c. influences health.
   d. influences treatment.
   e. All of the above

2. According to the *kāla bheda*, which of the following does not belong?
   a. *Muhūrta*
   b. *Pakṣha*
   c. *Pariṇāma*
   d. *Ṛtu*
   e. *Saṁvatsara*

3. What are the names of the two *ayanas*?
   a. *Akṣhi* and *nimeṣha*
   b. *Dakṣhiṇa* and *uttara*
   c. *Visarga* and *ādāna*
   d. Both B and C
   e. All of the above

4. Which three factors influence the effects felt from the eternal world?
   a. *Agni*, *Vāyu*, *Soma*
   b. *Uṣhṇa*, *Laghu*, *Śhīta*
   c. *Vāta*, *Pitta*, *Kapha*
   d. *Vāyu*, *Tejas*, *Pṛthvi*
   e. None of the above

5. *Ahorātri* refers to
   a. *anta*, *madhya*, *ādhi*.
   b. *chaya*, *prakopa*, *praśhamanā*.
   c. day and night.
   d. stages of digestion.
   e. All of the above

6. Why is it important to understand latitude, longitude, geographical zones, climate and weather for practical application of Āyurveda?
   a. Not all environments are like the subcontinent of India.
   b. The understanding offers a more accurate picture in a client assessment.
   c. They provide clues to the possible seasonal patterns in a particular region.
   d. All of the above
   e. None of the above

7. What does *ṛtu sandhi* indicate?
   a. Classically, it is the last week of the current *ṛtu* and the first week of the new *ṛtu*.
   b. Diet and habits should slowly shift to the upcoming season.
   c. It is the joint between the seasons.
   d. Through gradual transition, one avoids disorders caused by *asātmya*.
   e. All of the above

8. Suśhruta states in the *ṛtu lakṣhaṇas* for *grīṣhma* that
   a. herbs and shrubs dwindle.
   b. sun rays scorch the earth.
   c. the river water levels reduce.
   d. the southwest wind is unpleasant.
   e. All of the above

9. In *hemanta*, which *doṣha* is in *chaya*? What is the state of *agni*? Which *pañcha mahābhūtas* are expressing themselves?
   a. *Kapha*; *uttama*; *ākāśha* and *vāta*
   b. *Kapha*; *uttama*; *pṛthvi* and *ap*
   c. *Pitta*; *avara*; *tejas* and *ap*
   d. *Vāta*; *avara*; *pṛthvi* and *tejas*
   e. None of the above

10. Classically, human strength increases
   a. during *ādāna kāla*
   b. during *dakṣhināyana*
   c. during *uttara kāla*
   d. in the summertime
   e. All of the above

CRITICAL THINKING

1. Would *ādāna* and *visarga kāla* always occur at the same time around the world? Explain your reasoning.
2. Compare and contrast the concepts of *kāla* and *pariṇāma*.
3. Does *deśha* influence the presentation of *ṛtu*? Why?
4. How can knowledge of latitude and longitutde improve assessment skills?
5. Compare and contrast *ahorātri* and *ṛtu lakṣhaṇas*.

References

https://en.wikipedia.org/wiki/Hindu_calendar

A History of Science in World Cultures: Voices of Knowledge By Scott L. Montgomery, Alok Kumar, pages 103-104 (https://books.google.com/books?id=kkLeCQAAQBAJ&pg=PA103#v=onepage&q&f=false)

The Hindu Religious Year By Muriel Marion Underhill, page 32 (https://books.google.com/books?id=Fb9Zc0yPVUUC&pg=PA32#v=onepage&q&f=false)

UNIT II

Internal factors that influence health

Chapter 5 : Sātmya and charya

KEY TERMS

abrahmacharya	brahmacharya	okasātmya	vihāra
āchāra	charya	rātricharya	vṛtta
adhāraṇīya vegas	dinacharya	ṛtucharya	vṛtti
asātmya	nidrā	sātmya	

The application of *sātmya* applies to almost every aspect of health in Āyurveda. Review the details of *sātmya* in Chapter two for an explanation of classical definitions, original references and *sātmya bheda*. The classifications of *sātmya* are key to understanding the Āyurvedic perspective of *svastha* as they demonstrate how important *sātmya* is in all aspects of health and how it creates the big picture of holistic health.

This chapter covers the classical recommendations for *sātmya* in terms of the *āhāra* and *vihāra* that can be used to train an individual for promoting overall *svastha*. Because *sātmya* can apply to virtually all factors that influence *svastha*, this chapter will cover those topics which relate more closely to *charya*, or daily routines and regimens. *Sātmya* will also be covered in each subsequent chapter of this volume where appropriate for the chapter's main topic.

CLASSICAL REVIEW

The assessment of *sātmya* is based on the two main criteria: it must promote health and do so with long-term, regular use. For any food, behavior or activity to be considered *sātmya*, it must promote an individual's *svastha* when used regularly.

In cases where items may appear to be *sātmya* but are actually not, they are considered *okasātmya*. Assessing *sātmya* is done in the Clinical Svastha Assessment through all factors individually. Classically, the outcome of each factor assessed for *sātmya* can be measured as *uttama*, *madhyama* or *avara*, indicating the value of the factor towards promoting overall *svastha*.

Applying sātmya

A variety of recommendations for maintaining and promoting healthy *sātmya* can be found in several contexts in classical literature. These can be most broadly categorized as:

- *Rasa* — flavor profiles
- *Dinacharya* — daily routines
- *Ṛtucharya* — seasonal routines

With all recommendations, keep in mind that *sātmya* is inherently a flexible concept which is measured in a personalized manner for each individual. All methods of applying *sātmya* may be approached from a generalized perspective, and then customized as required for each individual.

Punarvasu Ātreya creates consensus at the conclusion of a debate on *sātmya* by stating that it requires a completely personalized approach.

येषामेव हि भावानां संपत् संजनयेन्नरम् ।
तेषामेव विपद्व्याधीन्विविधान्समुदीरयेत् ॥
च. सू. २५।२९

Yeṣhāmeva hi bhāvānāṁ saṁpat saṁjanayennaram |
Teṣhāmeva vipadvyādhīnvividhānsamudīrayet ||

Cha. Sū. 25/29

Yeṣhāmeva hi bhāvānāṁ (The very same foods) saṁpat (that may be used in a wholesome manner) saṁjanayennaram (to promote healthy growth of individuals) teṣhāmeva (can also be) vipad (in their opposite, or unwholesome state) vyādhīn vividhān samudīrayet (the specific causes for various diseases).

The main purpose of *sātmya* is to fulfill the goal of *dhātu sāmya*. To utilize this effectively on a general, daily basis, each individual should tailor their foods, habits and routines to offset the detrimental effects of the *guṇas* found in their local environment, season, baseline state and current state.

देशकालात्मगुणविपरीतानां हि
कर्मणामाहारविकाराणां च क्रियोपयोगः
सम्यक्, सर्वातियोगसन्धारणम्,
असन्धारणमुदीर्णानां च गतिमतां,
साहसानां च वर्जनं, स्वस्थवृत्तमेतावध्दातूनां
साम्यानुग्रहार्थमुपदिश्यते || ८

च. शा. ६।८

Deśhakālātmaguṇaviparītānāṁ hi
karmaṇāmāhāravikārāṇāṁ cha
kriyopayogaḥ samyak,
sarvātiyogasandhāraṇam,
asandhāraṇamudīrṇānāṁ cha
gatimatāṁ, sāhasānāṁ cha varjanaṁ,
svasthavṛttametāvaddhātūnāṁ
sāmyānugrahārthamupadiśhyate || 8

Cha. Śhā. 6/8

Svastha vṛttam (Svastha Vṛtta, the study and practice of promoting all aspects of health) upadiśhyate (is taught) etāvad (as this:) dhātūnāṁ sāmya (that *dhātu sāmya*, or equilibrium of the supportive structures of the body) ānugraha (be the goal [of the practice]) artham (which is achieved through these [following methods]).

Guṇa-viparītānāṁ (The characteristics that are opposite to) deśha (the environment), kāla (seasons), ātma (the individual's unique nature) vikārāṇāṁ cha (and the disease) kriya-upayogaḥ (should be utilized in all therapeutic manners) samyak (in their proper methods of application) hi karmaṇām (as activities, routines, habits,) āhāra (food).

Sarva (All things) atiyoga (in excess) sandhāraṇam (should be restrained or limited), asandhāraṇam ([except] that which should not be restrained [ie, the *adhāraṇīya vegas*]) udīrṇānāṁ cha gati matāṁ (which should be allowed to go out on their own as [the science states] is best); sāhasānāṁ cha (and extending one's self beyond ones capacity) varjanaṁ (causing injury [should also be avoided]).

Charaka provides the same explanation and recommendations in Cha. Vi. 3/36.

Both Charaka and Suśhruta discuss the targeted use of *rasa* in the context of *sātmya*. Charaka assesses *rasa* usage and measures it on a scale of *avara*, *madhyama* and *uttama* in Cha. Vi. 1/20.

Rasa sātmya	Proper, proportional use
Avara	1 *rasa*
Madhyama	2 – 5 *rasas*
Uttama	6 *rasas*

Suśhruta advises that the *rasa* which promotes *sukha* for an individual when used regularly is to be considered *sātmya* (Su. Sū. 35/39-40).

For seasonal maintenance of *svastha*, Charaka recommends that the practices of expelling the *doṣhas* in a safe and controlled manner be adopted on an annual basis.

हैमन्तिकं दोषचयं वसन्ते प्रवाहयन्
ग्रैष्मिकमभ्रकाले| घनात्यये वार्षिकमाशु
सम्यक् प्राप्नोति रोगानृतुजान्न जातु || ४५
च. शा. २।४५

Haimantikaṁ doṣhachayaṁ vasante
pravāhayan graiṣhmikamabhrakāle |
Ghanātyaye vārṣhikamāśhu samyak
prāpnoti rogānṛtujānna jātu || 45
Cha. Śhā. 2/45

Haimantikaṁ doṣha-chayaṁ (The *doṣhas* which have undergone *chaya* during winter) vasante pravāhayan (should be sent forward [ie, eliminated appropriately] in the spring). Graiṣhmikam-abhrakāle (Those [*doṣhas*] of the summer) ghanātyaye (are to be collected and expelled) vārṣhikamāśhu (during the early rainy season, and those of the rains during the next season [ie, *śharat*]). Samyak prāpnoti (When this is properly achieved), rogānṛtujānna jātu (individuals are not afflicted by seasonal disorders).

Season of *doṣha chaya*	Season of *śhodhana*
Hemanta Early winter	*Vasanta* Spring
Grīṣhma Summer	*Prāvṛt* Early rains
Varṣhā Late rains	*Śharat* Second summer

Managing okasātmya and asātmya

Classical recommendations state that foods or practices which are *okasātmya* or *asātmya* should be removed from an individual's regular routine. This should be done in a carefully controlled manner as long as the benefits outweigh the potential risks.

Charaka describes the methodology for gradually removing *okasātmya* and *asātmya* items in Cha. Sū. 7/36-37. He proposes that the inappropriate item be removed one quarter at a time and simultaneously replaced with one quarter of an appropriate, *sātmya* item.

This method follows a schedule that can be extended for as long as needed to allow the individual sufficient time to acclimate to the new item or habit. Suśhruta agrees with this statement and adds in Su. Chi. 24/97 that one-sixteenth or one-fourth of the habit can be progressively replaced to allow for an easier transition. Vāgbhaṭa provides a similar explanation in AH Sū. 7/48-49. Review Chapter Two for a discussion of *sātmya* and its appropriate management.

Charya

The term *charya* is used classically to refer to any type of regular routine, regimen or schedule that is intended to promote *svastha*. *Charya* is synonymous with *vṛtta*, *vṛtti* and *āchāra*. *Āchāra* also implies good conduct and proper ethical behavior.

The activities of *charya* may be adjusted at any time according to the individual's need, the season, and any other prioritized factor. The regular diets included in *charya* are referred to as *āhāra* while the habitual activities are often termed *vihāra*.

The purpose of adhering to *charya* is to prevent disease and promote *svastha*. Bhāvamiśhra states this at the beginning of the chapter on *dinacharya*:

मानवो येन विधिना स्वस्थस्तिष्ठति सर्वदा ।
तमेव कारयेद्वैद्यो यतः स्वस्थ्यं सदेप्सितम्
|| १

दिनचर्यां निशाचर्यामृतुचर्यां यथोदिताम् ।
आचरन्पुरुषः स्वस्थः सदा तिष्ठिति नान्यथा ॥

भा. प्र. पू. ५।२

Mānavo yena vidhinā svasthasthiṣhṭhati sarvadā |
Tameva kārayedvaidyo yataḥ svasthyaṁ sadepsitam || 1
Dinacharyāṁ niśhācharyāmṛtucharyāṁ yathoditām |
Ācharanpuruṣhaḥ svasthaḥ sadā tiṣhṭhati nānyathā ||

BP Pū. 5/2

Mānavo yena vidhinā (The methods and regimens for people) svasthas-thiṣhṭhati (to maintain their health) sarvadā (consistently and regularly) tameva kārayed-vaidyo (must be properly instructed by the *vaidya*) yataḥ svasthyaṁ sadepsitam (so that health can be preserved).

Yathoditām (These methods are explained here [in this science] and include) dinacharyāṁ (daily routines), niśhācharyām (nightly routines and) ṛtucharyāṁ (seasonal routines). Ācharan puruṣhaḥ (Adhering to these *āchara* [behaviors and routines]) svasthaḥ sadā tiṣhṭhati nānyathā (allows people to always maintain their health).

The following sections review the classical recommendations and guidance on *dinacharya*, *niśhācharya* (or *rātricharya*) and *ṛtucharya*. The original information is intended for the Indian subcontinent, its culture, seasons and people. The underlying theories and principles can be extracted from this information and applied globally.

Dinacharya

The concept of *dinacharya* exists in all major classical texts. *Dinacharya* is a foundation for personal, preventive health care that can be performed regularly and relatively easily to avoid disorders and diseases.

A thorough review of classical literature reveals that routines and recommendations for *dinacharya* can be widely customized to meet the needs of the individual. The classical texts include comprehensive lists of therapies and treatments that can be performed at home by the individual as needed. While some of these activities are meant to be performed daily, others are best done in certain seasons, or for a limited period of time under the guidance of a qualified Āyurvedic professional.

Several of the more complex therapies included in *dinacharya* are smaller, lighter versions of *upakrama*, or external therapeutic treatments. Therefore, they can have a more pronounced effect on the body and the *doṣhas* when applied for longer periods of time.

It is important that these types of therapies be instructed carefully and the results be monitored regularly. Self-monitoring is often simple and effective after sufficient education and experience to understand when to start or stop applying the therapy.

The following table includes a review of the *dinacharya* listed in major classical references. These recommendations may be customized to the individual in sequence, duration, timing and applicable factors.

The more complex activities listed here will be discussed in Volume 4 along with their indications, contraindications, general methods and procedures. Basic routines that can be advised today will be discussed in the last section of this chapter.

Recommended classical *dinacharya* activity	Cha. Sū. 5/	Su. Chi. 24/	AH Sū. 2/	BP Pū. 5/
Brāhma-muhūrta uttiṣhṭhate Waking up approximately one hour and thirty-six minutes before sunrise		✓ (no specific time)	✓	✓
Mala visarjana Evacuating the wastes (bladder and bowels)				✓
Mala-mārga śhauca Cleaning the orifices of the waste channels				✓
Añjana Collyrium	✓	✓	✓	✓
Uṣhaḥ pāna Drinking water at daybreak				✓
Ambu nasya Passing water through the nose (jala neti)				✓
Dhūmapāna Inhaling smoke	✓		✓	
Nasya Instilling nasal drops	✓		✓	✓
Danta dhāvana Brushing the teeth	✓	✓	✓	✓
Jihva lekhana Scraping the tongue	✓	✓		✓
Tāmbūla patra (dhāryamāṇa āsyena) Chewing mouth freshner, usually betel leaf (Piper betel)	✓	✓	✓	✓
Gaṇḍūṣha Filling the mouth with liquid (usually oil)	✓	✓	✓	✓
Mukha prakṣhālana Washing the face		✓		
Mūrdni taila (*śhiro abhyaṅga*) Applying oil to the head (in any of the four standard methods of *abhyaṅga*, *śhirodhāra*, *basti*, *pichu*)	✓	✓	✓	✓
Keśha prasādhanī Brushing or combing the hair		✓		✓

Karṇa tarpaṇa Refreshing oil application for the ears	✓	✓	✓	✓
Śharīra abhyaṅga Applying oil to the body	✓	✓	✓	✓
Seka Pouring water over the body		✓	✓	
Avagāha Soaking in a bathtub				✓
Vyāyāma Physical training, exercise		✓	✓	✓
Udvartana Dry powder massage, body rub		✓	✓	✓
Snāna Washing the body, showering, bathing	✓	✓	✓	✓
Anulepana Anointing; application of thin paste		✓		✓
Nirmala ambara dhāraṇa Wearing clean clothes	✓	✓	✓	✓
Gandha mālya Use of fragrance and garlands	✓	✓	✓	
Ratnābharaṇa dhāraṇa Use of jewelry and precious stones	✓	✓	✓	✓
Mukha ālepa Anointing the face; application of paste for the face		✓		✓
Pāda and mala-mārga śhauca Regular cleaning of the feet and excretory pathways	✓	✓	✓	✓
Pāda abhyaṅga Applying oil to the feet and massaging		✓		✓
Keśha, śhmaśhru, nakha-adi kalpana Regular trimming and doing the hair, beard, nails, etc	✓	✓	✓	✓
Uṣhṇīṣha Wearing a turban		✓		✓
Pādatra dhāraṇa Regular use of proper footwear	✓	✓	✓	✓

Chatra dhāraṇa Regular use of an umbrella	√	√	√	
Daṇḍa dhāraṇa Regular use of a walking stick	√	√	√	
Vyajana Fanning		√		
Saṁvāhana Gentle, pleasant, sensual massage		√		√
Sadvṛttta Proper behavior, conduct, actions		√	√	

Sadvṛttta is a significant topic that is discussed by all authors to promote proper, ethical behavior in all aspects of personal, professional and public relationships. These recommendations are usually spread across several chapters throughout each *saṁhitā*. Because the practice of *sadvṛttta* is intended to promote an individual's state of *sattva*, it will be covered in detail in Chapter nine.

Rātricharya

Rātricharya and *niśhācharya* are synonymous terms both indicating the routines and regimens to be followed at night before going to sleep. The few activities mentioned are only recorded in Bhāva Prakāśha, Pūrvakhanda, chapter 5, following the details on *dinacharya*.

Sleep hygiene may be considered with *rātricharya*.

Recommended classical *rātricharya* activity	Cha.	Su.	AH	BP Pū. 5/
Rātri bhojana Dinner				√
Maithuna Sexual intercourse				√
Nidrā Sleep				√

Rtucharya

Regular adherence to *ṛtucharya* is considered one of the primary aspects of preventive healthcare in classical Āyurveda. Proper dietary choices, lifestyle routines and self care during each season promotes health and prevents disease. It allows an individual to manage their *doṣhas* appropriately, support *agni*, increase *bala* and *ojas*, and maximize *āyus* while remaining synchronized with the natural ebbs and flows of the external environment and time.

Charaka begins his explanation of *ṛtucharya* with a statement that highlights its importance.

तस्याशिताद्यादाहाराद्बलं वर्णश्च बर्धते ।
यस्यर्तुसात्म्यं विदितं चेष्टाहारव्यपाश्रयम् ।
च. सू. ६।३

Tasyāśhitādyādāhārādbalaṁ varṇaśhcha vardhate |
Yasyartusātmyaṁ viditaṁ cheṣhṭāhāravyapāśhrayam || 3
Cha. Sū. 6/3

Tasyāśhitādyād (The appropriate use of all types of eatables), āhārād (foods and diets), vardhate (increases) balaṁ (the strength), varṇaśhcha (and complexion) yasya (of those individuals) rtu-sātmyaṁ (who are accustomed to the season's) viditaṁ (routines of) cheṣhṭa (activities), āhāra ([and] food), vyapāśhrayam (through regular application).

Use the references in the following chart to review the classical explanations and recommendations for *ṛtucharya*.

Ṛtu	Charaka	Suśhruta	Aṣhṭāṅga Hṛdaya	Bhāva Prakāśha
Hemanta	Cha. Sū. 6/9-18	Su. Chi. 24/103-109	AH Sū. 3/7-16	BP Pū. 5/316, 329
Śhiśhira	Cha. Sū. 6/19-21		AH Sū. 3/17	BP Pū. 5/317, 330
Vasanta	Cha. Sū. 6/22-26	Su. Chi. 24/103-109	AH Sū. 3/18-25	BP Pū. 5/317, 331-332
Grīṣhma	Cha. Sū. 6/27-32	Su. Chi. 24/103-109	AH Sū. 3/26-41	BP Pū. 5/318, 333
Prāvṛt		Su. Chi. 24/103-109		
Varṣhā	Cha. Sū. 6/33-40	Su. Chi. 24/103-109	AH Sū. 3/42-44	BP Pū. 5/318, 322-325
Śharad	Cha. Sū. 6/41-48	Su. Chi. 24/103-109	AH Sū. 3/49-54	BP Pū. 5/316, 326-328

The natural cycles of *doṣha chaya*, *prakopa* and *praśhamana* occur due to changes in the environment with each season and can never be completely avoided by residents of any location. The goals of *ṛtucharya* are to minimize the negative impacts of the *doṣhas* on the individual and prevent the need for *śhodhana* at the end of each of the *doṣha-prakopika ṛtus*.

It is helpful to compile the significant statements from all authors and review these key points about *ṛtucharya* to better comprehend the underlying principles. Use the following tables to review consolidated information. Source references are color-coded by text.

Color-coded references			
Cha. Sū. 6/9-48	Su. Sū. /	AH Sū. 3/	BP Pū. 5/

Ṛtu sātmya (Recommendations for general health during the ṛtu)						
	Śhiśhira	Vasanta	Grīṣhma	Varṣhā	Śharad	Hemanta
Rasas to favor	Madhura	Kaṭu	Madhura	Madhura	Madhura	Madhura
	Amla	Tikta		Amla *	Tikta	Amla
	Lavaṇa	Kaṣhaya		Lavaṇa *	Kaṣhaya	Lavaṇa
				Kaṭu		
				Tikta		
				Kaṣhaya		
Āhāra mātra	++			Moderate	Moderate	++
Āhāra guṇas to favor	Uṣhṇa	Laghu	Śhīta	Snigdha *	Laghu	Guru
	Guru	Rūkṣha	Drava	Laghu	Śhīta	Snigdha
	Snigdha	Uṣhṇa	Snigdha	Śhuṣhka (dry)	Rūkṣha	Uṣhṇa
			Laghu	Śhīta (end)	Uṣhṇa	

* Note that the indication for *amla* and *lavaṇa rasas* is specifically mentioned for days with complete cloud cover. Their extra usage during these times helps promote *agni*. (Cha. Sū. 6/37, AH Sū. 3/47)

Color-coded references			
Cha. Sū. 6/9-48	Su. Sū. /	AH Sū. 3/	BP Pū. 5/

Ṛtu sātmya (Recommendations for general health during the ṛtu)						
	Śhiśhira	Vasanta	Grīṣhma	Varṣhā	Śharad	Hemanta
Primary āhāra	Māṁsa, kṣhīra, ikṣhu, vasā, taila	Yava, godhūma	Jāṅgalā mṛga and pakṣhi, mantha, ghṛta-paya śhāli meals	Jāṅgalā māṁsa, purāṇā yava, godhūma, śhāli, mixed with kṣhaudra	Śhāli, mudga, sitā, āmalaki, paṭola, madhu, jāṅgalā māṁsa	Māṁsa, kṣhīra, ikṣhu, vasā, taila
Primary vihāra	Abhyaṅga, svedana, uṣhṇa		Candana, pearls, gardens, moonlight	Moderate; rūkṣha upakrama		Abhyaṅga, svedana, uṣhṇa
Nidrā		Avoid divā svapna	Divā svapna	Avoid divā svapna	Avoid divā svapna	
Maithuna	As desired, with a well-developed woman	Young girl	Abstinence	Abstinence		As desired, with a well-developed woman
Vyāyāma	¼ capacity	½ capacity	Avoid	Avoid	Gentle	½ capacity

Hemanta Ṛtucharya Āhāra Food for early winter		Cha. Sū. 6/9-48	AH Sū. 3/	BP Pū. 5/
Sātmya for the season				
	Gorasa Cow's milk products	✓		
	Ikṣhu-kṛti Sugarcane products	✓		
	Vasā Fat from animal meat or muscle	✓		
	Taila Oils	✓		
	Nava odana Freshly harvested grains, especially rice	✓		
	Uṣhṇa toya Hot water	✓		
Śhūkadhānya				
	Nava anna Freshly harvested grains, especially rice	✓	✓	✓
	Godhūma Wheat		✓	✓
	Piṣhṭa Flour		✓	✓
	Śhāli The group of rices			✓
Śhamīdhānya				
	Māṣha Urad dal, black gram (*Vigna mungo*)		✓	✓
Māṁsa				
	Snigdha, amla, lavaṇa rasa Meat soups prepared with oil, sour and salt	✓		
	Snigdha rasa pala puṣhṭa Meat soup from fully grown animals cooked with fat		✓	
	Audaka māṁsa Meat of aquatic animals	✓		

	Ānupa māṁsa Meat of marshy animals	√		
	Bileśhayāna (bhūmiśhayā) māṁsa Meat of burrow animals	√		
	Prasahā māṁsa Meat of predatory animals	√		
	Bhṛtā All meats prepared as dishes	√		√
Madya				
	Madirā All types of alcohol, in general	√		
	Sīdhu Sugarcane alcohols	√		
	Gauḍama Alcohol made from jaggery		√	
	Accha surā The clear portion of beer		√	
	Surā Beer		√	
Ambu				
	Uṣhṇa toya Hot water	√		
Gorasa				
	Gorasa Cow's milk products	√		
Ikṣhuvikāra				
	Ikṣhu-kṛti Sugarcane products	√	√	√
Āhārayogin				
	Madhu Honey	√		
	Vasā Fat of meat or muscle	√	√	

	Taila Oils, in general	✓	✓	
	Tila Sesame, sesame oil (*Sesamum indicum*)			✓

Hemanta Ṛtucharya Vihāra Activities for early winter		Cha. Sū. 6/9-48	AH Sū. 3/	BP Pū. 5/
Upakrama				
	Abhyaṅga Oil body massage	✓		
	Abhyaṅga with *vātaghna taila* Oil body massage with formulated oils to reduce vāta		✓	
	Abhyaṅga Oil body massage (with *lavaṇa taila*)			✓
	Utsādana Skin brightening massage with formulated powders	✓		
	Mūrdhni taila Oil head massage	✓	✓	
	Jentāka svedana Sauna	✓		
	Svedana Sweating		✓	
	Vimārdana Flexibility body massage		✓	
	Pādāghāta Invigorating body massage applied by the feet		✓	
Vyāyāma				
	Niyuddha kuśhala sārdha Training exercises (fighting, wrestling) to half capacity		✓	
	Śhrama Exertion to the point of fatigue or exhaustion			✓
Bāhya				
	Ātapa Exposure to sun	✓	✓	✓
Gṛha				
	Uṣhṇa bhūmi-gṛha Reside in warm homes	✓		
	Uṣhṇa garbha-gṛha Reside in warm, central rooms of dwellings, buildings	✓		

	Yāna, śhayana, āsana saṁvṛtaṁ Vehicle seats, beds, seats should be covered with thick, warm blankets	✓		
	Uṣhṇa-svabhāva, laghu prāvṛta śhayana Sleeping blankets should be naturally warm and light, like thick sheets of cotton, leather, silk, wool or tree bark		✓	
	Aṅgāra-tāpa santapta garbha-bhūveśhma chāriṇa Staying in inner rooms of dwellings heated by charcoal fires		✓	
Maithuna				
	Niṣheveta maithuna Sexual intercourse as desired; ideally at night after drinking alcohol with a healthy woman	✓	✓	
	Snigdha, sukha strī Loveable, satisfying woman			✓
Personal care				
	Guru, uṣhṇa vāsa Thick, warm clothes	✓		✓
	Aguru sadā Daily use of agarwood (*Aquilaria agallocha*)	✓		
	Kaṣhaya snāna Bath or shower with astringent *dravyas*		✓	
	Kuṅkuma, kastūri Application of saffron (*Crocus sativus*), musk from the musk deer (*Moschus moschiferus*)		✓	
	Aguru dhūpana Smoke bath with agarwood (*Aquilaria agallocha*)		✓	
	Pādatrāṇa Daily use of footwear		✓	
	Śhaucha-kārya sukha-udaka Water for cleaning (the excretory orifices) should be comfortable (in temperature)		✓	
	Kastūri, vara kuṅkuma, aguru yutā uṣhṇa ambu śhaucha Bath water heated properly with musk from the musk deer (*Moschus moschiferus*), good, high quality saffron (*Crocus sativus*), agarwood (*Aquilaria agallocha*)			✓

Hemanta Ṛtucharya Contraindications Contraindications for early winter	Cha. Sū. 6/9-48	AH Sū. 3/	BP Pū. 5/
Annapānāni vātalāni laghūni cha Food and drinks that increase *vāta* and are light	✓		
Pravāta Strong wind, stormy weather	✓		
Pramita āhāra Inadequate quantity of food	✓		
Udamantha Watery, diluted gruel	✓		

Hemanta Ṛtu Dinacharya Daily routine for early winter	Cha. Sū. 6/9-48	AH Sū. 3/	BP Pū. 5/
Wake up, evacuate wastes		✓	
Abhyaṅga with *vātaghna taila* Oil body massage with formulated oils to reduce *vāta*		✓	
Mūrdhni taila Oil head massage		✓	
Vimārdana Flexibility body massage		✓	
Niyuddha kuśhala sārdha Training exercises (fighting, wrestling) to half capacity		✓	
Pādāghāta Invigorating body massage applied by the feet		✓	
Kaṣhaya snāna Bath or shower with astringent *dravyas*		✓	
Kuṅkuma, kastūri Application of saffron (*Crocus sativus*), musk from the musk deer (*Moschus moschiferus*)		✓	

	Aguru dhūpana Smoke bath with agarwood (*Aquilaria agallocha*)		✓	
	Prāta bubhukṣhita Full breakfast (with appropriate foods)		✓	✓
	Uṣhṇa-svabhāva, laghu prāvṛta śhayana Sleeping blankets should be naturally warm and light, like thick sheets of cotton, leather, silk, wool or tree bark		✓	
	Niṣheveta maithuna Sexual intercourse as desired; ideally at night after drinking alcohol with a healthy woman		✓	

Śhiśhira

All recommendations for *śhiśhira* are the same as *hemanta*. In particular, the routines should be followed even more because of the increase in dryness during *śhiśhira* due to its concurrence with the beginning of *ādāna kāla*.

Charaka provides a few specific contraindications for the season.

Śhiśhira Ṛtucharya Contraindications Contraindications for late winter		Cha. Sū. 6/9-48	AH Sū. 3/	BP Pū. 5/
	Kaṭu, tikta, kaṣhaya rasa Pungent, bitter, astringent flavors	✓		
	Vātalāni Anything that increases any form of *vāta*	✓		
	Laghu Anything light	✓		
	Śhīta anna, pāna Cold meals and drinks	✓		

	Vasanta Ṛtucharya Āhāra Food for spring	Cha. Sū. 6/9-48	AH Sū. 3/	BP Pū. 5/
Śhūkadhānya				
	Yava Barley (*Hordeum vulgare*)	✓		
	Godhūma Wheat (*Triticum aestivum*)	✓		✓
	Purāṇa yava Aged barley (*Hordeum vulgare*)		✓	
	Purāṇa godhūma Aged wheat (*Triticum aestivum*)		✓	
	Ṣhaṣhtika śhāli The group of rices that mature in sixty days			✓
	Bahu śhāli bheda Various types of rice from the group of rice			✓
Śhamīdhānya				
	Yava sahita mudga Barley (*Hordeum vulgare*) mixed or made with moong dal or green gram (*Vigna radiata*)			✓
Māṁsa				
	Śhārabha Elk	✓		
	Śhāśha Rabbit	✓		
	Eṇa Antelope	✓		
	Lāva Common quail	✓		
	Kapiñjala Grey partridge	✓		
	Jāṅgalā, śhūlya bhuk Meat of desert animals, food roasted on an open flame		✓	✓

Madya				
	Nirgada sīdhu, mādhvīka (*mārdhvīka*) Non-poisonous sugarcane alchohol, wines	✓		
	Nirgada āsava, ariṣhṭa, sīdhu, mārdhvīka Non-poisonous fermented infusions, sugarcane alcohol, wines		✓	
Ambu				
	Sahakāra Mango juice prepared with fragrant, delicious flavors		✓	
	Mādhava Honey water		✓	
	Śhṛṅgavera, sāra, madhu, jalada ambu Water boiled or prepared with ginger (*Zingiber officinale*), asana (*Pterocarpus marsupium*), *sāra*, honey, or mustā (*Cyperus rotundus*)		✓	
Āhārayogin				
	Kṣhaudra *Kṣhaudra* honey		✓	✓

Vasanta Ṛtucharya Vihāra Activities for spring		Cha. Sū. 6/9-48	AH Sū. 3/	BP Pū. 5/
Upakrama				
	Vamana Therapeutic emesis	✓		✓
	Tīkṣhṇa vamana, nasyādya Strong therapeutic emesis, therapeutic nasal instillation and other therapies		✓	
	Nasya Therapeutic nasal instillation			✓
	Udvartana Skin brightening massage with formulated powders	✓	✓	✓
	Dhūma Therapeutic smoking	✓		
	Kavala-graha Therapeutic mouth wash	✓		
	Añjana Therapeutic collyrium	✓		
	Ghāta (*pādāghāta*) Invigorating body massage applied by the feet		✓	
	Abhaya (*harītakī*) *cha madhu* Myrobalan (*Terminalia chebula*) and honey as a lickable paste			✓
	Kaphaghna kavala Therapeutic mouth wash with *kapha*-reducing *dravyas*			✓
	Candana, kuṅkuma, aguru-kṛta lepa Therapeutic body pastes with sandalwood (*Santalum album*), camphor (*Cinnamomum camphora*), agarwood (*Aquillaria agallocha*)			✓
Vyāyāma				
	Vyāyāma Exercise	✓	✓	✓
Bāhya				
	Goṣhṭhi, kathābhi citrābhi madhyāhna Enjoyable afternoons with friends, playing games in gardens,		✓	

	cool breeze, fountains			
Personal care				
	Sukha ambu śhauca vidhi Frequent washing and cleaning with comfortably warm water	√		
	Candana, aguru Regular use of sandalwood (*Santalum album*), agarwood (*Aquillaria agallocha*)	√		
	Snāna Baths, showers		√	
	Karpūra, chandana, aguru, kuṅkuma anulipta application of light pastes of camphor (*Cinnamomum camphora*), sandalwood (*Santalum album*), agarwood (*Aquillaria agallocha*) or saffron (*Crocus sativus*)		√	

Vasanta Ṛtucharya Contraindications Contraindications for spring	Cha. Sū. 6/9-48	AH Sū. 3/	BP Pū. 5/
Guru Anything heavy	✓	✓	
Snigdha Anything unctuous, oily	✓	✓	✓
Śhīta Anything cold		✓	
Amla, madhura Anything sour and/or sweet	✓	✓	✓
Dadhi Curd, yogurt			✓
Durjara Hard-to-digest foods			✓
Avaśhyāya Dew, mist			✓

Vasanta Ṛtu Dinacharya Daily routine for spring		Cha. Sū. 6/9-48	AH Sū. 3/	BP Pū. 5/
	Śhleṣhma ulbaṇa After controlling *kapha doṣha* through appropriate *upakrama*		✓	
	Snāna Bath, shower		✓	
	Karpūra, chandana, aguru, kuṅkuma anulipta application of light pastes of camphor (*Cinnamomum camphora*), sandalwood (*Santalum album*), agarwood (*Aquillaria agallocha*) or saffron (*Crocus sativus*)		✓	
	Goṣhṭhi, kathābhi chitrābhi madhyāhna Enjoyable afternoons with friends, playing games in gardens, cool breeze, fountains		✓	

Grīṣhma Ṛtucharya Āhāra Food for summer		Cha. Sū. 6/9-48	AH Sū. 3/	BP Pū. 5/
Śhūkadhānya				
	Ghṛta, paya sa-śhāli anna Meals of *śhāli* rice prepared with ghee and milk	✓		
	Saktū lihyāt sa-śharkara Corn flour and sugar paste for licking	✓		✓
	Śhāli aśhnīyat jāṅgalā pala Meals of *śhāli* rice prepared with meat of desert animals		✓	✓
	Śhaśhāṅka kiraṇa bhakṣhya rajanya Corn-flour pastries fried in safflower oil eaten at night		✓	
Māṁsa				
	Jāṅgalā mṛga Deer from dry regions	✓		
	Jāṅgalā pakṣhiṇa Birds from dry regions	✓		
	Na ati ghana rasa *Māṁsa rasa* which is thin and easy to drink		✓	
Madya				
	Alpa na va madya In very small quantities or none at all	✓		
	Peya athavā subahu udaka Or if it is drunk, diluted with plenty of water	✓		
Ambu				
	Śhīta saśharkara mantha Churned drink prepared with sugar and cold water	✓		
	Rāga (stored in *nava mṛd*, fresh earthen jug) syrups and drinks which are sweet and spiced		✓	
	Khāṇḍava (stored in *nava mṛd*, fresh earthen jug) Mango juice, cooked, spiced and filtered		✓	
	Pānaka (stored in *nava mṛd*, fresh earthen jug) Fresh juice prepared with gentle flavors of spices		✓	✓
	Pañchasāra (stored in *nava mṛd*, fresh earthen jug)		✓	

	Five fruit juice, sweetened and spiced			
	Drava dravya Liquid forms of nourishment			✓
Gorasa				
	Rasālā Sweetened curd or yogurt		✓	✓
	Māhiṣha kṣhīra chandrana kṣhatra śhītala Buffalo's milk with sugar, cooled in the moonlight		✓	
	Kṣhīra ajāṅgalāni sitā Goat's milk added with sugar			✓
	Śhīta paya Cold milk, sweet drinks			✓
Ikṣhuvikāra				
	Sitā Sugar			✓

Grīṣhma Ṛtucharya Vihāra Activities for summer		Cha. Sū. 6/9-48	AH Sū. 3/	BP Pū. 5/
Bāhya				
	Śhīta kānana, jala kusuma cha Cool gardens, water fountains and flowers	✓	✓	
	Sugandha hima pānīya sicyamāna paṭāla Cloth sheets sprinkled with sweetly scented water are draped around to cool and humidify the air		✓	
	Śhītāṁśhu Coolness of moonlight			✓
Gṛha				
	Mukta-maṇi āsya, vyajana pāṇi-saṁsparśha chandana udaka śhītala While on a seat adorned with pearls and gems, fans and soft caresses cool with sandalwood-infused (*Santalum album*) water	✓		
	Gṛha su-aypa ghāra madhya dine During midday, stay in a home cooled by fountains and pleasant, cooling scents		✓	
	Divā śhītagṛhe nidrā Daytime naps in a cool house	✓		
	Niśhi chandrā śhuśhītala, chandana-digdhāṅga pravāte harmya-astake Stay in the coolness of moonlight, after applying chandana paste to the whole body, and sleep on an open terrace or rooftop	✓	✓	
Personal care				
	Malayaja Application of cold sandalwood paste (*Santalum album*)			✓

Grīṣhma Ṛtucharya Contraindications Contraindications for spring	Cha. Sū. 6/9-48	AH Sū. 3/	BP Pū. 5/
Lavaṇa, amla, kaṭu Salty, sour, pungent flavors	✓	✓	
Kaṭu, amla Pungent, sour flavors			✓
Kṣhāra Therapeutic alkalis			✓
Uṣhṇa Anything hot	✓		✓
Vyāyāma Exercise	✓		
Arkakara Exposure to sun rays		✓	✓
Madya Avoid alcohol or consume very small amounts, diluted with water		✓	
Śhrama Exhaustion			✓

Varṣhā Ṛtucharya Āhāra Food for monsoon	Cha. Sū. 6/9-48	AH Sū. 3/	BP Pū. 5/
Śhūkadhānya			
Bhojana-saṁskāra kṣhaudra Meals prepared with honey	✓		
Purāṇa yava Aged barley (*Hordeum vulgare*)	✓		
Purāṇa godhūma Aged wheat (*Triticum aestivum*)	✓		
Purāṇa śhāli Aged rice from the group of *śhāli* rice	✓		
Jīrṇa dhānya Aged grains		✓	
Śhāli The group of rice			✓
Yava Barley (*Hordeum vulgare*)			✓
Godhūma Wheat (*Triticum aestivum*)			✓
Māṁsa			
Jāṅgalā māṁsa Meat of animals from arid regions	✓	✓	✓
Rasa-kṛta Meat soups prepared by frying with oil and spices		✓	
Madya			
Kṣhaudrānvita chālpa mādhvīka (mārdhvīka), ariṣhṭa ambu vā Wines and fermented decoctions should be mixed with a little bit of *kṣhaudra* honey	✓		
Chira madhu ariṣhṭa Aged fermented decoctions prepared with honey		✓	

Ambu				
	Pāna-saṁskāra kṣhaudra Drinks prepared with *kṣhaudra* honey	√		
	Māhendra taptaśhīta vā kaupa sārasa eva vā Rain, well and pond water should be boiled	√	√	
	Kaupa, chyuta jala Drinking water should be sourced from deep wells, springs			√
Gorasa				
	Mastu with sauvarchala or pañchakola chūrṇa Whey with *sauvarcala* salt or the formulation of *pañchakola chūrṇa*		√	
	Dudhi uṣhṇa Hot milk, warmed dairy products		√	
Kṛtānna				
	Bhojya yūṣha saṁskṛta Soup and stew meals prepared with proper processing methods	√	√	

Varṣhā Ṛtucharya Vihāra Activities for monsoon		Cha. Sū. 6/9-48	AH Sū. 3/	BP Pū. 5/
Upakrama				
	Pragharṣha Dry rubbing, friction massage with formulated powders	√		
	Udvartana Skin brightening massage with formulated powders	√		
	Snāna Bath, shower	√		
	Śhodhana Therapies to expel the *doṣhas* (as appropriate) followed by *āsthāpana basti*		√	
	Svedana Therapeutic sweating		√	
	Mardana Friction massage		√	
Bāhya				
	Apāda chārī Avoid walking, travel in vehicles		√	
	Harmyapṛṣhṭe vased bhāṣhpa śhīta, śhītakara Reside in upper floors of homes, avoiding heat, cold and mist		√	
Gṛha				
	Akleda sthāna Reside in dwellings that are free from dampness	√		
Personal care				
	Gandha-mālyapara Apply fragrances and garlands	√		
	Laghu, śhuddha ambara Light, clean clothes	√		
	Satata dhūpita ambara Always apply fragrant smoke on clothing		√	

Varṣhā Ṛtucharya Contraindications Contraindications for spring	Cha. Sū. 6/9-48	AH Sū. 3/	BP Pū. 5/
Udamantha Watery, diluted *mantha*	✓	✓	
Avaśhyāya Dew and mist	✓		
Nādī jala Drinking water from rivers	✓	✓	
Vyāyāma Exercise	✓	✓	
Āṭapa Sun exposure	✓	✓	
Vyavāya Sexual intercourse	✓		
Pūrva pavana Direct breeze, wind blowing in one's face			✓
Vṛṣhṭi, gharma, hima Exposure to rain, heat (sun) and cold			✓
Śhrama Exertion			✓
Nadī-tīra Staying or residing near rivers			✓
Rūkṣha nitya Regular (daily) use of anything dry			✓

Śharad Ṛtucharya Āhāra Food for second summer		Cha. Sū. 6/9-48	AH Sū. 3/	BP Pū. 5/
Śhūkadhānya				
	Śhāli The group of rice	✓	✓	✓
	Yava Barley (*Hordeum vulgare*)	✓		✓
	Godhūma Wheat (*Triticum aestivum*)	✓		✓
Śhamīdhānya				
	Mudga Moong dal or green gram (*Vigna radiata*)	✓		✓
Māṁsa				
	Lāva Common quail	✓		
	Kapiñjala Grey partridge	✓		
	Eṇa Antelope	✓		
	Urabhra Sheep	✓		
	Śhārabha Elk	✓		
	Śhāśha Rabbit meat	✓		
	Jāṅgalā māṁsa Meat of animals from arid regions		✓	
	Svalpa pala jāṅgalā māṁsa Small quantities of meat of animals from arid regions		✓	
Śhaka				
	Paṭola Pointed gourd (*Trichosanthes diocia*)		✓	

Phala				
	Dhātrī *Āmalakī*, or Indian gooseberry (*Emblica officinalis* or *Phyllanthus emblica*)		✓	
Ambu				
	Nādī aṁśhūdaka Water from rivers and purified *haṁsodaka* water			✓
	Sara ambu kvathita Water from ponds, basins, boiled to be pre-digested and cooked with appropriate *dravya*			✓
	Haṁsodaka Purified *haṁsodaka* water for drinking	✓	✓	
Gorasa				
	Sarpi Ghee			✓
	Kṣhīra sa-sita milk with sugar			✓
	(Kvathita) paya Milk (cooked with appropriate *dravya*)			✓
Ikṣhuvikāra				
	Sitā Sugarcandy			✓
	Ikṣhva Sugarcane products			✓
	Aikṣhava paṭu rasa Sugarcane products with pungent (or slightly salty) flavors			✓
Kṛtānna				
	Mudga śhāli sahita Rice mixed or made with moong dal or green gram (*Vigna radiata*)			✓
Āhārayogin				
	Madhu Honey		✓	

Śharad Ṛtucharya Vihāra Activities for monsoon	Cha. Sū. 6/9-48	AH Sū. 3/	BP Pū. 5/
Upakrama			
Tikta sarpi pāna Drinking fats processed with bitter *dravyas*	✓	✓	
Vireka Therapeutic purgation	✓	✓	
Raktamokṣhaṇa Therapeutic blood-letting	✓	✓	✓
Balavanta virechana Therapeutic purgation according to strength			✓
Bāhya			
Pradoṣhe cha indu aśhmaya Evening moonlight	✓		✓
Sara krīḍana Water sports			✓
Su-hṛdā guṇeṣhu madhurā vācha Enjoyable, sweet conversations with friends			✓
Vyāyāma			
Viśhrama Rest, relaxation, deep breathing			✓
Personal care			
Haṁsodaka Purified *haṁsodaka* water for bathing	✓	✓	
Mālya Use of garlands	✓	✓	✓
Vimala vāsa Clean clothes	✓	✓	✓
Chandra cha chanda Use of camphor (*Cinnamomum camphora*) and chandana or sandalwood (*Santalum album*)		✓	✓

Śharad Ṛtu Dinacharya Daily routine for second summer		Cha. Sū. 6/9-48	AH Sū. 3/	BP Pū. 5/
	Pitta kopa jaya Control the aggravated *pitta*		✓	
	Kṣhudhita laghu anna When very hungry, eat light meals		✓	
	Haṁsodaka Use purified *haṁsodaka* water for all needs		✓	
	Saudheṣhu saudha-dhavalā chandrikā rajano-mukhe Spending evenings in terraces of grand mansions with white-painted rooftops under moonlight		✓	
	Chandana, *uśhīra*, *karpūra*, *mukta*, *vasana jvala* Use of sandalwood (*Santalum album*), Khus Khus grass (*Vetiveria zizanioides*), camphor (*Cinnamomum camphora*), pearls, and brilliant, sparkling clothes		✓	

Śharad Ṛtucharya Contraindications Contraindications for second summer	Cha. Sū. 6/9-48	AH Sū. 3/	BP Pū. 5/
Ātapa Exposure to sun	√	√	
Hima Exposure to cold			√
Vasā Fat of meat or muscle	√	√	
Taila Oils, in general	√	√	
Avaśhyāya Dew, mist	√	√	
Audaka māṁsa Meat of aquatic animals	√		
Ānūpa māṁsa Meat of marshy animals	√		
Kṣhāra Therapeutic caustic alkalis	√	√	
Dadhi Curd (homemade yogurt)	√	√	√
Prāgvāta Easterly wind	√	√	
Souhitya Excessive satiation with meals and food		√	
Tīkṣhṇa madya Strong alcohol		√	
Vyāyāma Exercise			√
Amla, kaṭu Sour, pungent flavors			√
Uṣhṇa, tīkṣhṇa Anything hot, sharp			√

Trayopastambha

The three main supports for complete *svastha* are *āhāra*, *nidra* and *brahmacharya* (or *abrahmacharya*). They contribute considerably to an individual's *sātmya*. These are also closely related to the diets, activities and behaviors that may be adjusted based on the environment and season.

These three constitute the foundations for complete health in Āyurveda. All classics include a strong emphasis on them and state that they are to be considered top priorities in establishing and maintaining *svastha* and *dhātu sāmya*.

Charaka and Vāgbhaṭa clearly list the *trayopastambha*. Vāgbhaṭa also highlights their importance by likening them to the solid foundation required to support a house.

However, Charaka and Vāgbhaṭa differ on their perspective of lifestyle. Charaka advises *brahmacharya* while Vāgbhaṭa indicates the opposite, or *abrahmacharya*. Both perspectives can be appropriately indicated at different stages of life.

त्रय उपस्तम्भा इति - आहारः, स्वप्नो, ब्रह्मचर्यमिति; || ३५

च. सू. ११।३५

Traya upastambhā iti - āhāraḥ, svapno, brahmacharyamiti; || 35

Cha. Sū. 11/35

Traya (The three) upastambhā (main, or primary supports [for a healthy life]) iti (are known as) – āhāraḥ (diet, or food), svapno (sleep), brahmacharyamiti (and adherence to living a restricted life).

आहारशयनाब्रह्मचर्यैर्युक्त्या प्रयोजितैः ।
शरीरं धायते नित्यमागारमिव धारणैः ॥ ५२

अ. हृ. सू. ७।५२

Āhāraśhayanābrahmacharyairyuktyā prayojitaiḥ | Śharīraṁ dhāyate nityamāgāramiva dhāraṇaiḥ || 52

AH Sū. 7/52

Āhāra (Diet, or food), śhayana (laying down, sleep), abrahmacharyair-yuktyā (and living a unrestricted life, in moderation) prayojitaiḥ (are the means to attain [*svastha*, *dhātu sāmya*, etc]). Śharīraṁ (The physical body) dhāyate (is supported by these) nityam-āgāramiva dhāraṇaiḥ (just as a house is supported [by a solid foundation]).

Trayopastambha Three main supports for complete health	Practically applied as
Āhāra	- Diet, in general - All consumed food - All consumed drinks
Nidrā	- Sleep, in general - Sleep schedule - Sleep habits
AND	
Brahmacharya	- Restricted life - Restriction of: • behavior • conduct • consumption • emotions • ethics • pleasures • senses • sexual intercourse
OR	
Abrahmacharya	- Unrestricted life

By utilizing the *trayopastambha* effectively, their benefits can impart strong, positive health outcomes. Charaka describes the results to expect and explains the requirements to achieve these results.

एभिस्त्रिभिर्युक्तियुक्तैरुपस्तब्धमुपस्तम्भैः शरीरंबलवर्णोपचयोपचितमनुवर्तते यावदायुःसंस्कारात् संस्कारमहितमनुपसेवमानस्य, य इहैवोपदेक्ष्यते || ३५

च. सू. ११।३५

Ebhistribhiryuktiyuktairupastabdham upastambhaiḥ śharīraṁ balavarṇopachayopachitamanuvartatey āvadāyuḥsaṁskārāt saṁskāram ahitamanupasevamānasya, ya ihaivopadekṣhyate || 35

Cha. Sū. 11/35

Ebhi-stribhir (Following) yukti (the proper) yuktair (application of) upastabdham (these supportive principles) upastambhaiḥ (of the *upastambha*, ie, *āhāra*, *nidrā* and *brahmacharya*), śharīraṁ (the physical body [which is prone to decay]) anuvartate (becomes endowed with) bala (physical strength [and *ojas*]), varṇa (color, complexion), upachaya (healthy growth) upachitam (all in a thriving manner). Yāvad (As long as) āyuḥ (throughout the course of life) saṁskārāt (the appropriate processes are followed) saṁskāram ahitam (and the unsuitable processes) anupasevamānasya (are not adopted in one's regular routine). Ya ihaiva upadekṣhyate (These methodologies are being explained here [in this chapter]).

The major outcomes to expect, identify and assess are:

- *Upachita bala* – strength, *ojas*
- *Upachita varṇa* – complexion
- *Upachita upachaya* – healthy growth

These three outcomes are commonly cited as strong indicators for several factors that directly impact *svastha*, including *agni*, *nidrā*, *vyāyāma* and others. The key to successful clinical application is the ability to differentiate the causative factors for the absence of any one of these and determine the appropriate plan of therapeutic intervention.

Āhāra

The relationships between *sātmya* and *āhāra* will be covered in detail in Chapter seven.

Nidrā

Review Volume two, chapter 22, on *nidrā* (sleep) for the fundamental mechanics of sleep and its classical explanations. In context of *sātmya*, proper *nidrā* for healthy individuals is the *bhūtadhātri* type, or that which naturally occurs by the onset of night itself. Several additional general recommendations are provided which are considered always beneficial except in unusual circumstances and disorders.

In general, the classics recommend that everyone adopt *nidrā* in a way which becomes *sātmya* based on known, health-promoting routines and regimens, including:

- Sleeping and waking up at approximately the same time daily
- Sleeping early at night, generally before 9pm, when the *tāmasika* effect is strongest
- Waking up before sunrise during the *brahma muhūrta*
- Avoiding sleep during the day, except in *grīṣhma ṛtu*

Suśhruta describes the benefits of *nidrā* when followed accordingly. He states that adhering to a regular sleep schedule will produce *dhātu sāmya*.

पुष्टिवर्णबलोत्साहमग्निदीप्तिमतन्द्रिताम् ।
करोति धातुसाम्यं च निद्रा काले निषेविता
॥ ८८

सु. चि. २४।८८

Puṣhṭivarṇabalotsāhamagnidīptimatandr
itām | Karoti dhātusāmyam cha nidrā
kāle niṣhevitā || 88

Su. Chi. 24/88

Puṣhṭi (A well-developed, properly
nourished, and healthy body), varṇa (proper
color and complexion), bala (strength [and
ojas]), utsāham (enthusiasm), agni-dīptim
(strong, well-functioning agni), atandritām
(lack of fatigue, tiredness or laziness), cha
(and) dhātusāmyam (dhātu sāmya, or
normal, healthy dhātus) karoti (are [each]
produced by) nidrā (sleep) kāle (at the proper
time) niṣhevitā (on a regular basis).

Charaka adds that nidrā is the root cause for
sukha. This key point indicates that proper
nidrā is absolutely vital to creating a
complete state of svastha.

देहवृत्तौ यथाऽऽहारस्तथा स्वप्नः सुखो मतः
| स्वप्नाहारसमुत्थे च स्थौल्यकार्श्ये विशेषतः
॥ ५१

च. सू. २१।५१

Dehavṛttau yathāhārastathā svapnaḥ
sukho mataḥ | Svapnāhārasamutthe cha
sthaulyakārśhye viśheṣhataḥ || 51

Cha. Sū. 21/51

Deha-vṛttau yatha (Just as the body is
regularly maintained and supported by)
āhāra (diet and food), tathā (so also)
svapnaḥ (sleep) sukho mataḥ (is responsible
for happiness and contentment). Svapna
(Sleep) āhāra samutthe (and diet or food)
cha sthaulya kārśhye viśheṣhataḥ (are the
specific [root] causes for the pathological
conditions of being overweight and

underweight).

Several approaches may be required to fully
and properly assess nidrā in an individual.
These may include assessments of the
current state of nidrā, along with a separate
determination of the individual's sātmya for
healthy nidrā.

To perform these assessments, begin by
analyzing the states of normal and abnormal
sleep, indications and contraindications
along with specific management protocols.

Normal sleep
Sleep is considered to be normal when an
individual is able to:

1. Fall asleep easily
2. Wake up naturally
3. Adhere to a regular schedule

Normal sleep is of two types based on the
time of occurrence which has the strongest
influence on the effects of sleep. The two
types of normal sleep include:

1. Rātri – sleeping at night
2. Divā – sleeping during the day

Sleeping at night is always considered ideal
for creating a stable routine and svastha
through sātmya. Only in exceptional
circumstances do recommendations call for
reversing this normal sleep schedule. See
the section on Management of sleep for an
explanation.

Vāgbhaṭa provides a straightforward
approach to achieving a healthy sleep
routine. He explains that normal sleep will
come easily to those who are not consumed
by sexual thoughts and behaviors. When one
is engaged in a lifestyle of restricted behavior
and genuinely content, they naturally fall
asleep around the same time each night.

ब्रह्मचर्यरतेर्ग्राम्यसुखनिःस्पृहचेतसः । निद्रा
सन्तोषतृप्तस्य स्वं कालं नातिवर्तते ॥ ६८

अ. हृ. सू. ७।६८

Brahmacharyaratergrāmyasukhaniḥspṛh achetasaḥ | Nidrāsantoṣhatṛptasya svaṁ kālaṁ nātivartate || 68

AH Sū. 7/68

Brahmacharya (Adherence to a restricted life), niḥspṛha ([and] indifference towards) ete grāmya sukha (pleasures of the material world) chetasaḥ (in one's genuine state of consciousness) nidrā santoṣha (promote sleep through true happiness [and which produces true happiness]) tṛptasya (which creates an overwhelming sense of contentment [in the individual]) svaṁ kālaṁ (at their proper time) nātivartate (neither too early or too late [each night]).

Suśhruta states that proper sleep produces significant positive outcomes for complete health. This assumes sleeping at night, avoiding sleep during the day and regularly following one's appropriate schedule.

अरोगः सुमना ह्योवं बलवर्णान्वितो वृषः ।
नातिस्थूलकृशः श्रीमान् नरो जीवेत् समाः शतम् ॥ ४०

सु. शा. ४।४०

Arogaḥ sumanā hyovaṁ balavarṇānvito vṛṣhaḥ | Nātisthūlakṛṣhaḥ śhrīmān naro jīvet samāḥ śhatam || 40

Su. Śhā. 4/40

Arogaḥ (Absence of disease), sumanā (pleasantness, happiness, beauty), hyovaṁ bala (physical strength [and *ojas*]), varṇānvito (accompanied with good color, or complexion) vṛṣhaḥ (and strong virility [are produced by proper sleep]). Na ati-sthūla-kṛṣhaḥ (One does not become overweight or underweight), śhrīmān (but instead becomes a well-disposed) naro (individual) jīvet (who lives) samāḥ (a proper life) śhatam (for one hundred years).

Suśhruta and Charaka clearly agree that normal sleep is a root cause for *sukha*, or happiness in life, and success.

Suśhruta further emphasizes that sleeping at night rather than during the day is the ideal method to follow habitually.

तस्मान्न जागृयाद्रात्रौ दिवास्वप्नं च वर्जयेत् ।
ज्ञात्वा दोषकरावेतौ बुधः स्वप्नं मितं चरेत् ॥ ३९

सु. शा. ४।३९

Tasmānna jāgṛyādrātrau divāsvapnaṁ cha varjayet | Jñātvā doṣhakarāvetau budhaḥ svapnaṁ mitaṁ charet || 39

Su. Śhā. 4/39

Tasmāt (Therefore), na (do not) jāgṛyād-rātrau (allow staying awake at night) cha (and) divāsvapnaṁ (then sleeping during the day) varjayet (to win over). Jñātvā (The learned scholars recognize that) doṣha-karāvetau (both of these increase the *doṣhas*) budhaḥ (and they know that) svapnaṁ (sleep) mitaṁ charet (should follow this regular schedule).

While the general recommendations to always follow a regular sleep schedule at night are practically seen to be effective in a large majority of the population, there are certain cases where individuals are unable to adhere to this routine for a variety of reasons.

When necessary, certain individuals are able to create a regular routine of staying awake at night and sleeping during the day. For these individuals, this schedule may become *okasātmya* or *sātmya* over time.

Suśhruta recognizes this phenomenon and states that for those who adapt their *sātmya* to a reversed schedule, no harm is caused.

(निद्रा सात्म्यीकृता यैस्तु रात्रौ च यदि वा दिवा ।)

दिवारात्रौ च ये नित्यं स्वप्नजागरणोचिताः ।
न तेषां स्वपतां दोषो जाग्रतां वाऽपि जायते
॥ ४१

सु. शा. ४।४१

(Nidrā sātmyīkṛtā yaistu rātrau cha yadi vā divā |)
Divārātrau cha ye nityaṁ svapnajāgaraṇochitāḥ | Na teṣhāṁ svapatāṁ doṣho jāgratāṁ vā ' pi jāyate || 41

Su. Śhā. 4/41

Nidrā sātmyī-kṛtā yaistu rātrau (When one's *sātmya* is habituated to staying awake during the night) cha yadi vā divā (and then sleeping during the day), divārātrau (and when this reversed schedule) cha ye nityaṁ (is followed regularly) svapna-jāgaraṇa (this method of sleeping and staying awake) uchitāḥ (becomes correct [proper, or *sātmya* for the individual]). Na teṣhāṁ svapatāṁ (Neither of these types of sleeping schedules) doṣho (create *doṣhas*) jāgratāṁ vā ' pi jāyate (by staying awake at night or sleeping during the day).

The key to developing a healthy reversed schedule is to practice it effectively so that it becomes *sātmya*, or healthy for that individual when continued and applied repeatedly. In these situations, it is highly likely that the individual will make several additional adjustments to their diet, lifestyle and other habits to accommodate and support the reversed sleeping schedule.

The bed, or sleeping surface, is also described by Suśhruta as it has a direct impact on the quality of an individual's sleep. The type of sleeping surface for sleeping at night compared to sleeping during the day can play a significant role in the production of positive or negative health outcomes.

When sleeping on a comfortable bed, Suśhruta states that one can expect better sleep that restores the body and mind.

श्रमानिलहरं वृष्यं पुष्टिनिद्राधृतिप्रदम् ।
सुखं शय्यासनं, दुःखं विपरीतगुणं मतम् ॥
८१

सु. चि. २४।८१

Śhramānilaharaṁ vṛṣhaṁ puṣhṭinidrādhṛtipradam | Sukhaṁ śhayyāsanaṁ, duḥkhaṁ viparītaguṇaṁ matam || 81

Su. Chi. 24/81

Śhrama-anila-haraṁ (Exhaustion and *vāta* are reduced), vṛṣhaṁ (virility), puṣhṭi (a well-developed, properly nourished, and healthy body), nidrā (sleep), dhṛti-pradam (and concentration improve) sukhaṁ (due to a comfortable) śhayya (bed) āsanaṁ (and seat). Duḥkhaṁ (An uncomfortable [bed and seat]) viparīta-guṇaṁ matam (produce the opposite *guṇas*, or results).

Divā svapna is defined by Suśhruta to cause deviation from one's normal state of health, assuming that regularly sleeping at night is *sātmya* for them.

विकृतिर्हि दिवास्वप्नो नाम; तत्र
स्वपतामधर्मः सर्वदोषप्रकोपश्च, ... ॥ ३८

सु. शा. ४।३८

Vikṛtirhi divāsvapno nāma; tatra svapatāmadharmaḥ sarvadoṣhaprakopaśhcha, ... || 38

Su. Śhā. 4/38

Divāsvapno nāma (*Divā svapna* or sleeping during the day is known as) vikṛtirhi (that which produces *vikṛti*, or a deviation from the normal, baseline state of health); tatra (and so) svapatām (this type of sleep [habit, or schedule]) adharmaḥ (is considered *adharma* or going against one's life purpose) sarva doṣha prakopa-śhcha (as it causes all *doṣhas* to go into a state of *prakopa*).

When practiced properly, however, *divā svapna* is an important component to maintaining *dhātu sāmya* according to Charaka. In order to achieve the beneficial results and outcomes of *divā svapna*, it must be applied properly.

धातुसाम्यं तथा ह्येषां बलं चाप्युपजायते |
श्लेष्मा पुष्णाति चाङ्गानि स्थैर्यं भवति
चायुषः || ४२

च. सू. २१।४२

Dhātusāmyaṁ tathā hyeṣhāṁ balaṁ chāpyupajāyate | Śhleṣhmā puṣhṇāti chāṅgāni sthairyaṁ bhavati chāyuṣhaḥ || 42

Cha. Sū. 21/42

Dhātu-sāmyaṁ (*Dhātu sāmya*) tathā hyeṣhāṁ (as well as one's) balaṁ (physical strength [and *ojas*]) chāpyupajāyate (are specifically supported [by following the correct regimens for *divā svapna*]). Śhleṣhmā (*Kapha*) puṣhṇāti (nourishes) chāṅgāni (all of the limbs of the body) sthairyaṁ bhavati (to produce stability) chāyuṣhaḥ (and longevity with high quality of life).

Classically, *divā svapna* was only indicated for everyone during summer season. The purpose of this is to directly offset the normal *vāta sañchaya* that occurs during this season in the Indian subcontinent. By sleeping for a short period during the day, people are able to restore their strength and reduce the negative effects of *ādāna kāla* and its extreme heat and dryness.

ग्रीष्मे त्वादानरूक्षाणां वर्धमाने च मारुते|
रात्रीणां चातिसङ्क्षेपाद्दिवास्वप्नः प्रशस्यते ||
४३

च. सू. २१।४३

Grīṣhme tvādānarūkṣhāṇāṁ vardhamāne cha mārute | Rātrīṇāṁ chātisaṅkṣhepāddivāsvapnaḥ praśhasyate || 43

Cha. Sū. 21/39-43

Grīṣhme (During summer), tu ādāna (because of the effects of *ādāna kāla*) rūkṣhāṇāṁ (dryness) vardhamāne (continuously increases little by little) cha mārute (along with the wind). Rātrīṇāṁ cha (And the nights) ātisaṅkṣhepāt (become shorter and shorter) divāsvapnaḥ (so sleeping during the daytime) praśhasyate (is therapeutic for everyone).

Rātri jāgaraṇa, staying awake at night, also has its own expected effects and outcomes. Suśhruta states that it is a direct cause for the same types of disorders seen as a result of improper *divā svapna*. However, when these same disorders are created by *rātri jāgaraṇa*, *vāta* and *pitta* are found to be the direct causative agents whereas *kapha* is the primary agent in *divā svapna*.

रात्रावपि जागरितवतां वातपित्तनिमित्तास्त
एवोपद्रवा भवन्ति ॥ ३८

सु. शा. ४।३८

Rātrāvapi jāgatiravatāṁ vātapittanimittāsta evopadravā bhavanti || 38

Su. Śhā. 4/38

Rātrāv-api jāgatiravatāṁ (And so staying awake at night) bhavanti (is the cause for) vāta pitta nimittāsta evopadravā (similar complications produced directly by *vāta* and *pitta*).

When *divā svapna* is indicated, Susruta states that sleeping for one *muhūrta* (approximately 48 minutes) is not prohibited. However, the wording of Susruta's recommendation implies that *divā svapna* may not be the first or best choice of management for these indications.

Whenever possible, more appropriate adjustments or accommodations should be attempted prior to advocating for *divā svapna*.

मुहूर्तं दिवास्वपनमप्रतिषिद्धम् ... । ३८

सु. शा. ४।३८

Muhūrtaṁ divāsvapanamapratiṣhiddham ... | 38

Su. Śhā. 4/38

Muhūrtaṁ (One muhūrta, or approximately 48 minutes) divā svapanam (of sleeping during the day) apratiṣhiddham (is not prohibited).

For those who have stayed awake late through the previous night, Suśhruta specifically recommends that they sleep the following morning for half of the time of missed sleep. However, Suśhruta does not explicitly state when this extra sleep must occur.

Vāgbhaṭa concurs with this and adds that the individual's normal meal should be skipped so that they can sleep for this extra time. Additional rules for indications and contraindications can also be considered in each situation.

रात्रावपि जागरितवतां जागरितकालादर्धमिष्यते दिवास्वपनम् । ३८

सु. शा. ४।३८

Rātrāvapi jāgaritavatāṁ jāgaritakālādardhamiṣhyate divāsvapanam | 38

Su. Śhā. 4/38

Rātrāvapi jāgaritavatāṁ jāgarita (For those who remained awake on the previous night), kālād-ardham (half of the time [that they remained awake]) iṣhyate (is allowed) divāsvapanam (for sleeping during the day).

असात्म्याज्जागरादर्धं प्रातः स्वप्यादभुक्तवान् ॥ ६५

अ. हृ. सू. ७।६५

Asātmyājjāgarādardhaṁ prātaḥ svapyādabhuktavān || 65

AH Sū. 7/65

Asātmyāt jāgarād (After remaining awake at night in an *asātmya* situation), ardhaṁ (half [of the total amount of time]) prātaḥ (on the following morning) svapyād (should be for sleeping) abhuktavān (avoiding eating the normal meal [during that time period]).

Finally, all authors provide comprehensive recommendations for contraindications of *divā svapna*. These are mentioned in Cha. Sū. 21/44-49, Su. Śhā. 4/38 and AH Sū. 7/60. Each individual recommendation is tabulated at the end of this section.

Abnormal sleep

Abnormal sleep is the opposite of normal sleep. It often presents in varying levels of seriousness and acuteness. Abnormal sleep can affect an individual in specific ways through diet, routines, seasonal and many other factors.

When abnormal sleep occurs, an individual may notice:

- Difficulty falling asleep
- Difficulty staying asleep
- Difficulty waking up
- Uncontrollable sleep
- Inability to adhere to a schedule

Most commonly, difficulty falling and staying asleep are seen as transient symptoms of deviation from normal health.

The classics provide a comprehensive list of potential causes for loss of sleep. Over a short-term period, some loss of sleep is generally not harmful for most individuals. However, the limit of acceptable sleep loss is highly variable.

When loss of sleep does produce a negative impact on health, the classics list the possibilities as *lakṣhaṇas* and specific disorders.

See the tabulated comparison at the end of this section for a complete review of causes and outcomes related to abnormal sleep.

Management of sleep

The recommendations for managing abnormal sleep and improving sleep quality in general both start by creating a sleep schedule and adhering to it. Any further attempts to improve sleep will generally be unsuccessful if the appropriate base schedule is not established first.

यथाकालमतो निद्रां रात्रौ सेवेत सात्म्यतः ।
... ६५

अ. हृ. सू. ७।६५

Yathākālamato nidrāṁ rātrau seveta sātmyataḥ | ... 65

AH Sū. 7/65

Yathā-kālam-ato (And so, the appropriate time) nidrāṁ (for sleep) rātrau (at night) seveta (must become habitual) sātmyataḥ (to develop [the sleep schedule to be] *sātmya*).

This applies to the majority of people and ideally is followed throughout one's lifetime with minor, expected variations for appropriate age categories. For example, children and the elderly are expected to sleep more, both at night and during the day.

In exceptional circumstances, there may be reasons to adopt an alternate sleep schedule for an individual. This is typically appropriate only for a specific period of time due to other factors, especially certain acute and emergency-related disorders. In very rare situations will there be a genuine need to permanently reverse the sleeping schedule. However, it can be done effectively for certain individuals if necessary.

More commonly, individuals experience periods of sleeplessness or too much sleep. Upon further investigation, these are often found to be related to an existing pathological condition, a seasonal change, or other relevant cause.

Management of sleeplessness and excessive sleep can be applied according to classical recommendations. With a holistic picture of the individual's complete state of expected *svastha*, their current state and their *sātmya*, a fully personalized approach can be tailored to meet their needs and requirements.

Bhāva Prakāśha reiterates much of the same information as the major authors for the entire topic of *nidrā* in a condensed format. He also integrates the effects of *nidrā* and *āhāra* along with several other activities that factor into daily routines for maintaining *svastha*. These explanations can be found in BP Pū. 5/202-212 and BP Pū. 5/300-302.

NORMAL SLEEP

Nidrā kāla niṣhevitā Results (benefits) of proper, habitual sleep	Cha. Sū. 21/36-38	Su. Chi. 24/88	AH Sū. 7/53	BP Pū. 5/301
Sukha Happiness, contentment	√		√	
Puṣhṭi A well-developed, properly nourished, and healthy body	√	√	√	√
Bala Strength and (*ojas*)	√	√	√	√
Vṛṣhatā Virility	√		√	
Jñāna Knowledge	√		√	
Jīvita Life	√		√	
Sukhāyuṣhā Satisfying, long life	√			
Varṇa Healthy complexion		√		√
Utsāha Enthusiasm		√		√
Agni dīpti Strong, well-functioning agni		√		√
Atandritā Lack of fatigue, tiredness or laziness		√		
Dhātu sāmya *Dhātu sāmya*, or normal state of equilibrium		√		

NORMAL SLEEP

Nidrā akāla niṣhevitā Results (negative effects) of improper, non-habitual sleep	Cha. Sū. 21/39-43	Su. Śhā. 4/	AH Sū. 7/53, 61
Duḥkha Sadness, discontent	✓		✓
Kārśhya Condition of being underweight, improperly nourished	✓		✓
Abala Lack of strength	✓		✓
Klībatā Impotence	✓		✓
Ajñāna Lack of knowledge	✓		✓
Jīvita na Loss of life	✓		✓
Sthaulya (Cha. Sū. 21/51) Condition of being overweight, over-nourished	✓		

Nidrā ayogya Contraindications for sleeping	Cha. Sū. 21/	Su. Śhā. 4/	AH Sū. 7/60
Viṣhārta Poisoned			✓
Kaṇṭha roga Diseases of the throat			✓

Divā svapna

Divā svapna yogya Indications for sleeping during the day	Cha. Sū. 21/39-43	Su. Śhā. 4/38, 48	AH Sū. 7/56-59	BP Pū. 5/203-204
For those who are exhausted by:				
Gīta Singing	✓			
Adhyayana Studying, especially practicing long recitations	✓			
Bhāṣhya Speaking			✓	
Madya nitya Alcoholics, or after taking alcohol	✓	✓	✓	✓
Strī Sexual intercourse	✓	✓	✓	✓
Karma Therapeutic treatments, especially *śhodhana*	✓	✓	✓	
Bhāra Carry heavy weight or loads	✓		✓	
Adhva Walking long distances	✓	✓	✓	✓
Vyāyāma Exercise				✓
Karśhita A weakened, emaciated state	✓	✓		
Ajīrṇa Indigestion	✓	✓	✓	
Rasājīrṇa A specific type of indigestion where a meal digests only after one full day				✓
Kṣhata-kṣhīṇa Chronic wasting disease of the chest, lungs and respiration	✓	✓		
Vṛddha Elderly	✓	✓	✓	✓

Bāla Young children	√	√	√	√
Abala Lack of physical strength	√		√	
Tṛṣhṇa Thirst	√	√	√	
Atīsāra Diarrhea	√	√	√	√
Śhūla Abdominal pain, discomfort	√	√	√	√
Śhvāsa Difficulty breathing	√		√	√
Hikka Hiccup	√	√	√	√
Māruta pīḍita Afflicted vāta, particularly being squeezed, distressed				√
Kṛśha Weak, thin, emaciated	√			
Abhighata Injured, beaten, assaulted, harmed	√		√	
Unmatta Intoxicated, insane, frantic, not in control of mental faculties	√		√	
Yāna Travel, especially by vehicle	√	√	√	
Vāhana Travel, especially by riding an animal		√		√
Prajāgara Staying awake at night	√			√
Krodha Anger	√		√	
Śhoka Grief, sadness	√		√	
Bhaya Fear	√		√	

Grīṣhme tu ādāna rūkṣhāṇa Summer, due to the dryness of *ādāna kāla*	✓		✓	
Kṣhīṇa Deficient (in any form)			✓	✓
Śhūla pīḍita Knotty abdominal pain			✓	
Divā svapna uchita Accustomed to sleeping during the day			✓	✓
Abhukta Not having consumed a meal recently		✓		✓
Medas, sveda, kapha, rasa, rakta kṣhīṇa Deficiency of *medas*, *sveda*, *kapha*, *rasa* or *rakta*		✓		
Kṣhīṇa kapha Deficient or reduced *kapha* (in any form)				✓

Divā svapna ayogya Contra-indications for sleeping during the day	Cha. Sū. 21/44-45	Su. Śhā. 4/38	AH Sū. 7/60	BP Pū. 5/202
Sarva ṛtu anyatra grīṣhma All seasons, except for summer	✓	✓		✓
Medasvina Having excessive bodily fat	✓		✓	
Sneha nityā Accustomed to consuming any kind of fat daily	✓		✓	
Śhleṣhmalā Predisposed to a predominance of *kapha*	✓		✓	✓
Śhleṣhma rogiṇa Suffering from disorders of *kapha*	✓			
Dūṣhīviṣhārtā Suffering from *dūṣhī viṣha* poisoning			✓	

Akāla divā svapna Results of improper sleeping during the day	Cha. Sū. 21/46-47	Su. Śhā. 4/38	AH Sū. 7/61
Due to doṣha prakopa:			
Halīmaka Advanced form of the disease *pāṇḍu*	✓		
Śhira śhūla Headache	✓		✓
Śhiro gaurava Heaviness of the head		✓	
Staimitya Stiffness, rigidity	✓		✓
Guru gātratā Heaviness of the limbs	✓		
Aṅgamarda Squeezing pain in the bodily limbs	✓	✓	
Agnināśha Extinction of *agni*	✓		

Agni daurbalya Weakness of *agni*		✓	✓
Pralepo hṛdayasya Feeling of a slimy layer or covering over the heart	✓		
Śhophā Swelling, intumescence	✓		✓
Ārochaka Loss of appetite accompanied with indigestion	✓	✓	
Hṛllāsa Regurgitating hiccup	✓		✓
Pīnasā Nasal drip, usually starting as a clear fluid	✓		✓
Pratiśhyāya Head cold		✓	
Ārdhāvabhedakā Headache in half of the head	✓		
Koṭha A type of skin disorder	✓		
Āruḥ piḍakā A type of skin disorder, presenting as painless	✓		
Kaṇḍū Itching	✓		
Tandrā Drowsy	✓		
Kāsa Cough	✓	✓	
Śhvāsa Difficulty breathing		✓	
Galāmayā Disorders of the neck and throat	✓		
Smṛti buddhi pramoha Early stages of loss of consciousness in the memory and power of intelligence	✓		
Saṁrodha srotas Proper blockage of the *srotas* (exudative networks)	✓		✓

Jvara Fever	✓	✓	✓
Indriya asāmarthya Improper association of senses with their respective objects	✓		
Viṣha vega pravarta(rdha)nam Exacerbation and advancement of the stages of toxic poison	✓		
Moha Loss of consciousness			✓

Rātri jāgaraṇa

Rātri jāgaraṇa yogya Indications for staying awake at night	Cha. Sū. 21/28	Su. Śhā. 4/48	AH Sū. 7/60	BP Pū. 5/300
Kapha Presence of *kapha doṣha*		✓		✓
Medas Presence of *vaikṛta medas*		✓		
Viṣha Presence of poison		✓	✓	✓
Sthaulya Condition of being overweight, over-nourished	✓			
Kaṇṭha roga Disorders of the throat			✓	

Rātri jāgaraṇa Results of staying awake at night	Cha. Sū. 21/	Su. Śhā. 4/88	AH Sū. 7/
Vāta, pitta nimitta upadrava The same complications as *divā svapna*, except that they are produced due to *vāta* and/or *pitta*		✓	

SLEEP LOSS

Nidrā nāśha hetu Causes for loss of sleep	Cha. Sū. 21/55-57	Su. Śhā. 4/42	AH Sū. 7/
Kāyasya, śhirasa (*vireka, chhardana*) Elimination of the *doṣhas* from the body and head (therapeutic purgation, therapeutic emesis)	✓		
Bhaya Fear	✓		
Chintā Worry	✓		
Krodha Anger	✓		
Dhūma Smoke	✓		
Vyāyāma Exercise	✓		
Rakta mokṣhaṇa Blood-letting	✓		
Upavāsa Intentional restriction of basic desires to promote health	✓		
Asukha śhayyā Uncomfortable bed	✓		
Sattva audārya Predominance of *sattva*	✓		
Tamas jayaḥ Control over *tamas*	✓		
Kāryaṁ kālo vikāra As the result of time and disease	✓		
Vāyu prakṛti *Vāta* predominant *prakṛti*	✓	✓	
Pitta Presence of *pitta doṣha*		✓	
Manas tāpāt		✓	

Overheating the mind			
Kṣhaya Deficient, reduced (in any form)		✓	
Abhighāta Injury, trauma		✓	

Management of sleep

Nidrā sātmya General management for healthy sleep	Cha. Sū. 21/	Su. Śhā. 4/	AH Sū. 7/65
Yathākālamato nidrām̐ rātrau seveta Adhere to a habitual schedule to sleep at the appropriate time every night			✓

Akāla nidrā chikitsā Management of improper sleep schedule	Cha. Sū. 21/	Su. Śhā. 4/	AH Sū. 7/61
Upavāsa Intentional restriction of basic desires to promote health			✓
Vamana Therapeutic emesis			✓
Svedana Therapeutic sweating			✓
Nāvana (*nasya*) Therapeutic nasal instillation of a specific type and method			✓

Nidrā nāśha chikitsā Management for loss of sleep	Cha. Sū. 21/52-54	Su. Śhā. 4/43-46	AH Sū. 7/66-68
Regular, consistent usage of:			
Abhyaṅga Oil massage	✓	✓	✓
Utsādana Skin brightening massage with formulated powders	✓		
Udvartana Dry powder massage, body rub		✓	✓
Snāna Bath, shower	✓		✓
Mūrdha, karṇa, akṣhi tarpaṇa Refreshing oil application for the head, ears and eyes			✓
Mūrdhni taila niṣhevaṇa Regular application of oil on the scalp (using all four methods of *abhyaṅga*, *śhirodhāra*, *basti* and *pichu*)		✓	

Rasa Soups			✓
Grāmya, ānūpa, audakā rasa Meat soup prepared from domesticated animals, animals from wet regions or aquatic animals	✓		
Śhālyannaṁ sadadhi Meals of *śhāli* rice mixed with curd (homemade yogurt)	✓		
Śhāli, godhūma piṣhṭānna bhakṣhya, ikṣhu saṁskṛta *Śhāli* and wheat prepared as chewable pastries, mixed with sugarcane		✓	
Madhura, snigdha bhojana, kṣhīra māṁsa rasādi Sweet and unctuous meals prepared with milk, meat soup, etc		✓	
Rasa bileśhayānā cha viṣhkirānā Chicken soup		✓	
Kṣhīra Milk	✓		✓
Dadhi Curd (homemade yogurt)			✓
Sneha Fats, oils	✓		
Madya Alcohol	✓		✓
Drākṣha, asita ikṣhu dravya, niśhi Preparations (juice) of grapes and brown sugar at night		✓	
Manaḥ-sukham Satisfied, pleasant state of mind	✓		
Manaso anuguṇā gandhāḥ śhabdāḥ Fine scents and pleasant sounds to satisfy the mind	✓		
Saṁvāhanāni Gentle, pleasant, sensual massage	✓	✓	
Chakṣhuṣha tarpaṇaṁ lepaḥ śhiraso vadanasya cha Refreshing paste or ointment application for the eyes, head and face	✓		
Svāstīrṇaṁ śhayanaṁ veśhma One's own comfortable bed and home	✓		

Śhayana, āsana, yānāni mṛdu Soft bed, seats and vehicles for travel		√	
Sukha kāla tathochita Favorable, regular sleeping schedule	√		
Kāntā bāhula tāśhleṣha Great comfort of one's wife			√
Nirvṛtiḥ kṛtakṛsyatā Satisfaction in that which one has accomplished			√
Mano anukūlā viṣhayā kāma Enjoying the objects of the mind as much as possible			√

Ati nidrā chikitsā Management for excessive sleep	Cha. Sū. 21/21-28	Su. Śhā. 4/47	AH Sū. 7/62-63
Sthaulya chikitsā Management protocols for conditions of being overweight, over-nourished	√		
Vamana hita saṁśhodhana Accustomed elimination of the *doṣhas*, especially therapeutic emesis		√	
Laṅghana Therapeutic reduction methods		√	√
Rakta mokṣhaṇa Blood-letting		√	
Mano vyākulanāni Deeply engaging mental thoughts, work, activity		√	
Tīkṣhṇa chardana Strong, sharp therapeutic emesis			√
Añjana Collyrium			√
Nāvana (nasya) Therapeutic nasal instillation of a specific type and method			√
Chintā Worry			√
Vyavāya Sexual intercourse			√

Śhoka Grief, sadness			✓
Bhī Fear			✓
Krodha Anger			✓

Brahmacharya and abrahmacharya

Brahmacharya and *abrahmacharya* are the two major types of lifestyles in traditional Vedic and Hindu cultures. They align with the classical Āyurvedic *puruṣhārthas* and the stages of life dominated by each.

Following a lifestyle of *brahmacharya* requires that the individual restrict their enjoyment and indulgence in material pleasures. The first appropriate time frame for this is considered to be childhood into adulthood, as one is practicing *dharma*. During the phase of *dharma*, the expectation is to prioritize study, focus on learning and prepare to practice that which he or she will do for the remainder of their life. Practicing *brahmacharya* during this stage of life provides valuable training that can serve the individual for the remaining stages.

Adhering to *brahmacharya* lays a primary importance on abstinence and the control of the sense organs. The restrictions on enjoyment and indulgence are meant to train the child and adolescent on how to control their own desires by learning when and how to limit their behaviors and activities. During this very impressionable stage of life, these lessons can provide an excellent foundation for mental stability and personal satisfaction in later years.

Once the responsibilities for *dharma* have been fulfilled, the individual moves into the phase of *artha* where they learn to gain the means to provide for themselves and others. Continuing in the lifestyle of *brahmacharya* helps limit their indulgence in activities which would reduce their chances of success later in life.

After achieving the skills required to maintain *artha*, individuals are then considered ready for *kāma*, or the stage of enjoyment of the fruits of their labor. Classically, this signals the appropriate time for marriage and starting their own family. During this stage, the lifestyle of *abrahmacharya* is appropriate. The individual is expected to enjoy the intimacy of their marital relationship, caring for their children and providing for the family. *Abrahmacharya* means that the individual is actively engaged in the material world for themselves and others, and that they do not strictly limit their enjoyment of material pleasures through their sense organs, emotions and sensual desires.

The phase of *kāma* lasts for the majority of life. As the end of life approaches, one transitions into the final stage of *mokṣha* to prepare for the transition of death. During this stage, the practice of *brahmacharya* is normally followed again.

Brahmacharya and *abrahmacharya* can be followed with varying degrees of strictness. True practice of *brahmacharya* according the classical Vedic traditions is a complex topic which is beyond the scope of this textbook. The Āyurvedic classics describe one's behavior, their manner of conducting themselves in public and private, personal ethics and similar characteristics. These are described under various categories and in different contexts according to each author.

Adhering to *brahmacharya* and *abrahmacharya* during the appropriate stages of life is classically considered to be a conscious choice made by the individual and their family. This behavior is often strongly influenced by their religious community and society.

These choices generally intend to do what is believed to be best for the family and society, and then the individual. This approach is not always be appropriate for certain individuals. Determining the level of rigidity or flexibility within the scope of these practices often requires complex decisions that directly impact the individual and societal norms.

Review the classical descriptions of activities and behaviors that are considered to be appropriate for *brahmacharya* directly from the source texts. Note the contextual placement of each description to understand the author's perspective on the topic. The primary goal of *brahmacharya* is control over the senses and limitation of pleasures, with sexual indulgence being the primary focus.

Additional concepts related to personal behavior, conduct and general ethics will be discussed in Chapter nine as they relate to the state of health for *sattva*. A few references are included here as they are closely related to the practices of *brahmacharya* and *abrahmacharya*.

Brahmacharya and abrahmacharya Descriptions of restricted and unrestricted lifestyles	Cha.	Su.	AH	BP
Dhāraṇīya vega Controllable urges	Cha. Sū. 7/26-30		AH Sū. 4/24	
Sadvṛtta Codes of conduct, personal ethics	Cha. Sū. 8/18-34		AH Sū. 2/19-48	BP Pū. 5/235-260
Brahmacharya Restricted sexual intercourse		Su. Chi. 24/111-113		
Abrahmacharya General conduct for sexual intercourse			AH Sū. 7/69-76	BP Pū. 5/266-299
Hita vyavāya Proper sexual intercourse and indications		Su. Chi. 24/130-132		
Ahita vyavāya Improper sexual intercourse and contraindications		Su. Chi. 24/114-130		

Adhāraṇīya vegas

The *adhāraṇīya vegas* include the natural urges of the body which should never be restricted or withheld. Whenever any of the following urges naturally present themselves, they should be allowed to be released easily and appropriately.

Certain *sadvṛtta*, or rules of personal conduct, dictate that certain urges be controlled in front of respected individuals and in social gatherings. In these situations, individuals should excuse themselves appropriately whenever possible to tend to their bodily needs as a first priority.

Understanding how an individual controls their *adhāraṇīya vegas* on a regular basis provides significant insight into their state of health and *sātmya*. Each of the *adhāraṇīya vegas* is related to specific disorders that can be produced when the urge is withheld too long, too frequently or in any other detrimental manner.

The following tables summarize the *adhāraṇīya vegas* mentioned in classical literature, the disorders that result from their inappropriate restriction and their general protocols for management.

Note Vāgbhaṭa's specific explanation of *śhvāsa* in AH Sū. 4/14. He states that it is "श्रमश्वासाद्विधारितात्" (*śhrama śhvāsād vidhāritāt*) which indicates labored breathing caused by exhaustion produced through any form of exertion.

Adhāraṇīya vega	Relieving reflexes not to be withheld	Cha. Sū. 7/3	Su. Utt. 55/4	AH Sū. 4/1	BP Pū. 5/8-10
Mūtra	Urine	✓	✓	✓	✓
Purīṣha / viṭ	Stool, feces	✓	✓	✓	✓
Vāta	Flatus	✓	✓	✓	✓
Udgāra	Burp, eructation	✓		✓	
Kṣhut	Hunger	✓	✓	✓	
Pipāsa / tṛṭ	Thirst	✓	✓	✓	
Chhardi / vami	Vomit, regurgitation	✓	✓	✓	
Kṣhavathu	Sneeze	✓	✓	✓	
Jṛmbha	Yawn	✓	✓	✓	
Kāsa	Cough		✓		
Niḥśhvāsa / śhvāsa	Heavy, deep or labored breathing, inhalation, especially on exertion	✓	✓	✓	
Bāṣhpa / aśhru	Crying, tears	✓	✓	✓	
Retasa	Ejaculation, orgasm	✓	✓	✓	
Nidrā	Sleep	✓	✓	✓	

Mūtra nigraha roga Disorders due to withholding the urge to urinate	Cha. Sū. 7/6	Su. Utt. 55/	AH Sū. 4/4	BP Pū. 5/10
Basti-mehanayoḥ śhūla Pain in the area of the urinary bladder and penis	✓			✓
Basti, meḍra, vaṅkṣhaṇa vedanā Agonizing pain in the bladder region, penis and groin			✓	
Mūtrakṛchchhra Difficulty in urination	✓			✓

Mūtra nigraha roga Disorders due to withholding the urge to urinate	Cha. Sū. 7/6	Su. Utt. 55/	AH Sū. 4/4	BP Pū. 5/10
Śhiro-ruja Headache	✓			✓
Vināma vaṅkṣhaṇa Bending of the body around the groin indicating pain	✓			✓
Ānāha Abdominal distention, bloating	✓			✓
Aṅga bhaṅga Painful feeling in the limbs as if they are breaking			✓	
Aśhmarī Urinary calculi			✓	
Prāya rogā Additional disorders of vāta and *purīṣha nigraha*			✓	
Mūtra nigraha roga chikitsā Management of disorders of withheld urination	Cha. Sū. 7/7	Su. Utt. 55/	AH Sū. 4/5-7	BP Pū.
Sveda Sweating	✓		✓	
Avagāha Tub bath	✓		✓	
Abhyaṅga Oil massage	✓		✓	
Avapīḍaka sarpi *Avapīḍaka* (a type of *nasya*), with ghee	✓			
Trividha bastikarma All three types of *basti* protocols	✓		✓	
Varti Rectal suppositories			✓	
Prāgbhakta ghṛta pāna Therapeutic consumption of ghee before a meal			✓	

Purīṣha nigraha roga Disorders due to withholding the urge to defecate	Cha. Sū. 7/8	Su. Utt. 55/	AH Sū. 4/3	BP Pū. 5/8
Pakvāśhaya śhūla Abdominal pain in the area of the *pakvāśhaya*	✓			✓
Śhira-śhūla Headache	✓		✓	
Vāta, varcha apravartana Retention of flatus, feces	✓			✓
Piṇḍika udveṣhṭa Ball-shaped contractions, usually muscular cramps	✓		✓	
Ādhmāna Abdominal distension	✓			
Āṭopa Abdominal distension with gurgling				✓
Parikarttikā Sharp, shooting or cutting pain in the rectum or anus			✓	✓
Ūrdhva vāta, purīṣha āsya Upward moving *vāta*, stool (or its components) coming out through the mouth			✓	✓
Pratiśhyāya Head cold			✓	
Hṛdayasya uparodhana A sensation or feeling of blockage in and around the heart			✓	
Purīṣha nigraha roga chikitsā Management of disorders of withheld defecation	Cha. Sū. 7/9	Su. Utt. 55/	AH Sū. 4/5-7	BP Pū.
Sveda Sweating	✓		✓	
Abhyaṅga Oil massage	✓		✓	
Avagāha Tub bath	✓		✓	
Varti Rectal suppositories	✓		✓	
Basti karma	✓		✓	

Therapeutic enemas				
Hita pratihate varcasyannapāna pramāthi cha Appropriate food and drink which promotes bowel movements	✓		✓	

Vāta nigraha roga Disorders due to withholding the urge for flatus	Cha. Sū. 7/12	Su. Utt. 55/	AH Sū. 4/2	BP Pū. 5/
Saṅga viṇ, mūtra, vāta Blockage, retention of feces, urine, flatus	✓		✓	✓
Ādhmāna Abdominal distension	✓			✓
Vedana Pain	✓		✓	✓
Klama Exhaustion, fatigue	✓		✓	✓
Jaṭhare vātajāśhchānye rogā Disorders of or in the *jaṭhara* (abdominal cavity) caused due to *vāta*	✓			✓
Gulma A disease characterized by a pathological cluster of *doṣhas* in the abdomen			✓	
Udāvarta Upward movement of *vāta*			✓	
Dṛṣhṭi vadha Loss of vision			✓	
Agni vadha Loss of *agni*			✓	
Hṛd roga Heart disorders			✓	
Vāta nigraha roga chikitsā Management of disorders of withheld flatus	Cha. Sū. 7/13	Su. Utt. 55/	AH Sū. 4/5-7	BP Pū.
Sneha vidhi All therapeutic protocols to produce oleation	✓			
Sveda vidhi All therapeutic protocols to produce sweating	✓		✓	
Varti Rectal suppositories	✓		✓	
Vātānulomana bhojana cha pāna Meals and drinks that produce *vātānulomana*	✓			

Basti Therapeutic enemas	✓		✓	
Abhyaṅga Oil massage			✓	
Avagāha Tub bath			✓	

Udgāra nigraha roga Disorders due to withholding the urge for eructations	Cha. Sū. 7/18	Su. Utt. 55/	AH Sū. 4/8	BP Pū.
Hikka Hiccup	√			
Śhvāsa Difficulty breathing	√			
Aruchi Lack of appetite	√		√	
Kampa Tremors	√		√	
Vibandha hṛdaya, uras Tightness, a binding sensation around the heart and in the chest	√		√	
Ādhmāna Abdominal distension			√	
Kāsa, hidmā Cough, hiccups			√	
Udgāra nigraha roga chikitsā Management of disorders of withheld eructations	Cha. Sū. 7/18	Su. Utt. 55/	AH Sū. 4/8	BP Pū.
Hikkāyās-tulya auṣhadha Medicines used in the management of *hikka* (hiccups)	√		√	

Kṣhut nigraha roga Disorders due to withholding the urge for eating	Cha. Sū. 7/20	Su. Utt. 55/	AH Sū. 4/11	BP Pū. 5/99
Kārśhya Condition of being underweight, improperly nourished	√		√	
Daurbalya Weakness, lack of strength	√			
Vaivarṇya Discoloration of complexion indicating *asvastha*	√			

Aṅgamarda Squeezing pain in the bodily limbs	√			√
Aruchi Lack of appetite	√		√	√
Bhrama Dizziness	√		√	
Aṅga-bhaṅga Feeling as if the limbs are being broken			√	
Glāni Exhaustion			√	
Śhūla Abdominal pain, discomfort			√	
Śhrama Exhaustion, fatigue				√
Tandrā Inattentiveness due to exhaustion				√
Lochana daurbalya Weakness of the eyes				√
Dhātu dāha Burning sensation of the *dhātus*				√
Bala kṣhaya Reduction of strength				√
Kṣhut nigraha roga chikitsā Management of disorders of withheld eating	Cha. Sū. 7/20	Su. Utt. 55/	AH Sū. 4/11	BP Pū.
Snigdha, uṣhṇa, laghu bhojana Unctuous, hot, light meals	√			
Laghu, snigdha, uṣhṇa, alpa bhojana Light, unctuous, hot and small meals			√	

Pipāsa nigraha roga Disorders due to withholding the urge for drinking fluids	Cha. Sū. 7/21	Su. Utt. 55/	AH Sū. 4/10	BP Pū. 5/100
Kaṇṭha, āsya śhoṣha Dryness of the throat and oral cavity	✓			✓
Bādhirya Deafness, loss of hearing	✓		✓	
Śhravaṇa avarodha Obstruction of the sense of hearing by covering				✓
Śhrama Exhaustion, fatigue	✓			
Sādo hṛdi Weakness, exhaustion of the heart	✓			
Śhoṣha Wasting, drying, shrivelling up of the body			✓	
Rakta śhoṣha Drying up or wasting of *rakta*				✓
Aṅgasāda Weakness, exhaustion of the bodily limbs			✓	
Sammoha Loss of consciousness			✓	
Bhrama Dizziness			✓	
Hṛd gadā Disorders of the heart			✓	✓
Pipāsa nigraha roga chikitsā Management of disorders of withheld thirst	Cha. Sū. 7/21	Su. Utt. 55/	AH Sū. 4/10	BP Pū.
Śhīta tarpaṇa Refreshing, strengthening, building protocols primarily using cold	✓			
Śhīta sarva vidhi hita All types of cooling measures are appropriate			✓	

Chhardi nigraha roga Disorders due to withholding the urge for vomiting	Cha. Sū. 7/14	Su. Utt. 55/	AH Sū. 4/17	BP Pū.
Kaṇḍū Itching	✓		✓	
Koṭhā A type of skin disorder	✓		✓	
Aruchi Lack of appetite	✓			
Vyaṅga Freckles	✓		✓	
Śhotha (Śhvayathu) Swelling	✓		✓	
Pāṇḍu Group of disorders with paleness, pallor or discoloration of complexion as the primary feature	✓		✓	
Jvara Fever	✓		✓	
Kuṣhṭha Group of skin disorders	✓		✓	
Hṛllāsa Regurgitating hiccup	✓			
Vīsarpa A type of skin disorder that spreads quickly	✓		✓	
Akṣhi (roga) (Disorders of the) eyes			✓	
Kāsa Cough			✓	
Śhvāsa Difficulty breathing			✓	
Chhardi nigraha roga chikitsā Management of disorders of withheld vomitus	Cha. Sū. 7/15	Su. Utt. 55/	AH Sū. 4/18	BP Pū.
Pracchardana Therapeutic emesis	✓			
Dhūma	✓		✓	

Therapeutic smoking				
Laṅghana Therapeutic reduction methods	√			
Rakta mokṣhaṇa Blood-letting	√		√	
Rūkṣha anna, pāna Dry foods and drinks	√		√	
Vyāyāma Exercise	√		√	
Vireka Therapeutic purgations	√		√	
Gaṇḍūṣha Filling the mouth with liquid (usually oil)			√	
Anāhāra Not consuming food			√	
Gaṇḍūṣha, anāhāra, rūkṣha bhuktvā, tad udvama (?) Each performed in sequence, then inducing vomiting			√	
Sa-kṣhāra lavaṇa taila, abhyaṅga Oil massage with oil prepared with alkali and salt			√	

Kṣhavathu nigraha roga Disorders due to withholding the urge for sneezing	Cha. Sū. 7/16	Su. Utt. 55/	AH Sū. 4/8	BP Pū.
Manyāstambha Disorders due to stiffness of the neck	√		√	
Śhira śhūla Headache	√		√	
Arditā Half-side facial or body paralysis	√		√	
Ārdhāvabhedakā Headache in half of the head	√			
Daurbalya indriya Weakened senses	√		√	

Kṣhavathu nigraha roga chikitsā Management of disorders of withheld sneezes	Cha. Sū. 7/17	Su. Utt. 55/	AH Sū. 4/9	BP Pū.
Urdhva jatru abhyaṅga Oil massage above the clavicular region	√			
Sveda Sweating (above the clavicular region)	√			
Dhūma Therapeutic smoking	√			
Nāvana *Nāvana* type of *nasya*	√			
Hita vātaghnam-ādya Appropriate foods and methods to reduce *vāta*	√			
Ghṛta cha uttara-bhaktika Consumption of ghee after a meal	√			
Tīkṣhṇa dhūma Strong therapeutic smoking			√	
(Tīkṣhṇa) añjana (Strong) collyrium			√	
(Tīkṣhṇa) ghrāṇa nāvana (Strong) use of a specific type of *nasya* (nasal instillation)			√	
Avana arka vilokena Gazing at the sun on the horizon			√	
Sneha, svedau cha śhīlayet Regular use of both *sneha* and *sveda*			√	

Jṛmbha nigraha roga Disorders due to withholding the urge for yawning	Cha. Sū. 7/19	Su. Utt. 55/	AH Sū. 4/15	BP Pū.
Vināma Distortion, bending of the body, crookedness	✓			
Akṣhepa Convulsions	✓			
Saṅkocha Contractions (of the muscles, body)	✓			
Supti Numbness	✓			
Kampa Tremors	✓			
Pravepana Trembling	✓			
Kṣhavathu roga Disorders listed resulting from withholding sneezing			✓	
Jṛmbha nigraha roga chikitsā Management of disorders of withheld yawns	Cha. Sū. 7/19	Su. Utt. 55/	AH Sū. 4/15	BP Pū.
Sarva vātaghna auṣhadha All medicines used to control *vāta*	✓		✓	

Kāsa nigraha roga Disorders due to withholding the urge for coughing	Cha.	Su. Utt. 55/	AH Sū. 4/13	BP Pū.
Rodha, vṛddhi śhvāsa Obstructed, increased respiration			✓	
Aruchi Lack of appetite, desire for food			✓	
Hṛd āmaya Disorders of the heart			✓	
Śhoṣha Wasting, drying, shrivelling up of the body			✓	
Hidmā Hiccups			✓	
Kāsa nigraha roga chikitsā Management of disorders of withheld coughs	Cha.	Su. Utt. 55/	AH Sū. 4/13	BP Pū.
Kāsa vidhi All therapies for cough			✓	

Niḥśhvāsa nigraha roga Disorders due to withholding the urge for deep breathing	Cha. Sū. 7/24	Su. Utt. 55/	AH Sū. 4/14	BP Pū.
Gulma A disease characterized by a pathological cluster of *doṣhas* in the abdomen	✓		✓	
Hṛdroga Heart diseases	✓		✓	
Sammohā Loss of consciousness	✓		✓	
Śhrama Exhaustion, fatigue	✓			
Niḥśhvāsa nigraha roga chikitsā Management of disorders of withheld deep breathing	Cha. Sū. 7/24	Su. Utt. 55/	AH Sū. 4/14	BP Pū.
Viśhrāma Rest	✓		✓	
Vātaghna kriyā hitā All appropriate treatments for controlling *vāta*	✓		✓	

Bāṣhpa nigraha roga Disorders due to withholding the urge for crying	Cha. Sū. 7/22	Su. Utt. 55/	AH Sū. 4/16	BP Pū.
Pratiśhyāya Head cold	√			
Akṣhiroga Eye disorders	√			
Hṛdroga Heart diseases	√			
Aruchi Lack of appetite	√		√	
Bhrama Dizziness	√		√	
Pīnasa Rhinorrhea, runny nose			√	
Akṣhi, śhiro, hṛd ruj Pain in the eyes, head, heart			√	
Manyāstambha Disorders due to stiffness of the neck			√	
Gulma A disease characterized by a pathological cluster of *doṣhas* in the abdomen			√	
Bāṣhpa nigraha roga chikitsā Management of disorders of withheld crying	Cha. Sū. 7/22	Su. Utt. 55/	AH Sū. 4/16	BP Pū.
Svapna Sleep, rest	√		√	
Madya Consumption of alcohol	√		√	
Priyā kathā Pleasing, enjoyable conversations and stories	√		√	

Retasa nigraha roga Disorders due to withholding the urge for ejaculation, orgasm	Cha. Sū. 7/10	Su. Utt. 55/	AH Sū. 4/19	BP Pū.
Meḍhre vṛṣhaṇayoḥ śhūla Pain in the penis and testicles	✓		✓	
Aṅgamarda Squeezing pain in the bodily limbs	✓			
Hṛdi Pain in or around the heart	✓		✓	
Vibaddha mūtra Retention of urine	✓		✓	
Śhukra sravaṇa Seminal discharge			✓	
Śhvayathu Swelling			✓	
Jvara Fever			✓	
Aṅga-bhaṅga Feeling as if the limbs are being broken			✓	
Vṛddhi Inguinal, scrotal hernia			✓	
Aśhma Stones (urinary, seminal)			✓	
Ṣhaṇḍatā Impotence			✓	
Retasa nigraha roga chikitsā Management of disorders of withheld ejaculation, orgasm	Cha. Sū. 7/11	Su. Utt. 55/	AH Sū. 4/20	BP Pū.
Basti Therapeutic enema			✓	
Abhyaṅga Oil massage	✓		✓	
Avagāha Tub bath	✓		✓	
Madirā Wine	✓			

Charaṇāyudhāḥ Chicken	✓		✓	
Śhāli *Śhāli* rice	✓		✓	
Paya Milk	✓			
Nirūha A type of *basti* (therapeutic enema)	✓			
Śhasta maithuna Regular sexual intercourse	✓		✓	
Surā Beer			✓	
Basti śhuddhi kara, siddha bhajet kṣhīra Urinary bladder cleanses using medicines prepared with milk			✓	

Nidrā nigraha roga Disorders due to withholding the urge to sleep	Cha. Sū. 7/23	Su. Utt. 55/	AH Sū. 4/12	BP Pū. 5/101
Jṛmbha Yawning	√		√	√
Aṅgamarda Squeezing pain in the bodily limbs	√		√	√
Tandrā Inattentiveness due to exhaustion	√			√
Śhiro roga Disorders of the head	√			
Śhiro gaurava Heaviness of the head				√
Akṣhi gaurava Heaviness of the eyes	√		√	√
Moha Loss of consciousness			√	
Mūrdha gaurava Heaviness of the head			√	
Ālasya Lassitude, laziness			√	
(Na) anna pāka Lack of digestion of food				√
Nidrā nigraha roga chikitsā Management of disorders of withheld sleep	Cha. Sū. 7/23	Su. Utt. 55/	AH Sū. 4/12	BP Pū.
Svapna Sleep, rest	√		√	
Saṁvāhana Gentle, pleasant, sensual massage	√		√	

KEY PRINCIPLES

The key principles that underlie *sātmya* are fundamental, classical principles with a practical degree of flexibility. They may be adapted and applied to any individual in any environment. Review these principles and their clinical applications.

Principle #1: Determining sātmya

The determination of *sātmya* is made based on its type (*sātmya*, *okasātmya* or *asātmya*) and its application (ideal baseline and current usage). To qualify as *sātmya*, two specific conditions must be met.

Sātmya must

- promote an individual's *svastha*
- and do so when used regularly

These requirements can be assessed in the context of application of *sātmya* with any factors that influence *svastha*.

When both of these requirements are not met, yet the factor appears to promote *svastha* for the individual, it should be considered *okasātmya* instead. And when any factor regularly influences an individual's *svastha* in a detrimental way, it is *asātmya*.

Type	Result
Sātmya	Always 1. Promotes *svastha* 2. When used regularly
Okasātmya	1. Sometimes promotes *svastha* 2. Not used regularly
Asātmya	1. Promotes *asvastha* 2. May be used regularly or irregularly

The application of *sātmya* may be considered in the context of any factor influencing *svastha*. *Rasa sātmya* is a good example that demonstrates adaptation to individually customized, health-promoting factors that regularly produce positive outcomes.

Determining the ideal baseline often requires having a complete, holistic understanding of the individual, their current state of svastha and habitual routine.

Many activities and behaviors that influence *svastha* have common *sātmya* recommendations that are applicable to all generally healthy individuals. These include:

- *Charya*
- *Āhāra*
- *Nidrā*
- *Abrahmacharya*
- *Adhāraṇīya vegas*

The key is to differentiate the ideal baseline for the individual that should be their normal level of *sātmya* from their current state for the same factor. Then the difference between the two can be determined and managed appropriately to promote *sātmya*.

Principle #2: Promoting sātmya

The promotion of *sātmya* is directly dependent on the determination of *sātmya* in Principle #1 based on its type, baseline and current status.

Once these are determined, an effective management plan can be created to shift the current state of *sātmya* closer toward the baseline with the goal of reaching and maintaining the baseline permanently.

Every management plan to promote *sātmya* must take the following into consideration:

- Schedule
- Key *guṇas*
- Quantum

The schedule for replacing *okasātmya* or *asātmya* with *sātmya* should always consider the duration of the habit, the mental state of the individual to change, available options, ease or difficulty of the change and potential risk factors. Not every situation will result in a positive health outcome through changing *sātmya*, and it is imperative that this be considered before making any recommendations.

Once the decision is made, the general classical schedule for implementing the change should be considered. General guidelines recommend that the individual substitute the *okasātmya* or *asātmya* factor by one quarter or less with a *sātmya* factor.

The time between changing substitution intervals may be as short as a few days to much longer periods or weeks, months or even years in certain cases. The final determination for each of these factors is completely dependent upon the individual, their state of mind, contraindications, and any restrictions or limitations that must be accommodated.

While the decision to effect the change ultimately lies with the individual, the recommendations provided must follow known guidelines. At times, this can present conflicts for the individual which must be managed accordingly. Any potential risks must always be disclosed. As a general rule, recommendations outside of normal guidelines should not be made unless all potential risks have been identified and properly mitigated.

The speed of the process may vary widely in practice. The individual's unique response must be confirmed through regular, ongoing assessment of *svastha* on all levels. With regular monitoring, adjustments and advancements in the substitution schedule may continue.

Promoting *sātmya* also requires a strong foundation in application of the rules of appropriate *guṇas* for the individual. Recall that the general rule to promote *sātmya* for an individual relies on utilizing *guṇa viparīta*, or opposite *guṇas*, based on the individual's:

- *Deśha*
- *Kāla*
- *Ātma*
- *Vikāra*

In order to effectively determine the individual's ideal baseline for *sātmya*, a thorough assessment of these factors must be completed. Then *guṇa viparīta* can be applied appropriately.

For an individual who remains in the same *deśha*, they naturally become accustomed to the related effects of the *kāla* and *ṛtu* in that location. By default, these are supposed to become *sātmya* for the individual, assuming that their remaining factors are functioning normally, that they are in a general state of *svastha* and that they make appropriate accommodations through diet and lifestyle.

In certain situations, an individual's own nature can predispose them to *sātmya* in peculiar or particular ways. This is said to be due to *ātma*. In cases of *vikṛti*, or deviation from *svastha* with the presence of *vikāra*, the individual may also be subject to changes in their *sātmya* which are appropriate for the disorder(s).

After taking each of these into account at any given point in time, the individual's *sātmya guṇas* and their associated *viparīta guṇas* can be determined. Ideally, these should remain generally similar for one's lifespan. However, that is only possible when the individual maintains all baseline factors within their normal ranges for *deśha*, *kāla*, *ātma* (or *prakṛti*) and *vikāra*. Any change to these, including common events such as moving to a different geographical region, or experiencing a deviation from normal health, can cause the individual's predisposition for their baseline *sātmya* to also change.

Once the requirements of schedule and key *guṇas* have been determined, the management of the change must be planned. This requires consideration from many angles in order to determine the appropriate methodology for the individual. Any potential obstacles to compliance must be identified as quickly as possible, and the individual's preferences and limitations must be taken into account in order to increase their chance of success to change their *sātmya* and maintain it.

Once the initial boundaries are identified, primary and secondary options can be compared. These are categorized based on approach, as:

1. *Samyak kriya-upayoga*
2. *Samyak karma*
3. *Samyak āhāra*

Kriya-upayoga consists of the therapeutic interventions that are appropriate for the individual's unique circumstance, their goal for promoting *sātmya* and any restrictions that may be applicable. *Karma* includes all activities, routines and habits and *āhāra* includes all dietary foods and drinks consumed internally to support the body.

As Punarvasu Atreya explains to a group of scholars in Cha. Sū. 25/29, the very same factors produce health or disease according to their usage. This is particularly relevant in the context of *sātmya*.

Finally, the quantum of the change required to effect proper *sātmya* must be considered. In many clinical cases, the root cause for improper *sātmya* is often found to be an adherence to over-indulgence, over-nourishment or over-stimulation singly or in combination.

In these cases, the management for restoration of healthy *sātmya* is to simply withdraw from the overindulgent habit or factor without requiring that it be replaced with something else. As an interim step, replacement with something less harmful may aid the individual in adjusting to the new change.

The classical recommendation for this aspect of management lies in the recommendation that anything which is *atiyoga*, or used in excess, should be restrained or limited to a level which is not harmful or habit-forming.

The main challenge with the practical application of this rule is that many individuals are unaware of that specific moment when something that is usually good for them, or perceived to be good for them, begins to produce the opposite result.

For many people, the associations of "good" or "bad" effects lie completely with the *dravya* and the expectation that the *dravya* remains constant. This common misunderstanding requires clear explanation and re-education in order for one to gain independence and control over their constantly shifting state of health.

The exception to the rule of controlling excessive behavior is with the *adhāraṇīya vegas*, or the natural urges of the body. These should not be controlled or limited. When they manifest, they must be relieved as quickly as possible in the most appropriate manner.

One of the most pertinent classical recommendations to avoid in excess is extending one's self beyond their capacity, in any form. In many Western cultures today, this type of behavior is not only common, but expected.

A simple way to handle this through the application of *sātmya* is to encourage the individual to recognize the habit utilizing all of the details listed in this principle. A management plan can be created and implemented based on the individual's motivation to improve their state of *svastha*. Recognition of responsibility in the process is often the most important component for success.

SĀTMYA ASSESSMENT

A thorough assessment of *sātmya* requires determining the individual's ideal baseline and distinguishing their current state of *sātmya* across all major types. Each factor that influences *svastha* should be assessed exclusively to the maximum extent possible, and then an overall assessment should be concluded based on the results.

Determining whether any food, activity or behavior is *sātmya*, *okasātmya* or *asātmya* for an individual requires observing the effects and outcomes in the person when the item is used or practiced regularly for a long duration of time.

Typically, at least one year of regular usage is needed to see the outcomes while maintaining stability all other factors. This is challenging, and often impossible, for many reasons. Compliance and consistency are typically the most common challenges.

Even when compliance is well-managed, the clinician must recognize that even the single change of maintaining *sātmya* over a longer duration will often contribute to improving *svastha*. This beneficial change alone can producing positive health outcomes and potentially reducing any existing *dhātu vaiṣhamya*.

When monitoring *sātmya* interventions, consistent assessments are critical to understanding and optimizing healthy outcomes.

Assessing ṛtucharya

Always complete the assessment of the individual's *ṛtu* before attempting to assess their *ṛtucharya*. Then, complete the table below with the individual's specific responses phrased as questions related to the current season only.

Question	Response for current season only
Primary *hita āhāra*	
Primary *hita vihāra*	
Primary *ahita āhāra*	
Primary *ahita vihāra*	
Specific likes, cravings	
Specific dislikes, aversions	
Estimated *hita āhāra*	
Estimated *hita vihāra*	

Assessing dinacharya

Complete the table below with the individual's specific responses phrased as questions related to their current routine in the current season.

Question	Response for current season only
Primary *hita vihāra*	
Primary *ahita vihāra*	
Specific likes, cravings	
Specific dislikes, aversions	
Estimated *hita vihāra*	

Assessing rātricharya

Complete the table below with the individual's specific responses phrased as questions related to their current routine in the current season.

Question	Response for current season only
Primary *hita vihāra*	
Primary *ahita vihāra*	
Specific likes, cravings	
Specific dislikes, aversions	
Estimated *hita vihāra*	

Assessing nidrā

Complete the table below with the individual's specific responses phrased as questions related to their current routine in the current season.

Question	Response for current season only
Primary *hita vihāra*	
Primary *ahita vihāra*	
Specific likes, cravings	
Specific dislikes, aversions	
Estimated *hita vihāra*	

Assessing abrahmacharya

Complete the table below with the individual's specific responses phrased as questions related to their current routine in the current season.

Question	Response for current season only
Primary *hita vihāra*	
Primary *ahita vihāra*	
Specific likes, cravings	
Specific dislikes, aversions	
Estimated *hita vihāra*	

Assessing overall sātmya

Complete the table below based on the individual's specific responses above. Determine which items fall into each category. For each item, gauge its level as *avara*, *madhyama* or *uttama*.

Question	Response for current season only
What is *sātmya*? As *avara*, *madhyama*, *uttama*	
What is *okasātmya*? As *avara*, *madhyama*, *uttama*	
What is *asātmya*? As *avara*, *madhyama*, *uttama*	

TEST YOURSELF

Learn, review and memorize key terms from this section.

abrahmacharya

āchāra

adhāraṇīya vegas

asātmya

brahmacharya

charya

dinacharya

nidrā

okasātmya

rātricharya

ṛtucharya

sātmya

vihāra

vṛtta

vṛtti

Chapter 5: Review

ADDITIONAL READING

Read and review the references listed below to expand your understanding of the concepts in this chapter. Write down the date that you complete your reading for each. Remember that consistent repetition is the best way to learn. Plan to read each reference at least once now and expect to read it again as you continue your studies.

References marked with (skim) can be read quickly and do not require commentary review.

CLASSICS		1st read	2nd read
Charaka	Cha. Sū. 5/, 6/		
Suśhruta			
Aṣhṭāṅga Hṛdaya	AH Sū. 2/, 3/		
Bhāva Prakāśha	BP Pū. 5/		

JOURNALS & CURRENT RESOURCES

QUESTIONS & ANSWERS

Record your questions for this chapter here for further research and discussion.

Question:

Answer:

Question:

Answer:

Question:

Answer:

SELF-ASSESSMENT

1. What two criteria does any food, behavior or activity have to meet in order to be considered *sātmya*?
   a. It must promote health when used long-term and must promote an individual's svastha when used regularly.
   b. It must fulfill the goal of *dhātu sāmya* and alleviate any aggravated *doṣhas*.
   c. It must be personalized to the individual and reduce the load of *āma* in the body.
   d. It must apply to all factors that influence *svastha* and be used sparingly.
   e. None of the above

2. *Hemanta ṛtu* is ideal for *śhodhana*.
   a. True
   b. False

3. Charaka's methodology for removing *okasātmya* and *asātmya* items is
   a. The item is to be removed 1/4 at a time and simultaneously replaced with 1/4 of an appropriate, *sātmya* item.
   b. The item is to be removed 1/16 at a time and simultaneously replaced with 1/16 of an appropriate, *sātmya* item.
   c. The item is to be removed 1/2 at a time and simultaneously replaced with 1/2 of an appropriate, *sātmya* item.
   d. The item should be removed immediately.
   e. None of the above

4. ______ is used classically to refer to any type of regular routine, regimen or schedule that is intended to promote *svastha*.
   a. *Charya*
   b. *Dinacharya*
   c. *Ṛtucharya*
   d. *Svastha*
   e. None of the above

5. *Divā svapna* is only indicated in which *ṛtu*?
   a. *Grīṣhma*
   b. *Hemanta*
   c. *Śhiśhira*
   d. *Vasanta*
   e. All of the above

6. The *trayopastambha* includes *āhāra*, *nidrā* and ____________ .
   a. *Abrahmacharya*
   b. *Brahmacharya*
   c. *Rātri jāgaraṇa*
   d. *Vyāyāma*
   e. Both A and B

7. *Puṣhti* is a result of _______ .
   a. Excessive exercise
   b. Improper sleep
   c. Less exercise
   d. Proper sleep
   e. Both B and C

8. The natural urges of the body which should never be restricted or withheld are called __________ .
   a. *Adhāraṇiya vegas*
   b. *Bhaya*
   c. *Dhāraṇiya vegas*
   d. *Krodha*
   e. None of the above

9. *Kāsa* and *śhvāsa* refer to
   a. Cough and difficulty breathing
   b. Headache and weakened senses
   c. Therapeutic purgations and not consuming food
   d. Therapeutic smoking and sweating
   e. All of the above

10. A thorough assessment of *sātmya* requires determining which of the following?
   a. A thorough understanding of an individual's *dinacharya*.
   b. The individual's ideal baseline and their current state of *sātmya* across all major types.
   c. The individual's specific likes and cravings
   d. All of the above
   e. None of the above

CRITICAL THINKING

1. Consider a case of an individual with cravings that promote their state of *svastha* versus one with opposite cravings. Explain an example and the inferences that could be drawn about their state of *svastha*.

2. Identify at least 3 examples of *sātmya*, *okasātmya* and *asātmya* in your life.

3. How does the management of *anidrā* and *ati nidrā* correlate to the doṣhas? How can this correlation provide insight to infer *nidāna* in practice?

4. Describe appropriate indications and life periods for practicing *brahmacharya* versus *abhramacharya*.

5. Which classical *ṛtu charya* guidelines and recommendations could be relevant in your geographical location? How, and why?

References

Chapter 6 : Prakṛti

KEY TERMS

avara
āyu
bala
bhautika prakṛti
darśhana
deha prakṛti
lakṣhaṇa
madhyama
mānasika prakṛti
prakṛti
pramāṇa
praśhna
saṁhanana
sāra
sparśhana
svabhāva
uttama
vikṛti

CLASSICAL REVIEW

An individual's *prakṛti* is perhaps one of the most prominent factors that can influence the state of *svastha*. Being set from the moment of conception, it remains stable throughout life and may only show signs of changing when the individual approaches death. The classics accept seven types of *deha prakṛti* based on combinations of *vāta*, *pitta* and *kapha*. The assessment of *deha prakṛti* includes two main aspects:

1. Identification of the individual's *deha prakṛti* type
2. General classification of the *deha prakṛti* type based on *uttama*, *madhyama* and *avara*

Vāgbhaṭa summarizes both of these concepts in the first chapter of Aṣhṭāṅga Hṛdaya.

शुक्रार्तवस्थैर्जन्मादौ विषेणेव विषक्रिमेः ॥ ९
तैश्च तिस्रः प्रकृतयो हीनमध्योत्तमाः पृथक् ।
समधातुः समस्तासु श्रेष्ठा, निन्द्या द्विदोषजाः ॥

अ. हृ. सू. १०

Śhukrārtavasthairjanmādau viṣheṇeva viṣhakrimeḥ ||
Taiśhcha tisraḥ prakṛtayo hīnamadhyottamāḥ pṛthak |
Samadhātuḥ samastāsu śhreṣhṭhā, nindyā dvidoṣhajāḥ ||

AH Sū. 1/9-10

Śhukra-ārtava sthair-janmādau (Both *śhukra* and *ārtava* [the male and female seeds of conception which are responsible for establishing the proportion of *doṣhas* in *prakṛti* from the very beginning of life] are born) viṣheṇeva viṣhakrimeḥ (just as poisonous worms arise from poison itself.) Taiśhcha tisraḥ prakṛtayo (And so the three [*doṣhas*] are created;) hīna-madhya-uttamāḥ pṛthak (when each one individually is predominant, it is considered on its own as *hīna*, *madhya* or *uttama* [weakest, moderate or strongest from *vāta*, *pitta* and *kapha*]). Samadhātuḥ (*Sama dhātu*, or the state of all three in equilibrium) samastāsu (is considered to be) śhreṣhṭhā (the best,) nindyā samastāsu (while that which is considered the worst) dvidoṣhajāḥ (is called *dvi-doṣhaja* or having two dominant *doṣhas*).

Based on this explanation, the seven types of *deha prakṛti* types are clearly defined and their general classification in relation to one another as *hīna*, *madhya* or *uttama* is implied. Both concepts are summarized in the following table.

	Hīna	Madhya	Uttama
Eka-doṣhaja	V	P	K
Dvi-doṣhaja (samsṛṣhṭa)	VK	VP	PK
Tri-doṣhaja (samadhātu)			VPK

Assessing *prakṛti*

A thorough *prakṛti* assessment includes the analysis of *prakṛti* from several key perspectives. These cover:

1. *Deha prakṛti*
2. *Bhautika prakṛti*
3. *Sāra*
4. *Mānasika prakṛti*

Each of these three is inherently connected to an individual's baseline, natural state. While *mānasika prakṛti* and its assessment is covered in Chapter nine with *sattva*.

Measurement of an individual's *pramāṇa* is also considered to be an indicative component of *prakṛti* according to Suśhruta in Su. Su. 35/14-15. However, this explanation is provided in the context of assessing *āyu* soon after birth. The measurements provided by Suśhruta for this assessment of *pramāṇa* are likely to be more accurate for individuals of Indian descent. Large, long-term studies need to be performed over various ethnic populations in the context of the classical Ayurvedic framework.

Considering this, *pramāṇa* assessment has been placed in this textbook with *bala* in Chapter eight. This follows Charaka's style more closely as *pramāṇa* assessment may be performed at any point in an individual's life. At different stages, *pramāṇa* may vary and is likely indicative of the current state of *saṁhanana*. The assessment in this context can also be used to investigate the individual's likely baseline for *pramāṇa*. See Chapter eight for complete details.

Assessment methodologies

Before assessing *prakṛti*, it is important to understand the context and specific methodologies that are often employed in the process. Many of the assessment parameters and their related questions may seem to repeat themselves with other areas of the overall Clinical Svastha Assessment. However, there are subtle yet key distinctions that can easily change the interpretation of the assessed parameters.

Initially, the Svastha Āchārya (SA) should ask themselves, "What is being assessed?" This is the first step to organizing and contextualizing the flow of the assessment. Multiple questions and answers are often required to fully understand each level and component during the early stages of practice.

Each response from the patient may provide more or less information than what is originally asked or sought. When additional key information is provided, it is the responsibility of the Svastha Āchārya (SA) to capture that and record it appropriately.

Contextualizing the *prakṛti* assessment

The first step of any *prakṛti* assessment is to set the context of the questions in the portion of the assessment. This guides the patient to responding in such a way which differentiates *prakṛti* from other factors in the overall assessment.

Specifically, this aids the clinician to perform the following.

1. Assess *prakṛti* versus *vikṛti*
2. Understand individual *svabhāva* (the natural state, or cause of being)
3. Recognize *prakṛti* as the *kāraṇa* which produces *kārya* (based on *kārya-kāraṇa bhāva*) as the current state of being

A successful *prakṛti* assessment will always determine whether the component being analyzed is natural for the individual. Is it their "fallback," or their constant tendency throughout life? Is it noticeable even during the best periods of health?

While many characteristics will be noticeable throughout life, they generally do not present an immediate health problem to the individual when other factors are maintained well enough to compensate.

Contextualizing questions in the *prakṛti* assessment typically requires that the clinician set boundaries on factors like *kāla*, *deśha* and *vaya* as a starting point. These boundaries help the patient specifically understand any types of pattern that are being investigated in specific periods of their life or throughout the entire duration.

When phrasing questions for *prakṛti* assessment, recall Vāgbhaṭa's statement explained at the beginning of this chapter (AH Sū. 1/9-10). Carefully consider the analogy of poisonous worms and notice how deeply it relates to the manifestation of an individual's *prakṛti*.

Darśhana, sparśhana, praśhna

Each assessment component will be analyzed using one or more of these three key methods of *parikṣha*:

1.	*Darśhana*	Observation
2.	*Sparśhana*	Palpation
3.	*Praśhna*	Communication

A basic understanding of these simple assessment methodologies provides a helpful guide to cover all possible approaches thoroughly.

Darśhana is observation, inspection or examination of the patient during the assessment without physical contact. It primarily relies on the sense of vision. Other senses such as smell and hearing may be employed secondarily. The sense of taste is generally not indicated classically for assessment.

Sparśhana requires manual application of the clinician's hands onto the physical body of the patient to perform palpation or tactual examination. It utilizes the sense of touch to examine the patient's physical body through superficial or deep palpation. *Sparśhana* is often employed to confirm information assessed through *darśhana*.

Praśhna is the direct communication between the patient and the clinician that conveys information vital to a successful assessment. *Praśhna* may also be translated as questioning, enquiring or asking. Questions asked by the clinician to the patient to assess any component fall under the methodology of *praśhna*.

Accurate application

The classical Āyurvedic medical compendia include many specific descriptions of *prakṛti* from multiple perspectives. These explanations were relevant for Āyurvedic clinical practice Indian subcontinent at that time.

Today, some of these explanations are still easy to understand and apply, while others are confusing or irrelevant. It is not possible to take the classical descriptions of *prakṛti* and apply them exactly from the classical texts throughout the modern world. *Prakṛti lakṣhaṇa* descriptions will be reviewed throughout this chapter considering this current obstacle.

Students and healthcare professionals are strongly encouraged to analyze each *prakṛti* assessment parameter to determine its applicability in their current environment. Sample questions and examples are provided for initial guidance.

Deha prakṛti

The *lakṣhaṇas* of *deha* (*doṣhaja* or *śharīrika*) *prakṛti* were covered extensively in Volume 2, Chapter 18. Review that chapter in full to prepare for the *prakṛti* assessment.

All major classical authors provide detailed descriptions of the *prakṛti lakṣhaṇas*. Many of the characteristics and descriptions are similar. Charaka and Suśhruta provide their own specific formats and methods to organize the *prakṛti lakṣhaṇas* for improved understanding and application.

The tables that follow cover each individual *deha prakṛti lakṣhaṇa* separately with references to their original quotations from Charaka and Suśhruta. Each *lakṣhaṇa* is grouped under a translated heading name that generally describes the *lakṣhaṇa* being assessed. Its methods of assessment (*darśhana*, *sparśhana* and *praśhna*) are listed with Charaka's classification *guṇa*.

Several examples are provided to guide the student through assessing the *lakṣhaṇa* using *darśhana*, *sparśhana* and *praśhna*. These starting points are helpful introductory methods that may be expanded and developed as practical clinical skills advance. The end of this chapter covers practical application methods for the level of practice as a Svastha Āchārya.

The assessment of each *prakṛti* is based primarily on Cha. Vi. 8/96-98 and Su. Śhā. 4/64-67. Similar statements from the two authors are grouped together under a general heading for the *lakṣhaṇa* assessed.

Vāta Prakṛti Assessment

Vāta prakṛti lakṣhaṇa	Weak bodily frame and build
Charaka's description	*Rūkṣha, apachita, alpa śharīrā* Dry, thin, weak body
Suśhruta's description	*Kṛśha* Weak
Guṇa(s)	*Rūkṣha*
Darśhana	Observe the bodily frame for proportion, overall development, state of nourishment and suppleness. Look specifically for the following signs. 1. Underdeveloped, disproportionate skeletal structure 2. Thin, weak skeletal structure, bones and components 3. Frail, dry physical appearance 4. Difficulty maintaining proper posture or stature
Sparśhana	Palpate the bodily limbs and joints superficially and deep. Examine the abdominal area, shoulder girdle, chest, ribs and neck. Note the following. 1. Skin texture, dryness, suppleness, elasticity 2. Skin quality, cracks around joints, lines, impressions 3. Depth and thickness of tissues 4. Depth of interior structures (vascular system, muscles, bones, organs) 5. Structural development, or lack thereof
Praśhna	Ask questions that investigate weakness in physical development or form. 1. Have you ever broken any bones? If so, please explain. 2. How do you usually put on weight? 3. How strong are/were you at your healthiest point in life? 4. How would you describe your physical frame? 5. How would you rate your stamina at your healthiest time of life? (low, medium, high) 6. How would you rate your stamina now? (low, medium, high)

Vāta prakṛti lakṣhaṇa	Voice quality and hoarseness
Charaka's description	*Pratata rūkṣha, kṣhāma, sanna-sakta jarjarasvarā* Constantly dry, weak (debilitated), low (sunk in), stuck, broken (hollow) voice
Suśhruta's description	N/A
Guṇa(s)	*Rūkṣha*

Darśhana	Listen to the speech, its production, qualities, continuation and ending point. Note all sounds produced, including changes in pitch, clearing the throat, coughs, cracks, etc. Listen specifically for the following. 1. Tone 2. Pitch 3. Control of consistent sound production, or lack thereof 4. Hoarseness, dryness, cracking, squeaking, roughness, feebleness, emptiness
Sparśhana	Optional. The throat may be superficially palpated during speech to observe vibrations and movement. Left and right sides of the larynx, neck and upper chest should be compared.
Praśhna	Ask questions that investigate weakness in the voice, throat and surrounding anatomical structures. 1. Do you ever notice difficulty speaking? 2. How long can you speak continuously with a moderate to loud voice? 3. Does your voice crack or change in pitch, tone or sound? 4. Do you feel like you have something stuck in your throat?

Vāta prakṛti lakṣhaṇa	Wakefulness, alertness
Charaka's description	*Jāgarūkā* Awake (alert, occupied)
Suśhruta's description	*Prajāgarūkaḥ* Always seems wide awake
Guṇa(s)	*Rūkṣha*
Darśhana	Observe the physical, energetic behaviors through the eyes, limbs, posture, respiration and fine muscular activity. Look specifically for the following signs. 1. Eyelids that are consistenly wide-open 2. Hyperactive eyeball movements, respiration, general movement 3. Twitching, constant muscular activity or movement 4. Appears tired but wired 5. Quick to act but actions, speech or behaviors are not well planned or executed
Sparśhana	Optional. Any areas of twitching or hyperactive physical movements may be superficially and deeply palpated. General palpation and examine observes neuro-muscular tension, pressure, sensitivity and reflexes.
Praśhna	Ask questions that investigate the level of wakefulness and alertness typically experienced. 1. Do you tend to sleep lightly? Are you easily awoken?

	2. Are you startled easily? 3. Are you able to maintain a consistent sleep schedule? 4. How well rested do you feel on a daily basis? 5. Do you experience bursts of energy or sustained energy?

Vāta prakṛti lakṣhaṇa	Gait, style or manner of walking
Charaka's description	*Laghu, chapala gati* Light, unstable, undirected gait
Suśhruta's description	*Drutagatiraṭano anavasthitātmā viyati cha* Walks quickly yet wanders without direction
Guṇa(s)	*Laghu*
Darśhana	Observe the style and manner of walking. If the patient is asked to walk under observation, note that this generally will not indicate their *gati* for purpose of *prakṛti*. If possible, observe their manner of walking in regular, daily scenarios. Look specifically for the following signs. 1. Initiation of stride 2. Pace and stride for consistency, length, speed 3. Completion of stride 4. Alignment, symmetry, leans or compensation
Sparśhana	Optional. Any asymmetry of the skeletal structure may be palpated to confirm or deny inconsistencies in gait. Muscular definition and joint arrangement may be palpated and compared from left to right.
Praśhna	Ask questions that encourage individual description of gait in regular, daily scenarios. Note that *vāta prakṛti* will have a natural tendency to be unobservant of their own behavior. 1. How do you usually walk through the [supermarket, park, various places]? 2. Do you tend to bump into things unexpectedly when you walk? 3. Do you enjoy strolling, wandering, meandering, etc? 4. How do you normally walk?

Vāta prakṛti lakṣhaṇa	Style or manner of movement
Charaka's description	*Laghu, chapala cheṣhṭa* Light, constantly moving, fidgeting physical movements and actions
Suśhruta's description	N/A

Guṇa(s)	*Laghu*
Darśhana	Observe the style and manner of general movements including sitting, standing, reaching, passing objects, etc. Whenever possible, note these movement mannerisms in regular, daily scenarios. Look specifically for the following signs. 1. Initiation of movement 2. Consistency, duration, speed and characteristics of movements 3. Completion of movement 4. Alignment, symmetry, leans or compensation
Sparśhana	Optional. Any asymmetry of the skeletal structure may be palpated to confirm or deny inconsistencies in movement. Muscular definition and joint arrangement may be palpated and compared from left to right.
Praśhna	Ask questions that encourage individual description of movement in regular, daily scenarios. Note that *vāta prakṛti* will have a natural tendency to be unobservant of their own behavior. 1. What do you notice about your own regular, daily movement and activity? 2. How would you describe your typical movements? 3. Do you feel you tend to be clumsy when moving?

Vāta prakṛti lakṣhaṇa	Style or manner of eating
Charaka's description	*Laghu, chapala āhāra* Light, unpredictable and constantly changing mannerisms and habits toward diet and food
Suśhruta's description	N/A
Guṇa(s)	*Laghu*
Darśhana	Optional. Observe the style and manner of eating. Look specifically for the following signs. 1. Activities, behaviors, mannerisms at the commencement of the meal 2. Behaviors while eating, chewing, swallowing 3. Activities, behaviors, mannerisms at the commencement of the meal 4. Speed of chewing, eating and completing the entire meal 5. Concentration on the meal, susceptibility to distractions, talking, etc
Sparśhana	N/A
Praśhna	Subjective descriptions provide the most information for this *lakṣhaṇa* due to restrictions on observation. Investigate the history of eating habits as

	thoroughly as current behaviors. The primary information sought here is related to how the individual eats, rather than what they eat. 1. How would you describe your typical dietary habits over the last [1, 3, 5, 10, 20] years? 2. During your healthiest period of life, what were your typical dietary habits? What was most enjoyable or disagreeable? 3. How would you describe your typical dietary habits now?

Vāta prakṛti lakṣhaṇa	Style or manner of speech
Charaka's description	*Laghu, chapala vyāhārā* Light, unstable, unpredictable, changing speech
Suśhruta's description	N/A
Guṇa(s)	*Laghu*
Darśhana	Listen to the style and manner of speech. Observe the content of speech, the speaker's mannerisms and consistencies. Listen carefully for tendencies to change what is said and how it is expressed. Look specifically for the following signs. 1. Activities, behaviors, mannerisms while formulating thoughts prior to speaking 2. Facial expressions, body language and behaviors while speaking 3. Listen for consistencies with the speech to vocal tone and expression 4. Observe the quantity and complexity of speech
Sparśhana	N/A
Praśhna	Optional. Subjective descriptions are often inaccurate. Questions that may produce valuable information typically allow subjective expression through descriptions of memories and past events. 1. Describe any experience where you had to give a speech, presentation or demonstration in front of an audience. 2. Describe conversations with your friends, family or significant other. 3. How would you describe your style of speech? 4. How would you describe your ability to express yourself through speech?

Vāta prakṛti lakṣhaṇa	Instability of the joints
Charaka's	*Anavasthita sandhi*

description	Unstable, unsteady joints
Suśhruta's description	N/A
Guṇa(s)	*Chala*
Darśhana	Observe the joints as the patient moves. Notice the manner in which the joints support the physical body and allow for movement on an individual level and throughout the body. Look specifically for the following signs. 1. Range of movement 2. Alignment and posture 3. Degrees of flexion, extension and neutral position, hyperextension and restricted extension 4. Stability and instability of the joints when bearing weight 5. Apparent strain on the joints in various positions
Sparśhana	Palpate the joints and areas around them superficially and deep. Examine the joint structure in neutral, extended and flexed positions. With the patient relaxed, move the joint through its normal range of motion. Note the same items above, and the following. 1. Density and quality of tissues surrounding and supporting the joint 2. Tension of tissues surrounding the joint through the range of motion 3. Flaccidity, laxity or mobility of joint components
Praśhna	Ask questions that investigate weakness in joint form and function. 1. How do your joints usually feel after walking or moving around for longer than normal? 2. Do you usually carry anything heavy? If so, how? 3. Do your joints tend to hyperextend easily or feel "loose?"

Vāta prakṛti lakṣhaṇa	Instability of the eyes and sight
Charaka's description	*Anavasthita akṣhi* Unstable, unsteady eyes
Suśhruta's description	Atiśh-cala-dṛṣhṭir Eyes and gaze move too much
Guṇa(s)	*Chala*
Darśhana	Observe the eyeballs and their movements. Look specifically for the following signs. 1. Constant, consistent movement of the eyeballs 2. Constantly changing focus or attention on visual objects 3. Tics, spasms, hyperactivity of the eyeballs

Sparśhana	N/A
Praśhna	Optional. Ask questions about sight and attention to visual objects. Note that these subjective answers are generally not very accurate. 1. Do you tend to look around a lot, or have trouble focusing visually on a single object? 2. Do you ever notice a sense of twitching or spasms inside or around your eyes?

Vāta prakṛti lakṣhaṇa	Instability of the eyebrows
Charaka's description	*Anavasthita bhrū* Unstable, unsteady eyebrows
Suśhruta's description	N/A
Guṇa(s)	*Chala*
Darśhana	Observe the eyebrows, their movements and any changes in skin texture in the surrounding areas. Look specifically for the following signs. 1. Constant, consistent movement of the eyebrows 2. Constant changes in facial expressions with exaggerated eyebrow movements 3. Tics, spasms, twitching of the eyebrows 4. Appearance of fine lines, wrinkles, depressions or any changes in the skin that indicate regular movement of the area and regular positions of the eyebrows.
Sparśhana	Optional. If the patient experiences an uncontrollable twitching sensation or other fine, repetitive movements around the eyebrow, these may be palpated if they present during assessment. 1. Gently apply the posterior surface of two or three fingers to the patient's eyebrow and forehead region where the twitching is present. Confirm its presence and note any specific characteristics.
Praśhna	Ask questions about the eyebrows, facial expressions and any sensations of movement. 1. Do you notice if you tend to make facial expressions? 2. Have you noticed any sensations of movement or twitching around your forehead or eyebrows?

Vāta prakṛti lakṣhaṇa	Instability of the jaw
Charaka's description	*Anavasthita hanu* Unstable, unsteady jaw
Suśhruta's description	*Danta-khādī* Grinds their teeth
Guṇa(s)	*Chala*
Darśhana	Observe the entire jaw line and surrounding areas of the cheeks and upper region of the throat as the patient speaks, chews, swallows, moves and remains in a resting position. Ask the patient to open and close the mouth completely several times. Look specifically for the following signs. 1. Uneven, unstable or irregular movements in the mandibular joints and mandible while opening or closing the mouth 2. Note any irregularities in dental alignment that may contribute to or cause instability in the jaw 3. Spasms, twitching or clicking in or around the surface of the mandibular area 4. Presence of movement of the mandibular joints when they would normally be in a resting state 5. Grinding the teeth
Sparśhana	Palpate the areas on and around the mandible and mandibular joints. Start superficially and gently move deeper to examine the stability of the joints. Ask the patient to open and close the mouth then bite down while palpating around the mandibular joints. Note the same items above, and the following. 1. Difference in range of motion between left and right sides 2. Thickness and quality of the joint components 3. Degrees of flexion and extension 4. Flexibility of range of left to right motion of the extended mandible 5. Strength of joint musculature in various ranges of motion
Praśhna	Ask questions about opening and closing the mouth, chewing, grinding the teeth or any other habitual movements of the jaw. 1. Does your jaw move around or out of place very easily? 2. Do you grind your teeth? 3. Do your teeth feel like they are aligned correctly? 4. Do you ever notice twitching or spasms around your jaw? 5. Do you feel tension in your jaw? 6. Do you wake with a tight jaw?" 7. Do you notice soreness, pain or other discomfort in your jaw or mandibular joints? 8. Do you notice clicking sounds or popping in your jaw?

Vāta prakṛti lakṣhaṇa	Instability of the lips
Charaka's description	*Anavasthita oṣhṭha* Unstable, unsteady lips
Suśhruta's description	N/A
Guṇa(s)	*Chala*
Darśhana	Observe the lips, their movements and any changes in skin texture in the surrounding areas. Look specifically for the following signs. 1. Constant, consistent movement of the lips 2. Constant changes in facial expressions with exaggerated lip movements 3. Tics, spasms, twitching of the lips 4. Appearance of fine lines, wrinkles, depressions or any changes in the skin that indicate regular movement of the area and regular positions of the lips
Sparśhana	Optional. If the patient experiences an uncontrollable twitching sensation or other fine, repetitive movements around the mouth or kips, these may be palpated if they present during assessment. 1. Gently apply the posterior surface of two or three fingers to the affected region where the twitching is present. Confirm its presence and note any specific characteristics.
Praśhna	Ask questions about the lips, facial expressions and any sensations of movement. 1. Do you notice if you tend to move your lips frequently even when you're not talking? 2. Have you noticed any sensations of movement or twitching around your mouth or lips?

Vāta prakṛti lakṣhaṇa	Instability of the tongue
Charaka's description	*Anavasthita jihvā* Unstable, unsteady tongue
Suśhruta's description	N/A
Guṇa(s)	*Chala*
Darśhana	Observing the tongue is easiest along with the jaw assessment. Ask the patient to open the mouth and extend (or "stick") the tongue out completely

	and hold it steady. Note movements, alignment, position, texture and other characteristics of the complete tongue. Look specifically for the following signs. 1. Constant, consistent movement of the tongue 2. Position and characteristics on left and right sides of the tongue 3. Spasms, twitching or other fine, uncontrollable movements
Sparśhana	N/A
Praśhna	Ask questions about the tongue and any sensations of movement. 1. Do you notice if you tend to move your tongue around often? 2. Have you noticed any sensations of movement or twitching on your tongue?

Vāta prakṛti lakṣhaṇa	Instability of the head
Charaka's description	*Anavasthita śhiraḥ* Unstable, unsteady head
Suśhruta's description	N/A
Guṇa(s)	*Chala*
Darśhana	Observe the head and neck region for regular or repetitive movements. Look specifically for the following signs. 1. Constant, consistent movement of the head 2. Adjustments, changes in focus or attention to objects 3. Movement of the hair, ears, nose or any other part of the head indicating fluctuations in the underlying musculature
Sparśhana	Optional. If the patient experiences an uncontrollable twitching sensation or other fine, repetitive movements anywhere on the head, these may be palpated if they present during assessment. 1. Gently apply the posterior surface of two or three fingers to the affected region where the twitching is present. Confirm its presence and note any specific characteristics.
Praśhna	Ask questions about the head and any sensations of movement. 1. Do you notice if you tend to move your head frequently? 2. Have you noticed any sensations of movement or twitching anywhere on your head?

Vāta prakṛti lakṣhaṇa	Instability of the shoulders and clavicular region
Charaka's description	*Anavasthita skandha* Unstable, unsteady shoulders and clavicular regions
Suśhruta's description	N/A
Guṇa(s)	*Chala*
Darśhana	Observe the entire region of the shoulder girdle, movements and any changes in skin texture in the surrounding areas. Look specifically for the following signs. 1. Constant, consistent movement of the shoulders 2. Position, alignment, tissue and muscular development of the shoulders and any variations between left and right sides 3. Visibility and depth of bones and skeletal structures 4. Range of motion of left and right joints and changes in alignment or posture during movement
Sparśhana	Palpate the areas on and around the shoulders and clavicular regions. Start superficially and gently move deeper to examine the stability of the joints. Ask the patient to raise and lower the arms or move the arms in any direction while palpating around the shoulder joints. Note the same items above, and the following. 1. Difference in range of motion between left and right sides 2. Thickness and quality of the joint components 3. Degrees of flexion and extension 4. Movement of the shoulder girdle while one joint is in motion 5. Strength of joint musculature in various ranges of motion
Praśhna	Ask questions about moving the shoulder joints and any characteristics noticed in the shoulders or clavicular regions. 1. Do your shoulders move around or out of place very easily? 2. Do you naturally feel strong or weak in your shoulders or upper body? 3. Have you typically experienced clicking, popping or misalignment in your shoulders?

Vāta prakṛti lakṣhaṇa	Instability of the hands
Charaka's description	*Anavasthita pāṇi* Unstable, unsteady hands
Suśhruta's description	N/A

Guṇa(s)	*Chala*
Darśhana	Observe the hands, their movements and any changes in skin texture in the surrounding areas. Look specifically for the following signs. 1. Constant, consistent movement of the hands 2. Any regular, repetitive movements of the hands, wrists or fingers that appear to be habitual 3. Appearance of fine lines, wrinkles, depressions or any changes in the skin that indicate regular movement of the area
Sparśhana	Palpate the hands in prone and supine positions. Flex and extend the fingers to examine range of motion. Begin superficially and move deeper to check for normal muscular reflexes, density and tone of tissues and the characteristics of the musculo-skeletal components. Note the same items above, and the following. 1. Exaggerated ranges of motion of any joints in the wrist, hands or fingers, and their comparison between left and right sides. 2. Ease of motion, flexion and extension of joints 3. Ability for stationary joints to remain immobile while other joints are in motion
Praśhna	Ask questions about the hands and any sensations of movement. 1. Do you notice if you tend to move your hands around frequently? 2. Do you normally rub your hands or fingers together, tap your fingers on a table, bite your nails, roll your fingers together, etc?

Vāta prakṛti lakṣhaṇa	Instability of the feet
Charaka's description	*Anavasthita pādāḥ* Unstable, unsteady feet
Suśhruta's description	N/A
Guṇa(s)	*Chala*
Darśhana	Observe the feet, their movements and any changes in skin texture in the surrounding areas. Look specifically for the following signs. 1. Constant, consistent movement of the feet 2. Any regular, repetitive movements of the feet, ankles or toes that appear to be habitual 3. Appearance of fine lines, wrinkles, depressions or any changes in the skin that indicate regular movement of the area
Sparśhana	With the patient seated or reclined in a relaxed and supported position, palpate the feet. Flex and extend the toes to examine range of motion. Begin

	superficially and move deeper to check for normal muscular reflexes, density and tone of tissues and the characteristics of the musculo-skeletal components. Note the same items above, and the following. 1. Exaggerated ranges of motion of any joints in the ankles, feet or toes, and their comparison between left and right sides. 2. Ease of motion, flexion and extension of joints 3. Ability for stationary joints to remain immobile while other joints are in motion
Praśhna	Ask questions about the feet and any sensations of movement. 1. Do you notice if you tend to move your feet around frequently? 2. Do you normally rub your feet or toes together, tap your feet or toes, roll your toes together, etc? 3. How steady do you usually feel when walking, jogging, running, etc? 4. Would you consider yourself accident prone? 5. Do you regularly slip, fall, trip, sprain your ankle, etc?

Vāta prakṛti lakṣhaṇa	Talkativeness
Charaka's description	*Bahu pralāpa* Abundance of talk
Susruta's description	*Pralāpī* Talks a lot unnecessarily
Guṇa(s)	*Bahu*
Darśhana	Observe the patient's behaviors, mannerisms and styles of expression during discussion. Look and listen specifically for the following signs. 1. Methods and patterns of answering questions 2. Descriptions of themselves, and accuracy of their perceptions with objective measurements 3. Repetitiveness in speech and explanations 4. Amount of explanation given compared to what is required 5. Word choice, sentence construction, train of thought, use of filler words and phrases ("like," "you know," etc)
Sparśhana	N/A
Praśhna	Ask questions to understand the patient's natural habits and patterns using speech as a mode of expression. 1. Have you always enjoyed long conversations with friends? 2. Do you normally talk with friends, family or relatives on a regular basis? 3. Do you enjoy giving speeches or speaking to an audience? What would be your ideal experience? 4. Do you generally have a lot to say?

Vāta prakṛti lakṣhaṇa	Visibility of superficial tendons
Charaka's description	*Bahu kaṇḍarā* Abundance of tendons
Susruta's description	N/A
Guṇa(s)	*Bahu*
Darśhana	Observe the areas around the neck, limbs and joints for easily visible, superficial tendons and supportive muscular structures. Look specifically for the following signs. 1. In neutral, flexed and extended positions, notice the changes in superficial tendon visibility 2. Amount and density of tendons in various areas of the body
Sparśhana	With the patient seated or reclined in a relaxed and supported position, palpate the neck, limbs and joints where tendons are superficially visible. Flex and extend the area while palpating superficially to examine changes in the depth, tension and position of the tendons without impeding them. Note the same items above, and the following. 1. Changes in depth of tendons and their comparison between left and right sides between relaxed and engaged activities 2. Any other structures impeding or interfering with the position of tendons
Praśhna	Ask questions about any prominent tendons and their normal appearance. 1. Have you noticed if your tendons always appeared this way? 2. Do you feel any tightness, pain, discomfort, inflammation, burning sensation, etc, around [this area]?

Vāta prakṛti lakṣhaṇa	Visibility of superficial veins
Charaka's description	*Bahu sirā pratānāḥ* Abundance of branches (networks) of veins
Susruta's description	*Dhamanītataḥ* With abundant veins visible through the skin
Guṇa(s)	*Bahu*
Darśhana	Observe bodily areas for easily visible, superficial veins. Look specifically for the following signs. 1. Visibility of a single vein or networks of veins in certain regions 2. Length, width and other characteristics of visible veins

	3. Comparison of visibility of veins between left and right sides
Sparśhana	With the patient seated or reclined in a relaxed and supported position, palpate the area where veins are superficially visible. Flex and extend the area while palpating superficially to examine changes in the length, width, depth and position of the veins without impeding them. Note the same items above, and the following. 1. Changes in visibility of veins and their comparison between left and right sides between relaxed and engaged activities 2. Any other structures impeding or interfering with the position of tendons
Praśhna	Ask questions about any prominent veins and their normal appearance. 1. Have you noticed if your veins always appeared this way? 2. Have you noticed any changes in the way your veins appear anywhere on your body?

Vāta prakṛti lakṣhaṇa	Initiates actions quickly
Charaka's description	*Śhrīghra samārambha* Quick initiation of actions
Susruta's description	N/A
Guṇa(s)	*Śhighra*
Darśhana	Observe actions, responses to questions and mannerisms during interactions. Look specifically for the following signs. 1. Constant, consistent interaction in discussions 2. Regular, habitual attempts to initiate actions or interactions 3. Indications throughout the patient's history of efforts to begin projects or activities, generate ideas or be quick to start anything
Sparśhana	N/A
Praśhna	Direct and indirect questions may be asked to gauge the patient's tendency to initiate actions. 1. Would you consider yourself a self-starter? 2. Do you enjoy starting new projects? 3. Do you tend to do new things easily? 4. Do you tend to do chores immediately? 5. Do you like to be the leader of the group?

Vāta prakṛti lakṣhaṇa	Reacts emotionally quickly
Charaka's description	*Śhrīghra kṣhobha* Quick initiation of emotions (irritation, agitation)
Susruta's description	N/A
Guṇa(s)	*Śhighra*
Darśhana	Observe the natural emotional demeanor under a variety of situations where the patient feels happy, sad, easy-going, stressed, angry, etc. Look specifically for the following signs. 1. Manner of reacting to situations that are easy or hard 2. Presence of short temper, quick response, irritation or other naturally quick reaction especially in situations where they feel frustrated 3. Self-awareness of the response and the ability to control it 4. Limitations on control
Sparśhana	N/A
Praśhna	Direct and indirect questions may be asked to gauge the patient's tendency to react emotionally. 1. Would you consider yourself quick to respond to situations emotionally? 2. Do you take time to think about the situation before responding emotionally or reacting? 3. Would you consider yourself having a short temper? 4. What do people generally say about your response to stressful situations?

Vāta prakṛti lakṣhaṇa	Becomes sick quickly
Charaka's description	*Śhrīghra vikārāḥ* Quick initiation of disease
Susruta's description	N/A
Guṇa(s)	*Śhighra*
Darśhana	An accurate assessment of this *lakṣhaṇa* generally requires consistent clinical observation of the patient over a longer period of time, such as 3 months or more. Observe the patient's response to a variety of causative factors that may cause illness. These factors may be specific to the individual or inflential over a larger group of people. Look specifically for the following signs.

	1. Quantum of instigating factor needed to cause the body to respond and produce illness. 2. Relative speed of contracting the illness compared to other individuals in the same environment or those exposed to similar causative factors.
Sparśhana	N/A
Praśhna	Ask questions about the patient's subjective impression and understanding of their tolerance and ability to resist illness. 1. Would you consider yourself to be the one who usually gets sick first? 2. What do people generally say about your tolerance to resist illness?

Vāta prakṛti lakṣhaṇa	Low cold tolerance
Charaka's description	*Śhītā sahiṣhṇavaḥ* Low tolerance for cold
Susruta's description	*Śhīta-dveṣhī* Hates cold
Guṇa(s)	*Śhīta*
Darśhana	Once the patient has acclimated to the environment and is at rest for at least 15 minutes, observe for outward signs of discomfort due to feeling cold. Look specifically for the following signs. 1. Discomfort due to shivering, pale complexion, contraction of the muscles and body 2. Heavier than normal clothing for the temperature and environment 3. Use of warm or hot comforts, rubbing hands together, attempts to generate heat
Sparśhana	N/A
Praśhna	Once the patient has acclimated to the environment and is at rest for at least 15 minutes, ask questions about the patient's subjective feeling of hot or cold. 1. Do you generally prefer hot or cold environments? 2. Does cold bother you? How, when and where? 3. Do you tend to feel cold quickly? 4. What is your ideal vacation climate or location? 5. How does your body handle cold weather? 6. Do you tend to have cold hands, feet or feel cold in any other part of your body? 7. Does your partner remark about your cold hands or feet? 8. Does air conditioning bother you? Why? 9. Do you prefer warm food and beverages instead of cold, frozen or iced?

Vāta prakṛti lakṣhaṇa	Contantly feels cold
Charaka's description	*Pratata śhītaka* Constantly feels cold
Susruta's description	N/A
Guṇa(s)	*Śhīta*
Darśhana	Once the patient has acclimated to the environment and is at rest for at least 15 minutes, observe for outward signs of discomfort due to feeling cold. Look specifically for the following signs. 1. Shivering, pale or bluish complexion, contraction of the muscles and body 2. Heavier than normal clothing for the temperature and environment 3. Use of warm or hot comforts, rubbing hands together, attempts to generate heat
Sparśhana	Once the patient has acclimated to the environment and is at rest for at least 15 minutes, gently palpate the patient's skin using the dorsal aspect of the clinician's hand and fingers. Compare temperature differences between the core of the body and extremities. Check the fingers, toes, neck, ears, eyes and cheeks. Observe the patient's reaction to touch and their response to the temperature of the clinician's hand.
Praśhna	Once the patient has acclimated to the environment and is at rest for at least 15 minutes, ask questions about the patient's subjective feeling of hot or cold. 1. Do you feel hot or cold now? 2. At what temperature do you generally feel comfortable? 3. When do you usually feel cold?

Vāta prakṛti lakṣhaṇa	Constantly shivering
Charaka's description	*Pratata udvepaka* Constantly shivering (trembling)
Susruta's description	N/A
Guṇa(s)	*Śhīta*
Darśhana	Once the patient has acclimated to the environment and is at rest for at least 15 minutes, observe for outward signs of shivering or trembling. Look specifically for the following signs. 1. Shivering, trembling, fine and gross contractions of the muscles of the

	body 2. Use of warm or hot comforts, rubbing hands together, attempts to generate heat
Sparśhana	Once the patient has acclimated to the environment and is at rest for at least 15 minutes, gently palpate the patient's skin using the dorsal aspect of the clinician's hand and fingers. Note any areas of shivering, muscular activity or goosebumps. Observe the patient's reaction to touch and their response to the temperature of the clinician's hand.
Praśhna	Once the patient has acclimated to the environment and is at rest for at least 15 minutes, ask questions about the patient's subjective feeling of shivering. 1. Do you feel shivering or trembling anywhere on your body now? 2. Do you usually shiver easily? When? 3. Have you always felt shivering easily when you get cold?

Vāta prakṛti lakṣhaṇa	Constantly feels stiff
Charaka's description	*Pratata stambha* Constant stiffness
Susruta's description	N/A
Guṇa(s)	*Śhīta*
Darśhana	Once the patient has acclimated to the environment and is at rest for at least 15 minutes, observe for outward signs of stiffness, tightness or contraction of the body. Look specifically for the following signs. 1. Stiffness, tightness or contracted states of the muscles of the body 2. Slow, difficult movements
Sparśhana	Once the patient has acclimated to the environment and is at rest for at least 15 minutes, gently palpate and examine the muscles and flexibility of the limbs. Note any areas of stiffness, hardness or inactivity. Observe the patient's reaction to touch and their response to the temperature of the clinician's hand.
Praśhna	Once the patient has acclimated to the environment and is at rest for at least 15 minutes, ask questions about the patient's subjective feeling of stiffness. 1. Do you feel stiffness anywhere on your body now? 2. Do you usually feel stiff easily? When? 3. Have you always felt stiff easily? 4. Does your stiffen change when you feel hot or cold?

Vāta prakṛti lakṣhaṇa	Roughness of head hair
Charaka's description	*Paruṣha keśha* Rough (stiff, hard) hair on the head
Susruta's description	*Alpa, rūkṣha keśhaḥ* Has scanty and dry hair on the head
Guṇa(s)	*Paruṣha*
Darśhana	Ask the patient to come for clinical assessment after shampooing their hair, and without applying conditioner or hair styling products. Observe the quality, texture, thickness and shine of the hair on the head. Look specifically for the following signs. 1. Overall dryness, roughness, hardness, texture and shine
Sparśhana	Gently examine the hair on the head to confirm characteristics noted through *darśhana*. Observe and feel individual hairs for quality, texture and roughness.
Praśhna	Ask questions about the patient's history of the hair on the head and its qualities, texture and roughness. 1. Does your hair naturally feel rough? 2. How would you describe your hair in its normal, natural state?

Vāta prakṛti lakṣhaṇa	Roughness of the beard
Charaka's description	*Paruṣha śhmaśhru* Rough (stiff, hard) beard
Susruta's description	*Alpa, rūkṣha śhmaśhru* Has scanty and dry beard
Guṇa(s)	*Paruṣha*
Darśhana	Ask the patient to come for clinical assessment after washing their beard and avoid applying any products. Observe the quality, texture, thickness and shine of the beard. Look specifically for the following signs. 1. Overall dryness, roughness, hardness, texture and shine
Sparśhana	Gently examine the beard to confirm characteristics noted through *darśhana*. Observe and feel individual hairs for quality, texture and roughness.
Praśhna	Ask questions about the patient's history of the beard and its qualities, texture and roughness.

	1. Does your beard naturally feel rough, stiff or hard? 2. How would you describe your beard in its normal, natural state? 3. How would you describe the way your beard and mustache usually grow?

Vāta prakṛti lakṣhaṇa	Roughness of bodily hair
Charaka's description	*Paruṣha roma* Rough (stiff, hard) bodily hair
Susruta's description	N/A
Guṇa(s)	*Paruṣha*
Darśhana	Ask the patient to come for clinical assessment after showering and avoid applying any products. Observe the quality, texture, thickness and shine of the hair on the body. Look specifically for the following signs. 1. Overall dryness, roughness, hardness, texture and shine
Sparśhana	Gently examine the hair on the body to confirm characteristics noted through *darśhana*. Observe and feel individual hairs for quality, texture and roughness.
Praśhna	Ask questions about the patient's history of the hair on the body and its qualities, texture and roughness. 1. Does the hair on your body naturally feel rough? 2. How would you describe your bodily hair in its normal, natural state?

Vāta prakṛti lakṣhaṇa	Roughness of the nails
Charaka's description	*Paruṣha nakha* Rough (stiff, hard) nails
Susruta's description	*Alpa rūkṣha nakha* Has scanty and dry nails
Guṇa(s)	*Paruṣha*
Darśhana	Observe the quality, texture, thickness, strength, cracks and shine of the fingernails and toenails.
Sparśhana	Examine the nails to confirm characteristics noted through *darśhana*. Observe and feel individual nails for quality, texture, strength and roughness.

Praśhna	Ask questions about the patient's history of the fingernails and toenails and their qualities, texture and roughness. 1. Do your fingernails or toenails naturally feel rough? 2. How would you describe your fingernails and toenails in their normal, natural state? 3. Do your fingernails or toenails crack or chip easily?

Vāta prakṛti lakṣhaṇa	Roughness of the teeth
Charaka's description	*Paruṣha daśhana* Rough (stiff, hard) teeth
Susruta's description	N/A
Guṇa(s)	*Paruṣha*
Darśhana	Observe the quality, texture, smoothness and shine of the teeth.
Sparśhana	N/A
Praśhna	Ask questions about the patient's history of their teeth and the qualities, texture and roughness. 1. Do your teeth naturally feel rough? 2. How would you describe your teeth in their normal, natural state?

Vāta prakṛti lakṣhaṇa	Roughness of the mouth (or face)
Charaka's description	*Paruṣha vadana* Rough (stiff, hard) mouth, lips (or face)
Susruta's description	N/A
Guṇa(s)	*Paruṣha*
Darśhana	Ask the patient to come for clinical assessment after showering, washing their face and avoiding application of any products. Observe the quality, texture, smoothness, sheen and complexion of the face and lips.
Sparśhana	Gently examine the face and lips to confirm characteristics noted through *darśhana*.
Praśhna	Ask questions about the patient's history of the face and lips and their

	qualities, texture, smoothness and roughness. 1. Do your face or lips naturally feel rough? 2. How would you describe your face and lips in their normal, natural state?

Vāta prakṛti lakṣhaṇa	Roughness of the hands
Charaka's description	*Paruṣha pāṇi* Rough (stiff, hard) hands
Susruta's description	*Sphuṭita kara carano* Prone to cracks in the hands
Guṇa(s)	*Paruṣha*
Darśhana	Ask the patient to come for clinical assessment after showering, washing their hands and avoiding application of any products. Observe the quality, texture, roughness, dryness and hardness of the hands. Look for any cracks, discontinuity in the superficial and deep surfaces of the skin especially around creases and on the palmar surface.
Sparśhana	Palpate and examine the hands to confirm characteristics noted through *darśhana*.
Praśhna	Ask questions about the patient's history of the hands and their qualities, texture, roughness and cracks. 1. Do your hands naturally feel rough? 2. How would you describe your hands in their normal, natural state? 3. Have your hands regularly been prone to dryness, roughness and cracks?

Vāta prakṛti lakṣhaṇa	Roughness of the feet
Charaka's description	*Paruṣha pādāḥ* Rough (stiff, hard) feet
Susruta's description	*Sphuṭita kara carano* Prone to cracks in the hands and feet
Guṇa(s)	*Paruṣha*
Darśhana	Ask the patient to come for clinical assessment after showering, washing their feet and avoiding application of any products. Observe the quality, texture, roughness, dryness and hardness of the feet. Look for any cracks,

	discontinuity in the superficial and deep surfaces of the skin especially around creases and on the soles.
Sparśhana	Palpate and examine the feet to confirm characteristics noted through *darśhana.*
Praśhna	Ask questions about the patient's history of the feet and their qualities, texture, roughness and cracks. 1. Do your feet naturally feel rough? 2. How would you describe your feet in their normal, natural state? 3. Have your feet regularly been prone to dryness, roughness and cracks? 4. Have you usually used closed or open footwear?

Vāta prakṛti lakṣhaṇa	Cracking of bodily limbs and parts
Charaka's description	*Sphuṭita aṅga, āvayavāḥ* Cracking of bodily limbs and parts
Susruta's description	N/A
Guṇa(s)	*Viśhada*
Darśhana	Observe the patient's physical body for discontinuity in the limbs and visible bodily parts. Look and listen specifically for the following signs. 1. Superficial and deep cracks in the skin around the joints 2. Insufficient support of joints and limbs due to musculo-skeletal abnormalities 3. Indications that internal bodily parts and organs are functioning abnormally which may indicate being "cracked or broken"
Sparśhana	Palpate and examine the bodily parts and limbs to confirm characteristics noted through *darśhana.*
Praśhna	Ask questions about the patient's history of the bodily parts and limbs, any cracks or sensations of slipping or displacement of structures from their normal anatomical locations. 1. Do your bodily parts and limbs tend to show cracks externally on the skin? 2. Have any of your bodily parts ever felt as though they slipped or moved out of their normal place?

Vāta prakṛti lakṣhaṇa	Producing sounds from joints
Charaka's description	*Satata sandhi-śhabda-gāmina* Constantly producing sounds from the joints when walking (moving around)
Susruta's description	N/A
Guṇa(s)	*Viśhada*
Darśhana	Observe the patient's physical body when engaged in any type of movement and listen for any sounds produced. Look and listen specifically for the following signs. 1. Cracking, popping or other sounds produced through any movement 2. General absence of pain, swelling or other symptoms 3. Slipping, slight diplacement or unstable movement of the joint
Sparśhana	Palpate and examine the joints to confirm characteristics noted through *darśhana*. Note any cracking, popping or other sounds which can be felt on the joint as it is in motion.
Praśhna	Ask questions about the patient's history of the joints in general and the affected joints. 1. Do your joints usually make sounds when you move? 2. Have your joints been affected by any other symptoms like pain or swelling along with the sounds produced? 3. Have the sound-producing joints generally felt unstable, or that they could easily slip out of place during movements?

Vāta prakṛti lakṣhaṇa	Unlucky, ugly
Charaka's description	N/A
Susruta's description	*Durbhagaḥ* Is unlucky, ugly
Guṇa(s)	N/A
Darśhana	Observe the patient for physical characteristics and behaviors that can cause them to be disliked and perceive that they are unlucky or ugly. Look for indicators of general happiness or contentment, physical symmetry, asymmetry, and abnormally large or small features in relation to the rest of their face or body. Observe their behavior in situations that result in optimism or pessimism. Track consistency in their mental stability and decision-making processes.

Sparśhana	N/A
Praśhna	Direct and indirect questions may be used to gauge the patient's tendency to react optmistically or pessimistically. Ask questions to elicit characteristics described above. 1. Do you tend to make decisions easily and stick to those decisions? 2. Do you tend to have a hard time making decisions? 3. Do you notice if you change your mind a lot? 4. Do you experience a lot of misfortune? 5. Do you tend to see the glass half full or half empty?

Vāta prakṛti lakṣhaṇa	Unreliable as a friend
Charaka's description	N/A
Susruta's description	*Adhṛtir, adṛdha sauhṛdaḥ* Unsteady, unreliable as a friend
Guṇa(s)	N/A
Darśhana	Observe the patient for physical characteristics and behaviors that indicate unsteadiness in commitment or unreliability. Observe their behavior in situations that require commitment and follow-through. Track consistency in their ability to be reliable.
Sparśhana	N/A
Praśhna	Direct and indirect questions may be used to gauge the patient's tendency to behave unreliably. Ask questions to elicit characteristics described above. 1. Do you have many close friends? 2. How would you describe your closest friends? 3. How do you usually stay in contact with your friends?

Vāta prakṛti lakṣhaṇa	Theivish
Charaka's description	N/A
Susruta's description	*Steno* Behaves like a thief
Guṇa(s)	N/A
Darśhana	Observe the patient for physical characteristics and behaviors that indicate

	tendencies to take things which do not belong to them. Watch eye movements carefully. Observe their behavior and mannerisms when presented with something of interest.
Sparśhana	N/A
Praśhna	Direct and indirect questions may be used to gauge the patient's tendency to take things which do not belong to them. Ask questions to elicit characteristics described above. 1. Have you ever stolen anything? 2. What would you do if you found a stranger's wallet on the ground?

Vāta prakṛti lakṣhaṇa	Malicious
Charaka's description	N/A
Susruta's description	*Krāthī* Behaves maliciously
Guṇa(s)	N/A
Darśhana	Observe the patient for physical characteristics and behaviors that indicate tendencies to behave maliciously and hurt themselves or others.
Sparśhana	N/A
Praśhna	Direct and indirect questions may be used to gauge the patient's tendency to behave maliciously, or hurt themselves or others. 1. Have you ever hurt anyone physically or emotionally? 2. Have you ever hurt yourself physically or emotionally? 3. Do you have a tendency to desire revenge? 4. If someone hurts you, do you have a right to hurt them back?

Vāta prakṛti lakṣhaṇa	Ungrateful
Charaka's description	N/A
Susruta's description	*Kṛtaghnaḥ* Ungrateful
Guṇa(s)	N/A
Darśhana	Observe the patient for physical characteristics and behaviors that indicate

	tendencies to be ungrateful, unthankful or unappreciative.
Sparśhana	N/A
Praśhna	Direct and indirect questions may be used to gauge the patient's tendency to ungrateful or unappreciative. 1. How do you show appreciation for the significant people in your life? 2. Do you volunteer or contribute to your community?

Vāta prakṛti lakṣhaṇa	Uncertain, disorganized
Charaka's description	N/A
Susruta's description	*Avyavasthitam* Uncertain, disorganized, unsettled
Guṇa(s)	N/A
Darśhana	Observe the patient for physical characteristics and behaviors that indicate tendencies to be disorganized, clumsy, confused, unconfident, anxious, apprehensive or uncertain about themselves.
Sparśhana	N/A
Praśhna	Direct and indirect questions may be used to gauge the patient's tendency to be disorganized, clumsy or anxious. 1. Describe how your organize your home or living space. 2. Describe how you organize your work space. 3. How do you tend to behave in social situations with new people? 4. How do you tend to behave in social situations with known friends?

Vāta prakṛti lakṣhaṇa	Unprosperous
Charaka's description	N/A
Susruta's description	*Manda ratna dhana* Slow [if at all to build up] precious jewels and wealth
Guṇa(s)	N/A
Darśhana	Observe the patient for characteristics, behaviors and attitudes that indicate that they consider themselves financially stable. Look beyond material wealth for signs that they have worked to create financial stability for themselves.

Sparśhana	N/A
Praśhna	Direct and indirect questions may be used to gauge the patient's financial stability through income, spending habits, savings, borrowing and prioritization of these. 1. How would you describe your current financial situation? 2. Have you had a tendency to save or spend? 3. Have you had a tendency to live beyond your means? 4. What are your future financial plans?

Vāta prakṛti lakṣhaṇa	Moaning
Charaka's description	N/A
Susruta's description	*Vilapati anibaddhaṁ* Constantly moaning
Guṇa(s)	N/A
Darśhana	Observe the patient for characteristics, behaviors and attitudes that demonstrate any tendency to moan as a response to anything disliked. Look for reactions that indicate avoidance, despondance, disinterest or evasion and corresponding physical cues, such as a sigh, moan, groan, change in posture, etc.
Sparśhana	N/A
Praśhna	Direct and indirect questions may be used to gauge the patient's tendency to be avoidant. However, it may be more reliable to observe for these characteristics through indirect questions that allow natural behaviors to express themselves. 1. Describe a difficult situation that you had to face recently. 2. As a child and teenager, how would you respond to being told to do chores? 3. How do you typically handle challenging responsibilities at work? 4. How do you typically handle challenging responsibilities at home?

Vāta prakṛti lakṣhaṇa	Jealous
Charaka's description	N/A
Susruta's	*Matsaryanāryo*

description	Jealous of others, never satisfied by others
Guṇa(s)	N/A
Darśhana	Observe the patient for characteristics, behaviors and attitudes that demonstrate any tendency to be jealous of others, or not be satisfied with their own things. Look for reactions that indicate interest, attention, attraction to, desire and corresponding physical cues, such as raised eyes or eyebrows, increased attention, change in posture, etc, in situations where they become interested.
Sparśhana	N/A
Praśhna	Direct and indirect questions may be used to gauge the patient's tendency to be jealous. However, it may be more reliable to observe for these characteristics through indirect questions that allow natural behaviors to express themselves. 1. Do you consider yourself to become jealous easily? 2. As a child and teenager, how would you respond to others having something that you didn't, and that you wanted? 3. What do you usually do to achieve or obtain things you want in life? 4. If you could have anything, what would it be?

Vāta prakṛti lakṣhaṇa	Music-lover
Charaka's description	N/A
Susruta's description	*Gandharvicittaḥ* Loves music
Guṇa(s)	N/A
Darśhana	Observe the patient for indications that they enjoy music, varieties of music, regularly listening to music, etc.
Sparśhana	N/A
Praśhna	Direct questions may be used to enquire about the patient's interest in music. 1. How frequently do you listen to music? 2. How does music make you feel? 3. What types of music do you prefer or avoid? 4. Do you play any instruments? If so, describe.

Vāta prakṛti lakṣhaṇa	Harsh
Charaka's description	N/A
Susruta's description	*Paruṣho* Harsh
Guṇa(s)	N/A
Darśhana	Observe the patient for characteristics, behaviors and attitudes that demonstrate any tendency to be harsh towards themselves or others. Look for reactions that indicate sharp reactions, criticism, sternness, hardness or strictness and corresponding physical cues, such as frowning, a defensive stance, change in posture, etc, in situations where they become harsh.
Sparśhana	N/A
Praśhna	Direct and indirect questions may be used to gauge the patient's tendency to be harsh or critical. However, it may be more reliable to observe for these characteristics through indirect questions that allow natural behaviors to express themselves. 1. Do you consider yourself to be hard on yourself or others? 2. When someone does something wrong, what do you do? 3. Would you consider yourself to be a good problem solver?

Vāta prakṛti lakṣhaṇa	Few friendships
Charaka's description	N/A
Susruta's description	*Sañchaya mitraḥ* Has very few friendships
Guṇa(s)	N/A
Darśhana	Observe the patient for characteristics, behaviors and attitudes that demonstrate any tendency to have friendships. Look for reactions that indicate they consider relationships to be important, or an significant part of their life, and corresponding physical cues, such as smiling, appearing happy, change in posture, etc, in situations where they discuss friendships.
Sparśhana	N/A
Praśhna	Direct and indirect questions may be used to gauge the patient's friendships. Their direct explanation must be considered reliable, espeically for eliciting a

	historical account of friendships. 1. Over the course of your life, how many friends did you typically have at any time? 2. How many friends do you still have from childhood? 3. How many friends have you made in the last 5 to 10 years?

Vāta prakṛti lakṣhaṇa	Anxiety in dreams
Charaka's description	N/A
Susruta's description	*Gacchati sambhrameṇa suptaḥ* Even in dreams he walks around agitated or anxious
Guṇa(s)	N/A
Darśhana	N/A
Sparśhana	N/A
Praśhna	Direct questions are most reliable to elicit an understanding of the patient's dreams. Enquire about specific examples, tendencies and themes. 1. Do you ever feel anxiety or fear in your dreams? 2. What are you usually doing in your dreams? 3. Do you often dream flying, falling, moving around or being active?

Vāta prakṛti lakṣhaṇa	Similarities to animals
Charaka's description	N/A
Susruta's description	*Āja, Gomāyu, Śhaśha, Ākhu, Uṣhṭra, Śhunāṁ, Gṛdhra, Kāka, Kharā* Behaves like a goat, jackal, rabbit, mouse or rat, camel, dog, vulture, crow, donkey or mule
Guṇa(s)	N/A
Darśhana	Observe the patient's characteristics, behaviors and attitudes. Look for similarities in any of the animals listed above.
Sparśhana	N/A
Praśhna	N/A

Bhautika prakṛti

Bhautika prakṛti lakṣhaṇas have been reviewed extensively in Volume 2, Chapter 18. Review that chapter in full as a preparatory resource for this portion of the *prakṛti* assessment.

Performing an assessment of an individual's *bhautika prakṛti* may be considered an confirmatory step in the overall *prakṛti* assessment. When the *deha prakṛti* portion is sufficient to conclusively determine an individual's *prakṛti*, the *bhautika* portion may not be required.

However, in many cases it is challenging to finalize an individual's *deha prakṛti* quickly and accurately especially during initial stages of clinical practice. To help determine a speculative *deha prakṛti*, the *bhautika prakṛti* can confirm or deny natural tendencies towards predominance of specific *bhūtas*.

To increase confidence in a final *bhautika prakṛti* determination, multiple *lakṣhaṇas* should be definitively assessed. The presence of a single *lakṣhaṇa* should not be considered sufficient for a final determination of a predominant *bhūta*.

The *lakṣhaṇas* listed in the following tables have been taken from classical descriptions in Cha. Śhā. 4/12 and Su. Śhā. 4/80. The basic assessment methods listed are categorized based on their application through *darśhana*, *sparśhana* and *praśhna*. The examples provided are intended to guide introductory clinical practice.

Note that *lakṣhaṇas* behave in a similar manner to *guṇas* as they tend to associate themselves in clusters or patterns of certain presentations.

Nābhasa Prakṛti Assessment

Nābhasa prakṛti lakṣhaṇas with nearest English equivalent	Assessment methods	
Su. Śhā. 4/80		
Śhuchir-atha Purity, cleanliness in all things	*Darśhana*	Observe for signs of genuine cleanliness in all aspects, including self-care, presentation, carriage, speech, behavior, mannerisms, etc.
	Sparśhana	N/A
	Praśhna	Enquire about personal care habits. Listen carefully to determine subjective accuracy. Compare subjective descriptions to observations.
Chira-jīvī A long life	*Darśhana*	Classically, these signs include a well-proportioned bodily frame and components, a generally healthy appearance and demeanor, more signs of the presence of healthy, well-developed *kapha* and fewer signs of the presence of *vāta doṣha*.
	Sparśhana	On manual examination, the quality, strength, depth and formation of tissues, skeletal structures and physical components may provide indicative clues.
	Praśhna	Review familial history to understand causes of death, ages and general levels of health of immediate and extended family members.
Khairmahadbhiḥ Large, hollow spaces in the cavities of the body	*Darśhana*	Observe the visible openings of the body including the nostrils, mouth and ears. Compare left to right sides and consider proportions in the size of the opening to the body.
	Sparśhana	Perform an abdominal examination superficially and deep. Compare organ sizes to relative space throughout the abdomen. Estimate proportionate sizing of cavity space to organ size.
	Praśhna	If appropriate, enquire about personal and other professional opinions of vaginal or anal opening sizes if the patient has had recent examinations of these areas.
Cha. Śhā. 4/12		
Śhabdaḥ Sound	*Darśhana*	Observe any sounds produced by the body.
	Sparśhana	Optional. If sounds are regularly produced by the joints,

		palpate the affected area for abnormality. Listen to sounds produced by the patient's body, if any, and the quality, tone and content of speech.
	Praśhna	Ask the patient if they notice that their body produces sounds often. If so, ask for details about patterns including where, when, frequency, quantity, etc.
Śhrotraṁ Sense of hearing, ears	*Darśhana*	Observe reactions to sounds at various levels, sensitivity to sound or other indicators.
	Sparśhana	N/A
	Praśhna	Enquire about history with sound exposure, subjective perception of sound compared to others or sensitivity. Ask for results of hearing tests.
Lāghavaṁ Lightness	*Darśhana*	Observe the physical body for signs that indicate thin, underdeveloped skeletal structure, bones and other components. Listen for hollowness in the voice.
	Sparśhana	On manual examination, the quality, strength, depth and formation of tissues, skeletal structures and physical components may provide indicative clues.
	Praśhna	Enquire about the patient's history of weight, weight gain and loss, specific areas of the body that tend to gain weight, bone density, and subjective perception of lightness, thinness or hollowness.
Saukṣhmyaṁ Minuteness	*Darśhana*	Observe all general characteristics for subtle nature and presentation. These may be easier to notice as the absence of gross manifestations of other signs.
	Sparśhana	On manual examination, grossly manifesting characteristics are often absent.
	Praśhna	Enquire about subjective perception to sensitivity. Look for variations in gross manifestations of signs and symptoms compared to sensitivity.
Viveka Discrimination, distinction, the power of separation	*Darśhana*	Observe the ability to discern and differentiate information in various situations and levels of complexity. Listen to subjective descriptions of interactions, problem solving and decision-making.
	Sparśhana	N/A
	Praśhna	Enquire about tendencies in handling problems, making decisions and personal strategies for determining answers.

Vāyavya Prakṛti Assessment

Vāyavya prakṛti lakṣhaṇas with nearest English equivalent	Assessment methods	
Cha. Śhā. 4/12		
Sparśhaḥ Sensation, tangibility	*Darśhana*	Observe for a tendency to naturally interact via touch, or ease in touch as a primary method for understanding objects and the external world. When possible, also observe the patient's ability to comprehend intangible and tangible objects or concepts.
	Sparśhana	N/A
	Praśhna	Ask the patient if they notice whether they use their sense of touch as a primary means of interacting with the external world.
Sparśhanaṁ The sense of touch	*Darśhana*	Observe reactions to touch at various levels, sensitivity to touch or other indicators.
	Sparśhana	Check sensitivity of reception of touch on various locations of the body using superficial and deep pressure.
	Praśhna	Enquire about history with touch exposure, subjective perception of touch compared to others or sensitivity.
Raukṣhyaṁ Dryness	*Darśhana*	Observe dryness in the physical body through the skin, eyes, mouth and hair. Also observe for dryness in demeanor, mannerisms, speech and habits.
	Sparśhana	Palpate and examine the patient's skin, eyes and oral cavity for signs of flaking, cracking, poor elasticity, thinness, etc.
	Praśhna	Enquire about overall tendencies to experience dryness in any of the above. Look for seasonal, annual and other patterns in presentation.
Preraṇaṁ Initiation, impulse	*Darśhana*	Observe the presence or absence of a natural impulse to initiate actions through physical action, speech and mental behavior.
	Sparśhana	N/A
	Praśhna	Enquire about personal history and behavior related

		to initiating activities. Listen for patterns that demonstrate repetitive starts without follow-through or completion.
Dhātuvyūhanaṁ Separation, distinction and development of the supportive systems of the body	*Darśhana*	Observe for variations in the *dhātus* being displaced, shifted into alternate positions, separated from the normal *dhātu* and other inconsistencies or asymmetries in normal physical structure.
	Sparśhana	Palpate and examine any *dhātus* or areas where diplacement, separation or abnormality may be present.
	Praśhna	Enquire about any history related to findings. Determine the onset, duration, normality and other characteristics.
Cheṣhṭāśhcha śhārīryaḥ And all actions of the body	*Darśhana*	Observe all actions of the physical body through voluntary and involuntary muscular activity, skeletal movement, respiration and any other physical movement. Correlate the characteristics of these with related *guṇas*.
	Sparśhana	Palpate and examine areas where physical activity may provide indication or correlation with related *guṇas*.
	Praśhna	Enquire about any history related to correlated findings. Determine the onset, duration, normality and other characteristics.

Āgneya Prakṛti Assessment

Āgneya prakṛti lakṣhaṇas with nearest English equivalent	Assessment methods	
Cha. Śhā. 4/12		
Rūpaṁ Visible form	*Darśhana*	Observe for a tendency to naturally interact with the external world through an understanding of form. Listen to personal descriptions of events and scenarios for a preference in usage or understanding of visible form, shape or structure.
	Sparśhana	N/A
	Praśhna	Ask the patient if they notice whether they use their sense of vision as a primary means of interacting with the external world. Ask them to describe details.
Darśhanaṁ The sense of sight	*Darśhana*	Observe reactions to various visual stimuli, sensitivity to light, movement or other indicators.
	Sparśhana	Visual sensitivity may be tested through the demonstration of different stimuli in brightness, contrast, movement, etc.
	Praśhna	Enquire about history of visual exposure, subjective perception of vision compared to others or sensitivity.
Prakāśhaḥ Shine, luster, brightness	*Darśhana*	Observe the general appearance, skin, complexion, eyes, expressions and character for signs of brightness, luster and glowing activity. These may present as sparks of ideas, creativity, enthusiasm, excitment or eagerness. Look for the texture, brightness, shine and sparkle of the eyes, especially the iris and pupils.
	Sparśhana	Optional. Palpate and examine the skin to better observe its complexion, brightness, sheen and luster.
	Praśhna	Enquire about history of general appearance and behavior of the same characteristics.
Pakti The capacity to digest	*Darśhana*	Observe immediate and long-term signs of strong digestive capacity. Assess the *jīrṇa āhāra lakṣhaṇas* for specific measurements.
	Sparśhana	Palpate and examine the physical body to correlate, confirm or deny signs of strong digestive capacity. Presence of warmth or heat on the bodily surface,

		pink or reddish complexion, perspiration, suppleness or softness may be present after consuming a large quantity of food or certain types of foods.
	Praśhna	Enquire about history of regular appetite along with the strong capacity to digest proportionately large quantities of food and meals. Ask about the typical responses, signs and other characteristics noticed after eating large portions of food or meals. Correlate with the *jīrṇa āhāra lakṣhaṇas*.
Uṣhṇyaṁ Heat	*Darśhana*	Observe the general appearance, skin and complexion of the central portion of the body compared to the extremities. Look for pink or reddish color indicating the quantity and quality of vascular supply and its ability to transfer heat to the extremities. Observe the patient's clothing in context of the external environmental temperature and their perceived level of comfort. When possible, perform observations during or immediately after activity and at rest.
	Sparśhana	When the patient has spent at least 15 minutes in a stable, comfortable environment at rest, palpate and examine the skin for temperature and perspiration using the dorsal aspect of the clinician's hand and/or fingers. When possible, compare the temperatures between the patient's abdominal regions including the superficial areas over and around the heart to multiple points of the extremities including fingers, toes, ears, nose and cheeks.
	Praśhna	Enquire whether the patient subjectively feels hot or cold in the current environment after spending at least 15 minutes in the room at rest. Ask about personal perception of heat generation over the patient's history.

Āpya Prakṛti Assessment

Āpya prakṛti lakṣhaṇas with nearest English equivalent	Assessment methods	
Cha. Śhā. 4/12		
Raso Flavor, taste	*Darśhana*	Observe for a tendency to naturally interact with the external world through an understanding of taste. Listen to personal descriptions of events and scenarios for a preference in usage or understanding of taste or flavor.
	Sparśhana	N/A
	Praśhna	Ask the patient if they notice whether they use their sense of taste as a primary means of interacting with the external world in literal and figurative contexts.
Rasanaṁ The sense of taste	*Darśhana*	Observe reactions to various flavors, sensitivity to flavors in varying degrees or other indicative responses.
	Sparśhana	N/A
	Praśhna	Enquire about history with taste, subjective perception of taste compared to others or sensitivities to specific flavors or foods.
Śhaityaṁ Coolness	*Darśhana*	Observe the general appearance, skin and complexion of the central portion of the body compared to the extremities. Look for a pale, whitish color or absence of pink or reddish color indicating the quantity and quality of vascular supply and its ability to transfer heat to the extremities. Observe the patient's clothing in context of the external environmental temperature and their perceived level of comfort. When possible, perform observations during or immediately after activity and at rest.
	Sparśhana	When the patient has spent at least 15 minutes in a stable, comfortable environment at rest, palpate and examine the skin for temperature and perspiration using the dorsal aspect of the clinician's hand and/or fingers. When possible, compare the temperatures between the patient's abdominal regions including the superficial areas over and around the heart to multiple points of the extremities including fingers, toes, ears, nose and cheeks.
	Praśhna	Enquire whether the patient subjectively feels hot or

		cold in the current environment after spending at least 15 minutes in the room at rest. Ask about personal perception of heat generation over the patient's history.
Mārdavaṁ Softness	*Darśhana*	Observe the physical body and mental disposition in terms of the softness. Physically, the overall appearance of the tissues is plump, not well-defined, lacking tone, flabby or spongy. In behavioral and mental disposition, the patient finds it difficult to make decisions and stick to them. They are very easily swayed by others and prefer not to be responsible.
	Sparśhana	Palpate and examine the quality, texture and softness of the bodily tissues for the same characteristics. Notice any sensitivity to touch.
	Praśhna	Enquire about physical form and structure of the body over the patient's history. Listen to subjective accounts of various situations and descriptions of their involvment, level of responsibility and behavior of the same characteristics.
Snehaḥ Unctuousness, oiliness, attachment	*Darśhana*	Observe the physical body, orifices and eyes for signs of natural, abundant lubrication and moisture.
	Sparśhana	Palpate and examine the quality, texture, supplness and moisture of the skin in several areas of the body. Compare areas exposed to higher degrees of the elements (such as hands and face) to other areas that are more often protected.
	Praśhna	Enquire about the need to use moisturizers in all forms. Ask about the quality and texture of areas if moisturizer is not used to determine the natural presence of *sneha*.
Kledaśhcha And moisture, stickiness	*Darśhana*	Observe for signs of production of moisture in the physical body and in mental disposition. Physically, there may be easy production of sweat, saliva, tears, urine, edema or other increase in bodily fluids. Mentally and emotionally the patient may tend to stickiness, attachment, easy flow of emotions, etc.
	Sparśhana	Palpate and examine the physical body for the same characteristics.
	Praśhna	Enquire about the history of the same characteristics.

Pārthiva Prakṛti Assessment

Pārthiva prakṛti lakṣhaṇas with nearest English equivalent	Assessment methods	
Su. Śhā. 4/80		
Sthira Stability	*Darśhana*	Observe for signs of stability in the physical body and mental disposition. Look and listen for indicators of steadfastness especially in difficult situations or under stress. Observe levels and abilities to coordinate complex movements and tasks, planning and mitigation of instability.
	Sparśhana	Palpate and examine the physical body to correlate or confirm stability of the skeletal frame, structure, bones, joints and binding tissues including the muscles and supportive structures.
	Praśhna	Enquire about long-term stability in physical and mental behaviors using the same characteristics.
Vipula-śharīraḥ A strong body	*Darśhana*	Observe for signs of strength in the physical body. Look and listen for indicators of strength generated by the individual alone in difficult situations or under stress. Observe the ability to physically overcome obstacles independently.
	Sparśhana	Palpate and examine the physical body to correlate or confirm strength of the skeletal frame, structure, bones, joints and binding tissues including the muscles and supportive structures.
	Praśhna	Enquire about long-term strength in physical behaviors using the same characteristics.
Kṣhamāvāñ Tolerance, patience, forbearance	*Darśhana*	Observe for signs of strength in mental disposition. Look and listen for indicators of strength generated by the individual alone in difficult situations or under stress. Observe the ability to mentally overcome obstacles independently.
	Sparśhana	N/A
	Praśhna	Enquire about long-term strength in mental behaviors using the same characteristics. Ask the patient to describe how they have handled stressful situations independently, with loved ones and in groups of various settings.

Cha. Śhā. 4/12		
Gandho Smells, odors	*Darśhana*	Observe for a tendency to naturally interact with the external world through an understanding of odors or smells. Listen to personal descriptions of events and scenarios for a preference in usage or understanding of odors or smells.
	Sparśhana	N/A
	Praśhna	Ask the patient if they notice whether they use their sense of smell as a primary means of interacting with the external world. Ask them to describe how their sense of smells works and its typical level of acuity.
Ghrāṇaṁ The sense of smell	*Darśhana*	Observe reactions to various odors, sensitivity to odors or other indicative responses.
	Sparśhana	N/A
	Praśhna	Enquire about history of the sense of smell, subjective perception of smell compared to others or sensitivity. Ask about any anatomonical or physiological defects in the nasal passages that may interfere with the sense of smell.
Gauravam Heaviness	*Darśhana*	Observe the physical body for heaviness and density in structure, actions and carriage. Look and listen for heaviness in mental disposition, emotions, speech and expressions.
	Sparśhana	Palpate and examine the physical body for density of tissues and relative heaviness of limbs.
	Praśhna	Enquire about long-term characteristics and behaviors indicating heaviness in all aspects.
Sthairyaṁ Stability	*Darśhana*	See *sthira* above.
	Sparśhana	
	Praśhna	
Mūrtiśhcheti And anything which takes on physical form	*Darśhana*	Observe the physical development of the body for fullness of structures and shapes.
	Sparśhana	Palpate and examine for the same characteristics.
	Praśhna	Enquire about the same characteristics. Ask the patient to describe the waste materials typically produced by their body.

Sāra

The assessment of *sāra* is based on the *sāra lakṣhaṇas* provided in Cha. Vi. 8/102-115 for the eight types. These include one type for each of the *sapta dhātus* and one for *sattva sāra*. Additionally, Charaka mentions *sarva sāra* which is the presence of all types of *sāra* in an individual. However, this is not considered as a ninth type.

Depending on which type is found to be present in an individual, certain characteristics and outcomes are to be expected. Suśhruta provides his perspective in Su. Sū. 35/16.

In practice, *sāra* assessment can be challenging to determine accurately from only a single clinical encounter. It is often better understood after a sufficient period of time that allows the clinician to observe the patient through a range of seasons and states of health.

The *sāra lakṣhaṇas* are explained in Volume 2, Chapter 20. They are listed here with their methods of assessment and expected outcomes. In order to accurately assess any state of *sāra*, the associated *dhātu(s)* should be in their optimal state for whatever period of time is necessary to allow the *lakṣhaṇas* to manifest properly. Subjective histories from the patient are generally insufficient alone to provide accurate assessments.

Traditional perspectives on *sāra* assessment are often considered to require proper, thorough *pañchakarma* prior to assessment to provide high accuracy in results. This is because classical *pañchakarma* resets internal physiology and allows the clinician to observe the natural, baseline state of the patient.

Review the *lakṣhaṇas*, their assessment methods and the expected outcomes based on their manifestation. Accurate assessments will find the correlation of multiple *lakṣhaṇas* and outcomes in higher levels of *sāra* such as *madhyama* or *uttama*.

Tvak Sāra Assessment

Assess the baseline strength of *rasa dhātu* as *avara* (*asāra*), *madhyama* or *uttama*.

Snigdha, śhlakṣhṇa, mṛdu, prasanna (tvak)
Skin is supple, smooth, soft and pleasing to look at

Darśhana	Observe the appearance of the skin for suppleness, smoothness, softness and pleasant appearance.
Sparśhana	Palpate and examine the skin for the same characteristics.
Praśhna	Enquire about the long-term characteristics of the skin and its durability.

Sūkṣhma, alpa, gambhīra, sukumāra loma
Bodily hair is very fine, less (sparse), deeply-rooted and delicate (pleasant to look at)

Darśhana	Observe the bodily hair for fineness (absence of thickness), density, visible strength, depth and construction of hair follicles and appearance.
Sparśhana	Palpate and examine the hair follicles for the same characteristics.
Praśhna	Enquire about the long-term characteristics of the hair follicles and their durability.

Saprabha eva cha tvak
And the skin is full of luster, glowing, brilliant

Darśhana	Observe the color, complexion, luster and appearance of the skin for proper sheen.
Sparśhana	Palpate and examine the skin for the same characteristics.
Praśhna	Enquire about the long-term characteristics of the skin and its durability.

Tvak sāra produces	Nearest English equivalent
• *Sukha* • *Saubhāgya* • *Aiśhvarya* • *Upabhoga* • *Buddhi* • *Vidya* • *Ārogya* • *Praharṣhaṇa* • *Ānya-āyuṣhyatvaṁ cha*	• Happiness, contentment • Good fortune, success, beauty • Prosperity, wealth, power • Pleasure, enjoyment, contentment through eating • Intelligence • Learned knowledge, wisdom • Absence of disease • Pleasure, excitement, sensual pleasure • And above all else, longevity, full lifespan, quality of life

Rakta Sāra Assessment

Assess the baseline strength of *rakta dhātu* as *avara* (*asāra*), *madhyama* or *uttama*.

Karṇa, akṣhi, mukha, jihvā, nāsa, oṣhṭha, pāṇi-pāda tala, nakha, lalāṭa, mehana - snigdha, rakta varṇa, śhrīmad-bhrājiṣhṇu
The ears, eye area, face, tongue, nose, lips, soles of the hands feet, nails forehead and genital organs are unctuous (thick, moist), reddish color, and sexy

Darśhana	Observe the appearance of the ears, eye area, face, tongue, nose, lips, soles of the hands feet, nails and forehead for suppleness and moisture, pink or red skin tones and an attractive appearance.
Sparśhana	Palpate and examine the same areas for these specific characteristics.
Praśhna	Enquire about the long-term characteristics of these areas of the body and their appearance.

Rakta sāra produces	Nearest English equivalent
• *Sukha* • *Uddhatāṁ medhāṁ* • *Manasvitvaṁ* • *Saukumāryam* • *Anati-balam* • *Akleśha-sahiṣhṇutvam* • *Uṣhṇāsahiṣhṇutvaṁ cha*	• Happiness, contentment • Arrogance, sharp mental state and intelligence • Magnanimity, wisdom • Delicate, tender body • Low degree of strength • Intolerance to stress, difficult situations, work • And intolerance to heat

Māṁsa Sāra Assessment

Assess the baseline strength of *māṁsa dhātu* as *avara* (*asāra*), *madhyama* or *uttama*.

Śhaṅkha, lalāṭa, kṛkāṭikā, akṣhi, gaṇḍa, hanu, grīvā, skandha, udara, kakṣha, vakṣha, pāṇi-pāda sandhaya - sthira, guru, śhubha, māṁsa-upacitā
The temples, forehead, nape of the neck, eye area, cheeks, jaw, neck, shoulders, abdomen, axillae, chest, joints of the arms and legs are stable, heavy, beautiful, and covered with well developed muscles

Darśhana	Observe the muscle tone and adjoining muscular structures in each location for stability, heaviness, density, development and pleasant appearance.
Sparśhana	Palpate and examine the musculature for the same characteristics.
Praśhna	Enquire about the long-term characteristics of the musculature and its durability.

Acchidra gātraṁ
Absence of hollow, empty, defective, faulty, undeveloped areas of the body

Darśhana	Observe the body for compactness of tissues and lack of under-developed, incompletely developed or empty-looking spaces.
Sparśhana	Palpate and examine the bodily tissues for the same characteristics.
Praśhna	Enquire about the long-term characteristics of the musculature and its development.

Gūḍha asthi, sandhi māṁsa upachita
Well-covered bones and joints by well-developed muscles

Darśhana	Observe the skeletal structure and joints for well-developed musculature, supportive joint structures and lack of bony protuberances.
Sparśhana	Palpate and examine the bones and joints for the same characteristics.
Praśhna	Enquire about the long-term characteristics of the skeletal structure and joints.

Māṁsa sāra produces	Nearest English equivalent
• *Kṣhamāṁ* • *Dhṛtimalaulyaṁ* • *Vittaṁ* • *Vidyāṁ* • *Sukham* • *Ārjavam* • *Ārogyaṁ* • *Balamāyuśhcha dīrghamācha*	• Tolerance, forbearance, patience • Steadiness, firm courage (self-control) • Acquisitions, property, wealth, money • Acquired knowledge, wisdom • Happiness, contentment • Honesty, sincerity, straight-forwardness • Absence of disease • Strength throughout one's long lifespan

Medo Sāra Assessment

Assess the baseline strength of *medo dhātu* as *avara* (*asāra*), *madhyama* or *uttama*.

Varṇa, svara, netra, keśha, loma, nakha, danta, oṣhṭha, mūtra, purīṣheṣhu viśheṣhataḥ sneho
The complexion, voice, eyeballs, hair on the head, body hair, nails, teeth, lips, urine and stools are unctuous (greasy, oily)

Darśhana	Observe each component for signs of naturally-produced lubrication.
Sparśhana	Palpate and examine the components for the same characteristics.
Praśhna	Enquire about the long-term characteristics of the components and lubrication.

Snigdha mūtra, sveda, svara
Unctuous or oily urine and sweat, and a smooth voice

Darśhana	Observe the components for presence of lubrication.
Sparśhana	Palpate and examine the components for the same characteristics.
Praśhna	Enquire about the long-term characteristics of the components and lubrication.

Bṛhat śharīra
Big, bulky body

Darśhana	Observe the appearance of the physical body, its size, bulk and proportions.
Sparśhana	Palpate and examine the body for the same characteristics.
Praśhna	Enquire about the long-term characteristics of the body and its size.

Āyāsa asahiṣhṇuta
Incapable of tolerating stress, work, difficulties

Darśhana	Observe the behaviors for signs of dislike or avoidance of stress and difficulty.
Sparśhana	On examination, note sensitivity to deep pressure or pain.
Praśhna	Enquire about the long-term behaviors in difficult situations.

Medo sāra produces	Nearest English equivalent
• *Vitta* • *Aiśhvarya* • *Sukha* • *Upabhoga* • *Pradānāni* • *Ārjavam* • *Sukumāra upachāratāṁ cha*	• Acquisitions, property, wealth, money • Prosperity, wealth, power • Happiness, contentment • Pleasure, enjoyment, contentment through eating • Generosity • Honesty, sincerity, straight-forwardness • Delicate tenderness in their approach and interactions

Asthi Sāra Assessment

Assess the baseline strength of *asthi dhātu* as *avara* (*asāra*), *madhyama* or *uttama*.

Pārṣhṇi, gulpha, jānu, aratni, jatru, cibuka, śhiraḥ, parva-sthūlāḥ, sthūla-asthi, nakha, dantāśhchā
The heels, ankles, knees, elbows, collar bones, chin, head, small joints (of the hands and feet), nails and teeth are thick-boned (strong, heavy)

Darśhana	Observe the thickness of each location, their comparative sizes, appearances (thin or thick), width, depth, hardness and compactness.
Sparśhana	Palpate and examine each location for the same characteristics.
Praśhna	Enquire about the long-term characteristics of the skeletal structure and joints.

Mahā śhiraḥ, skandha
Large (big) head and shoulder area

Darśhana	Observe the head, neck and shoulder girdle for well-developed skeletal structures, frame, width, overall size and proportion.
Sparśhana	Palpate and examine the head, neck and shoulder girdle for the same characteristics.
Praśhna	Enquire about the long-term characteristics of the frame size and proportions compared to siblings, close relatives and similar friends.

Dṛḍha danta, hanu, asthi, nakha
Strong teeth, jaw, bones and nails

Darśhana	Observe the skeletal structure, bones, teeth and nails for well-developed form, strength, resistance to injury, cracks or breaking.
Sparśhana	Palpate and examine the areas for the same characteristics.
Praśhna	Enquire about the long-term characteristics of each area and its strength.

Asthi sāra produces	Nearest English equivalent
• *Temaha utsāhāḥ* • *Kriyāvantaḥ* • *Kleśhasahāḥ* • *Sāra, sthira śharīrā* • *Bhavanti āyuṣhmantaśhcha*	• Extreme excitability, enthusiasm • A high degree of activity • High tolerance for stress • Solid, stable body • Longevity, a full lifespan, high quality of life

Majjā Sāra Assessment

Assess the baseline strength of *majjā dhātu* as *avara* (*asāra*), *madhyama* or *uttama*.

Mṛdvaṅgā balavantaḥ
The limbs are soft (supple) yet strong

Darśhana	Observe the limbs of the body for overall development, strength and suppleness.
Sparśhana	Palpate and examine the limbs of the body for the same characteristics.
Praśhna	Enquire about the long-term, regular characteristics of the limbs and their strength and suppleness.

Snigdha varṇa svarāḥ
The complexion and voice are unctuous (smooth)

Darśhana	Observe the overall complexion for characteristics of suppleness, elasticity, sheen and natural glow. Listen to the voice for smoothness, depth and absence of cracking or other sounds.
Sparśhana	Palpate and examine the skin for the same characteristics.
Praśhna	Enquire about the long-term characteristics of the skin and voice.

Sthūla dīrgha vṛtta sandhayaśhcha
The joints are thick (heavy, well-set), long and round

Darśhana	Observe the joints for size, shape and appearance. Look for signs of strength in the joints implying stability, depth, high density, roundness (being filled with supportive tissues and structures), length and proportionate size.
Sparśhana	Palpate and examine the joints for the same characteristics.
Praśhna	Enquire about the long-term characteristics of the joints.

Mahā śhiraḥ, skandha
Large (big) head and shoulder area

Darśhana	Observe the head, neck and shoulder girdle for well-developed skeletal structures, frame, width, overall size and proportion.
Sparśhana	Palpate and examine the head, neck and shoulder girdle for the same characteristics.
Praśhna	Enquire about the long-term characteristics of the frame size and proportions compared to siblings, immediate and distant family members and close friends.

Dṛḍha danta, hanu, asthi, nakha
Strong teeth, jaw, bones and nails

Darśhana	Observe the skeletal structure, bones, teeth and nails for well-developed form, strength, resistance to injury, cracks or breaking.
Sparśhana	Palpate and examine the areas for the same characteristics.
Praśhna	Enquire about the long-term characteristics of each area and its strength.

Akṛśha, uttama bala
Not (too) thin or lean, with high levels of strength

Darśhana	Observe the overall skeletal structure for development, size, proportions, width, density, stature and depth. Observe physical strength through weight-bearing activity to see the strength of the skeletal system, muscular system and coordinating abilities. Compare to siblings, immediate and distant family members and close friends.
Sparśhana	Palpate and examine the bones and joints for the same characteristics.
Praśhna	Enquire about the long-term characteristics of the skeletal structure and joints.

Snigdha, gambhīra svara
Smooth, deep voice

Darśhana	Listen to the voice for smoothness, depth and absence of cracking or other sounds.
Sparśhana	N/A
Praśhna	Enquire about the long-term characteristics of the voice.

Saubhāgya upapanna
Good fortune

Darśhana	Observe for characteristics of luck, good fortune or "being in the right place at the right time" on a regular, consistent basis.
Sparśhana	N/A
Praśhna	Enquire about the long-term characteristics of luck.

Mahā netra
Large eyes

Darśhana	Observe both eyes, the cranial sockets and frame, eyeballs, sclera and pupils for size, proportion, alignment, distance and their setting in the skull.
Sparśhana	Optional. Gently palpate or examine the areas around the eye sockets.
Praśhna	Enquire about the long-term characteristics of the eyes.

Majjā sāra produces	Nearest English equivalent
• *Dīrghāyuṣho* • *Balavantaḥ* • *Śhruta* • *Vitta* • *Vijñāna* • *Āpatya* • *Sammāna bhājaśhcha*	• Long lifespan • Excellent strength • Astute listening and comprehension • Acquisitions, property, wealth, money • Acquired scientific knowledge • Children • Recognition for honorable contributions

Śhukra Sāra Assessment

Assess the baseline strength of *śhukra dhātu* as *avara* (*asāra*), *madhyama* or *uttama.*

Saumyāḥ
A saumya appearance (soft, gentle, pleasing, with good looks)

Darśhana	Observe the overall physical structure, face, demeanor and mannerism for gentleness, pleasantness and attractive appearance.
Sparśhana	Optional. On manual examination of the body or limbs, note the overall softness of the body and ease in which the patient receives touch.
Praśhna	Enquire about general appearance, attractiveness and interest from the opposite (or same) sex throughout life. Listen to personal accounts of interaction with the opposite (or same) sex for descriptions that would indicate the presence of any of these characteristics.

Saumya prekṣhiṇaḥ
Soft, gentle look (of the eyes)

Darśhana	Observe the face and eyes carefully for signs or looks that indicate gentleness, attraction or interest.
Sparśhana	N/A
Praśhna	Enquire about interactions with the opposite (or same) sex and listen for descriptions that emphasize these characteristics.

Kṣhīra-pūrṇa-lochana
Eyes that look as though they are full of milk

Darśhana	Observe the eyes carefully for signs or looks that indicate moist sclera, large size and milkiness.
Sparśhana	N/A
Praśhna	N/A

Iva praharṣha bahulāḥ
Abundant interest, excitement

Darśhana	Observe behavior, demeanor and body language that imply interest or excitement towards intimacy.
Sparśhana	N/A
Praśhna	Optional. Enquire about interactions with the opposite (or same) sex and listen for descriptions that emphasize these characteristics.

Snigdha, vṛtta, sāra, sama-saṁhata, śhikharadaśhanāḥ, prasanna, snigdha, varṇa svara
Unctuous, round, strong, even (symmetrical), attractive, pleasant and smooth complexion and voice

Darśhana	Observe the complexion and voice for suppleness, well-roundedness (completeness), signs of being fully well-developed, strong and sweet, evenness and symmetry, attractiveness, pleasantness and smoothness.
Sparśhana	Palpate and examine the skin for the same characteristics.
Praśhna	Enquire about the long-term characteristics of the skin and voice.

Ābhrājiṣhṇavo
Alluring, charming, magnetic appearance (personality)

Darśhana	Observe personality, behavior, demeanor and body language that imply charm, magnetism and attraction.
Sparśhana	N/A
Praśhna	Optional. Enquire about interactions with the opposite (or same) sex and listen for descriptions that emphasize these characteristics.

Mahā-sphichaśhcha
Large buttocks

Darśhana	Observe the overall physical structure and proportionate size of the buttocks.
Sparśhana	N/A
Praśhna	Optional. Enquire about the long-term proportions of the physical structure.

Snigdha, saṁhata, śhveta asthi, danta, nakha
Supple, proportionate (compact, well-formed) and white bones, teeth and nails

Darśhana	Observe the bones, teeth and nails for characteristics of supplness, proportion, compactness and color, especially whiteness indicating thickness and supple development.
Sparśhana	Palpate and examine the bones and nails for the same characteristics.
Praśhna	Enquire about the long-term characteristics of the bones, teeth and nails.

Bahula kāma, prajaṁ
Abundant sexual desire and children

Darśhana	Observe and listen to personal descriptions of relationships, reproductive planning, children and related information.
Sparśhana	N/A
Praśhna	Enquire about the long-term behavioral patterns in intimate relationship, number of children and related information.

Śhukra sāra produces	Nearest English equivalent
• *Strīpriya* • *Upabhogā* • *Balavantaḥ* • *Sukha* • *Aiśhvarya* • *Ārogya* • *Vitta* • *Sammāna āpatya bhājaśhcha*	• Enjoys sexual pleasures (and women enjoy them) • Pleasure, enjoyment, contentment through eating • Excellent strength • Happiness, contentment • Prosperity, wealth, power • Absence of disease • Acquisitions, property, wealth, money • Recognition for honorable actions and many children

Sattva Sāra Assessment

Assess the baseline strength of *sattva* as *avara* (*asāra*), *madhyama* or *uttama*.

Smṛti-manto
Good memory

Darśhana	Observe the behavior, memory and confidence level in long, medium and short-term events. Listen for changes, irregularities or inconsistencies in personal accounts, histories or any other descriptions.
Sparśhana	N/A
Praśhna	Enquire about the long-term characteristics of the memory in a variety of situations (educational, professional, personal life, etc).

Bhakti-mantaḥ
Good dedication

Darśhana	Observe the behavior, commitment levels and dedication to completing activities even in difficult situations.
Sparśhana	N/A
Praśhna	Enquire about the long-term characteristics of commitment and dedication in various situations.

Kṛtajñāḥ
Appreciation, gratefulness

Darśhana	Observe the behavior, mannerisms, reactions, expectations and demeanor towards others and situations that are considered outside of one's control for genuine appreciation, gratefulness and respect.
Sparśhana	N/A
Praśhna	Enquire about the long-term characteristics of genuine appreciation, gratefulness and respect in various situations.

Prājñāḥ
Wisdom

Darśhana	Observe for innate responses and reactions to right versus wrong, as well as learned behaviors. Listen to personal descriptions that indicate ability to learn from previous mistakes and reliably correct behaviors.
Sparśhana	N/A

Praśhna	Enquire about the long-term characteristics, growth and application of wisdom in various situations.

Śhuchayo
Cleanliness, purity

Darśhana	Observe the natural inclinations towards cleanliness and purity in behavior, mannerisms and personality.
Sparśhana	N/A
Praśhna	Enquire about the long-term characteristics of cleanliness and purity in behavior.

Maha-utsāhā
Abundant enthusiasm

Darśhana	Observe the natural disposition for abundant enthusiasm. Listen for vocal tones, expressions and other indicators of enthusiasm.
Sparśhana	N/A
Praśhna	Enquire about the long-term characteristics of abundant enthusiasm in behaviors, activities and mannerisms.

Dakṣhā
Skill

Darśhana	Observe the level of skill in various areas and aspects of personal and professional life. Listen for indicators of ability to learn new skills and apply them.
Sparśhana	N/A
Praśhna	Enquire about the long-term abilities to learn and apply skills.

Dhīrāḥ
Courage, concentration of mind

Darśhana	Observe the natural inclination to remain committed, focused and concentrated on a goal with courage, self-assurance and determination.
Sparśhana	N/A
Praśhna	Enquire about the long-term characteristics of these behaviors.

Samara-vikrāntayo
Bravery, steadfast attitude in conflict

Darśhana	Observe the natural inclination to maintain bravery, confidence and steadfastness even in stressful, demanding or difficult situations where success is not immediately apparent.
Sparśhana	N/A
Praśhna	Enquire about the long-term characteristics of the same behaviors.

Dhinastyakta-viṣhādāḥ
Absence of sorrow

Darśhana	Observe the general demeanor, body language, personal outlook and tendency towards happiness or sorrow. Listen for indicators in personal accounts of behavior and changes in vocal tone.
Sparśhana	N/A
Praśhna	Enquire about the long-term characteristics of the same behaviors.

Suvyavasthita gati
Confident gait

Darśhana	Observe gait, stance, carriage, posture and presentation in walking, introducing one's self and other scenarios.
Sparśhana	N/A
Praśhna	Optional. Enquire about the long-term characteristics of posture and carriage.

Gambhīra buddhi
Depth of intellect

Darśhana	Observe the depth of intellect in various scenarios. Listen for patterns of limitations of intellectual capacity, relationship between intellectual application and interest in the subject and ability to apply intellect broadly, deeply and effectively in known and unknown situations.
Sparśhana	N/A
Praśhna	Enquire about the long-term characteristics of intellect in various situations of personal and professional life.

Cheṣhṭāḥ kalyāṇābhi niveśhinaśhcha
Engages in correct (benevolent) actions sincerely

Darśhana	Observe the natural inclination to choose actions in a variety of situations where proper action may be easy or difficult.
Sparśhana	N/A
Praśhna	Enquire about the long-term characteristics of behavior, decision-making and determination to engage in right action.

Śhauryopetaṁ
Endowed with heroism

Darśhana	Observe the overall personality, mannerisms and behaviors for indicators of heroism, the desire to help the underserved or others in need.
Sparśhana	N/A
Praśhna	Enquire about the long-term characteristics of behaviors indicating heroism in various situations.

Sattva sāra produces	Nearest English equivalent
• *Teṣhāṁ sva-lakṣhaṇair-evaguṇā vyākhyātāḥ*	• The *lakṣhaṇas* (as explained above) indicate the characteristics produced

Sarva Sāra Assessment

Assess the baseline strength of *sarva dhātu* as *avara* (*asāra*), *madhyama* or *uttama*.

Sarvaiḥ sārair upetāḥ puruṣhā bhavanti
Characteristics of all of the *sāras*, including *sattva sāra*

Darśhana	Observe and listen for indicators of all types of *sāras*.
Sparśhana	Palpate and examine the body for indicators of all types of *sāras*.
Praśhna	Enquire about the long-term characteristics of all types of *sāras*.

Atibalāḥ
Too much strength

Darśhana	Observe physical, mental and vocal indicators of strength and abilities beyond what is needed as a consistent pattern in various situations. This *lakṣhaṇa* is meant to assess the presence of excessive strength in a variety of capacitites rather than an outward demonstration of strength.
Sparśhana	N/A
Praśhna	Enquire about the long-term characteristics of strength in capacities beyond what is needed.

Parama sukha
The best (ultimate) level of happiness, contentment

Darśhana	Observe the behavior, personality, demanor and mannerisms for an extremely genuine state of contentment in all areas of life. This is not extreme happiness generated by force or an unnatural desire to be happy.
Sparśhana	N/A
Praśhna	Enquire about the long-term characteristics of disposition and contentment.

Yuktāḥ kleśha sahāḥ
Sensible tolerance for stress; knows limits and acts accordingly

Darśhana	Observe the natural ability to determine, measure and assess stressful situations accurately. Listen for the awareness of these situations and the ability to decide to engage or disengage appropriately according to one's own level of strength.
Sparśhana	N/A
Praśhna	Enquire about the long-term characteristics of discernment and decision-making

	in stressful situations. Ask about the individual's ability to understand and know their own limits physically and mentally in a variety of situations.

Sarvārambha iṣhvātmani jāta pratyayāḥ
Commences all desires with calculated ideas, plans thoroughly

Darśhana	Observe the natural tendencies to plan, analyze and carefully assess ideas before acting. Listen to personal accounts of behavioral patterns and the ability to learn from mistakes for self-development.
Sparśhana	N/A
Praśhna	Enquire about the long-term characteristics of ideas, decision-making and participation in various scenarios. Ask about self-development in relation to planning.

Kalyāṇa abhiniveśhinaḥ
Benevolent intentions

Darśhana	Observe the matural tendencies to act, behave and participate in various scenarios for the greater good.
Sparśhana	N/A
Praśhna	Enquire about the long-term characteristics of intentions when engaging in various scenarios. Ask about tendencies and behaviors within the immediate family and close friends.

Sthira samāhita śharīrāḥ
Stable, well-bound and well-built body

Darśhana	Observe the physical bodily frame and overall structure for build, size, proportions and compactness.
Sparśhana	Palpate and examine the physical body for the same characteristics.
Praśhna	Enquire about the long-term characteristics of the bodily frame and structure.

Susamāhita gatayaḥ
Well-coordinated movements

Darśhana	Observe the physical movements, coordination and motor skills in a variety of fine, medium and gross activities.
Sparśhana	N/A

Praśhna	Enquire about the long-term characteristics of coordination and motor skills. Ask about involvement in sports, dance or other activities where these skills are required.

Sānunāda snigdha gambhīra mahāsvarāḥ
Vocal sounds are smooth and deep with a great (bellowing) voice

Darśhana	Observe and listen to the tone, texture and use of the voice.
Sparśhana	N/A
Praśhna	Enquire about the long-term characteristics of the voice. Ask about involvement in singing and the style, depth and range.

Sarva sāra produces	Nearest English equivalent
• *Sukha* • *Aiśhvarya* • *Vitta* • *Upabhoga* • *Sammāna bhājomandajaraso* • *Manda vikārāḥ* • *Prāyastulya guṇa vistīrṇāpatyāśh chirajīvinaśhcha*	• Happiness, contentment • Prosperity, wealth, power • Acquisitions, property, wealth, money • Pleasure, enjoyment, contentment through eating • Recognition for honorable work • Slow to develop disease • Almost all of the same characteristics are found in their children who also experience long lives

KEY PRINCIPLES

Classical literature provides excellent resources for understanding *prakṛti* through assessments most appropriate for the Indian subcontinent, its people and culture. Ample descriptions and details are available to allow the student to gain a significant understanding of what is being assessed, why and how.

By thoroughly understanding these methodologies, the key principles of *prakṛti* assesment can be identified and extracted. These principles can then be associated to their related *guṇas* and *doṣhas*.

Performing a *prakṛti* assessment in a new environment with subjects of varied ethnic and cultural backgrounds can be customized to identify and measure the intended *guṇas* and *doṣhas* using appropriate methods. Different characteristics can be used where they are appropriate for the individual being assessed. These characteristics are looking for the same *guṇas* and *doṣhas* but asking the questions in a way which the individual will understand easily and relate to. This methodology will allow the patient's responses to elicit more accurate findings.

Outcomes of various *prakṛti* assessments may be categorized according to the predominant type based on *guṇa* and *doṣha* and the degree of presentation as *hīna*, *madhyama* or *uttama*.

Review the following summaries of the key principles from this chapter as guidance for practical application.

Principle #1: Contextualizing prakṛti assessment

Each type of *prakṛti* assessment must be performed in such a manner that allows it to be contextualized within the most accurately representative time period of the individual's life. Questions should be phrased based on the general, regular and repetitive behavior over the entire lifespan as well as within the healthiest period. Variations in responses can be analyzed and considered within the context of any other influencing factor(s).

Wherever comparisons to other individuals are helpful, immediate family members should be considered first. These include siblings, parents and children, followed by extended family members who are blood relatives. When none of these are available for comparison, individuals of similar ethnic backgrounds who have grown up and lived in similar conditions should be considered next.

Principle #2: Results of deha prakṛti assessment

A complete *deha prakṛti* assessment will result in a determination of the individual's *prakṛti*, an understanding of the implications and the degree of strength provided by that *prakṛti*.

Deha prakṛti is classified as one of seven types with a related degree of strength.

Deha prakṛti	Strength
Vāta	*Hīna*
Pitta	*Madhyama*
Kapha	*Uttama*
Vāta-Pitta	*Hīna*
Vāta-Kapha	*Madhyama*
Pitta-Kapha	*Uttama*
Vāta-Pitta-Kapha	*Uttama*

The final statements of each line in Cha. Vi. 8/96-98 state the relative degrees of each assessed type of *deha prakṛti*.

Additionally, the *guṇas* provided by Charaka may be analyzed to more accurately specify the outcome of the *deha prakṛti* assessment.

Principle #3: Results of bhautika prakṛti assessment

A complete *bhautika prakṛti* assessment will result in a determination of the primary and secondary *mahābhūtas* that comprise an individual's *prakṛti*. The presence of *lakṣhaṇas* for each *mahābhūta* can be assessed and measured in degrees of *avara*, *madhyama* or *uttama*.

When the primary *mahābhūtas* are determined, these can be correlated to the related *doṣha* to aid in confirming the *deha prakṛti*. See Su. Sū. 35/14-15.

Principle #4: Results of sāra assessment

A complete *sāra* assessment will result in a determination of the primary, predominant *sāra* for the individual. The maximum presence of *lakṣhaṇas* related to a single *sāra* is generally the determinant for assessment. See also Cha. Vi. 8/102-116 and Su. Sū. 35/17.

CURRENT PRACTICAL APPLICATION

The practical application of each type of *prakṛti* assessment should be performed in a logical, consistent manner to distinguish *prakṛti* from *vikṛti*. Each assessed parameter and its *parikṣha* method (*darśhana*, *sparśhana* and *praśhna*) should be recorded clearly and completely during the assessment.

Use the *prakṛti lakṣhaṇa* tables to identify and prioritize the *lakṣhaṇas* to assess. Record each question and answer asked during the assessment in as much detail as possible.

TEST YOURSELF

Learn, review and memorize key terms from this section.

avara

āyu

bala

bhautika prakṛti

darśhana

deha prakṛti

lakṣhaṇa

madhyama

mānasika prakṛti

prakṛti

pramāṇa

praśhna

saṁhanana

sāra

sparśhana

svabhāva

uttama

vikṛti

Chapter 6: Review

ADDITIONAL READING

Read and review the references listed below to expand your understanding of the concepts in this chapter. Write down the date that you complete your reading for each. Remember that consistent repetition is the best way to learn. Plan to read each reference at least once now and expect to read it again as you continue your studies.

References marked with (skim) can be read quickly and do not require commentary review.

CLASSICS		1st read	2nd read
Charaka	Cha. Vi. 8/		
Suśhruta	Su. Sū. 35/		
Aṣhṭāṅga Hṛdaya			
Bhāva Prakāśha			

JOURNALS & CURRENT RESOURCES

Reliability and validity in a nutshell   Katrina Bannigan and Roger Watson

Development and validation of a Prototype Prakriti Analysis Tool   Sanjeev Rastogi

https://www.stanfordchildrens.org/en/service/chest-wall/pectus-excavatum

QUESTIONS & ANSWERS

Record your questions for this chapter here for further research and discussion.

Question:

Answer:

Question:

Answer:

Question:

Answer:

SELF-ASSESSMENT

1. Which *deha prakṛti* type(s) are categorized under the *uttama* category?
   a. *Kapha*
   b. *Pitta*
   c. *Vāta-Pitta-Kapha*
   d. All of the above
   e. None of the above

2. Which *deha prakṛti* type(s) are categorized under the *hīna* category?
   a. *Vāta*
   b. *Vāta-Kapha*
   c. *Vāta-Pitta*
   d. Both A and B
   e. None of the above

3. *Darśhana*, *sparśhana* and *praśhna* correlate with which definitions?
   a. Communication, palpation and observation
   b. Observation, auscultation and percussion
   c. Observation, palpation and communication
   d. Palpation, observation and communication
   e. Percussion, auscultation and observation

4. Which *deha prakṛti* would most likely present with the *lakṣhaṇa* of *rūkṣha*?
   a. *Vāta*
   b. *Pitta*
   c. *Kapha*
   d. *Vāta-Pittaja*
   e. *Tri-doṣhaja*

5. Which *deha prakṛti* would most likely present with the *lakṣhaṇa* of *uṣhṇa-dveṣhī* (hates heat)?
   a. *Vāta*
   b. *Pitta*
   c. *Kapha*
   d. *Vāta-Kaphaja*
   e. *Tri-doṣhaja*

6. Which *deha prakṛti* is similar to animals like lions, horses, elephants, bulls, eagles and swans?
   a. *Vāta*
   b. *Pitta*
   c. *Kapha*
   d. *Vāta-Pittaja*
   e. *Tri-doṣhaja*

7. ________ is a product of *māṃsa sāra*.
   a. *Manasvitvaṁ* (magnanimity, wisdom)
   b. *Saukumāryam* (delicate, tender body)
   c. *Sukham* (happiness, contentment)
   d. All of the above
   e. None of the above

8. _________ is a product of *medo sāra*.
   a. *Bhavanti āyuṣhmantaśhcha* (longevity, a full lifespan, high quality of life)
   b. *Kriyāvantaḥ* (a high degree of activity)
   c. *Sāra, sthira śharīrā* (solid, stable body)
   d. *Vitta* (acquisitions, property, wealth, money)
   e. None of the above

9. _________ is a product of *majja sāra*.
   a. *Āpatya* (children)
   b. *Ārogya* (absence of disease)
   c. *Manasvitvaṁ* (magnanimity, wisdom)
   d. *Upabhogā* (pleasure, enjoyment, contentment through eating)
   e. All of the above

10. *Śhauryopetaṁ* (endowed with heroism) is a *lakṣhaṇa* categorized in
    a. *Majjā sāra*
    b. *Māṃsa sāra*
    c. *Medo sāra*
    d. *Sattva sāra*
    e. *Śhukra sāra*

CRITICAL THINKING

1. Consider the overlapping *guṇa* of *laghu* between *vāta* and *pitta*. How does this *guṇa* influence characteristics in *prakṛti*?

2. Consider the overlapping *guṇa* of *snigdha* between *pitta* and *kapha*. How does this *guṇa* influence characteristics in *prakṛti*?

3. Consider the overlapping *guṇa* of *śhīta* between *vāta* and *kapha*. How does this *guṇa* influence characteristics in *prakṛti*?

4. Compare and contrast the *prakṛti* assessment methods for *deha prakṛti* and *bhautika prakṛti*.

5. Identify example characteristics that demonstrate the reasoning for grading *prakṛti* strength as *hīna*, *madhyama* or *uttama*.

References

Chapter 7 : Agni and āhāra

KEY TERMS

agni
āhāra
āhāra śhakti
āhāra vidhi vidhāna
āma lakṣhaṇas
aṣhṭa āhāra vidhi viśheṣhāyatanāni
dvi-anna kāla
guru
jaraṇa śhakti
jīrṇa āhāra lakṣhaṇas
karaṇa
koṣhṭha parīkṣha
krūra koṣhṭha
laghu
madhyama koṣhṭha
mandāgni
mātra
mṛdu koṣhṭha
sama
sāma doṣha lakṣhaṇas
samāgni
saṁskāra
tīkṣhṇāgni
vaiṣhamya
viruddha āhāra
viṣhamāgni
viṣhamāśhana

Dietary habits and food choices are one of the most prominent aspects of holistic health management. In Western culture, these topics are currently in an exploratory phase among scientific and health-focused communities. New research and evidence provide a wealth of knowledge which contribute to the development of a comprehensive foundation for practice.

As part of this ongoing, developmental process, communication standards including terminology continue to evolve. In this chapter and throughout this textbook series, the terms used in dietary contexts will adhere to the following definitions and scope.

Diet, diet plan, diet protocol

A diet, diet plan or diet protocol includes all of the food and fluids that an individual consumes. It also covers any directions, rules, methods, restrictions or limitations for those food and fluids.

Dietary habits, routines, regimens

Dietary habits, routines and regimens include all aspects of implementing and adhering to a specific dietary protocol. When applied through Āyurveda, dietary habits, routines and regimens are always personalized for individuals.

Meal

A meal is a variety of foods prepared to sustain and appropriately nourish the individual. A proper meal, according to classical Āyurveda, includes the main portion of food properly cooked and accompanied by appropriate side items which may be uncooked.

A proper meal contains the correct quantities of various food types that are appropriate for the individual, the season, their stage of life, energetic demand, mental state, current pathology, state of *agni* and additional factors.

Proper measurement of a meal is done on the basis of digestive time due to all related factors. The correct quantity of a meal is that which takes 4 to 6 hours to properly digest. Determination of proper digestion is assessed using *lakṣhaṇas* detailed in this chapter.

Snack

A snack is a smaller quantity of food that should take 2 hours or less to digest properly. It may contain only a single food or a variety of foods. It may be cooked, but more often is is uncooked, raw, or cooked and naturally preserved, such as baked goods.

Food

Food includes all edible used for human consumption. Classically, food is categorized based on how it is consumed either as a meal, by drinking, licking, or chewing hard. It is also classified by its type or source, including grains, meat products, dairy, vegetables, fruits, condiments, sugar products, and others.

Each individual type of food has specific properties and actions when consumed. These base effects may be modulated by processing the food with other foods and by cooking it in different ways.

Water

Water is the fundamental fluid to support human health. Classically, it is categorized according to its source such as rain water, or from a lake, pond or stream.

Water must be treated appropriately to purify it for human consumption. This typically involved cooking it, and optionally boiling it with specific herbs. Optionally, herbs could be added after boiling to impart flavor, color and beneficial effects to promote digestion.

Classically, water is always cooked before consumption. Drinking water at various temperatures, such as hot, warm, cool or cold, produces specific effects in the body. Targeted use of water through cooking methods and temperature is a key component in dietary protocols.

Fluids, drinks

All fluids and drinks, other than properly treated water can support human health when used appropriately. Fluids have a base, liquid form and are typically created from expressed juice. Drinks are preparations that combine one or more fluids with additional ingredients to create a specific outcome having its own *guṇa* and *karma*.

Classically, other fluids and drinks would be used appropriately in specific seasons, pathologies or indicated situations. The proportion of total fluid intake to total food intake also varied according to these factors.

Fluids and drinks do not have a separate classification system but are considered similar to the products that produce them. They could be created from fruits, vegetables, herbs, or cooked food. They may contain any flavors, including sweeteners, depending on the intended effect.

Each individual type of fluid has specific properties and actions when consumed. These base effects may be modulated by processing the fluid with other fluids or foods and by cooking it in different ways to create a specific drink.

CLASSICAL REVIEW

Āhāra is often considered to be one of the most important factors in health. While this is certainly true, its practical implementation is more complex. What is eaten is not always as important as how it is eaten and how well it is digested, absorbed and assimilated. The classical approach to understanding and applying *āhāra* in an individual's state of *svastha* is quite different from standard Western paradigms. Many factors influence the final results and effects of *āhāra*, especially the state of *agni*.

Charaka hints at the critical relationship between *agni* and *āhāra* in the following *śhloka*.

बलमारोग्यमायुश्चप्राणाश्चाग्नौप्रतिष्ठिताः ।
अन्नपानेन्धनैश्चाग्निर्ज्वलतिव्येतिचान्यथा ॥
च. सू. २७।३४२

Balamārogyamāyuśhchaprāṇāśhchāgna upratiṣhṭhitāḥ |
Annapānendhanaiśhchāgnirjvalativyetic hānyathā ||

Cha. Sū. 27/342

Bala (Strength,) ārogya (complete absence of disease,) āyuśhcha (life and longevity, and) prāṇāśhcha (*vāta*, overall) agnaupratiṣhṭhitāḥ (all rely on *agni*). Annapāna (Food and drink) indhanaiśhcha (act as the fuel) agnir-jvalati (which ignite *agni* and allow it to burn;) vyetichānyathā (without these [food and drink], *agni* dwindles).

Because *agni* and *āhāra* are so closely related, they are almost always assessed together and in context of each other. This chapter explores the classical perspectives of how *agni* and *āhāra* contribute to a state of *svastha*. Before beginning this chapter, review *agni* and its mechanics of normal function in detail in Volume 2, Chapter five.

Āhāra and *nidrā* also have a key relationship that strongly influences the state of *agni*. Bhāva Prakāśha discusses this in BP Pū. 5/206 – 212.

Agni

Assessing *agni* in the context of *svastha* strives to determine how *agni* is behaving in its current state and predict how it should behave in its normal, healthy state. This involves determining and assessing all of the following:

- Any tendency toward a specific state of *sama* or *vaiṣhamya*
- The natural behavior of the *koṣhṭha*
- Normal intake and output behavior
- Ability to properly and completely digest consumed food
- Any tendency toward formation of *āma* due to incomplete digestion
- Habits, behaviors and factors that contribute to the state of *agni*

Assessing agni

While all factors of the individual's state of *agni* may be assessed during the short window of time of a standard assessment, they must also be understood in a manner which represents the normal, baseline state for that individual. This requires a deeper understanding of the patient's *prakṛti* as a baseline for predictive knowledge. Additionally, the clinician must be able to carefully determine and delineate secondary factors that may have a direct influence on normal *agni*.

For example, an individual who recently experienced a time period of satisfying sleep, proper physical activity and health-promoting dietary habits will be more likely to have an *agni* assessment that falls within their normal, healthy range.

Additionally, the baseline *agni* assessment can be performed in the context of the healthiest period of the individual's life. All questions during the assessment can be addressed to the specific time period in which the individual felt their healthiest, strongest or best.

Recall that *agni* may be assessed in any of four categories. Review their *lakṣhaṇas* and assessment methods in the following tables. The *lakṣhaṇas* described are expected to be present when that type of *agni* is predominant. The presence of *lakṣhaṇas* for a short period of time more likely indicates the current state of *agni*. And the presence of *lakṣhaṇas* as a regular habitual state over the course of life is more likely associated to the individual's baseline.

Sama Normal, healthy	*Vaiṣhamya* Abnormal, predominant *doṣha*	
Samāgni	*Viṣhamāgni*	Vāta
	Tīkṣhṇāgni	Pitta
	Mandāgni	Kapha

Samāgni Assessment

Samāgni lakṣhaṇas are described by Charaka in Cha. Chi. 15/3-5. These explain the proper functions of *agni* when it is operating in its normal, healthy state.

Samāgni Outcomes of normal digestion	Cha. Chi. 15/3-5			
Āyu Life, quality of life, lifespan	✓			
Varṇa Proper skin tone and complexion	✓			
Bala Strength	✓			
Svāsthya Complete state of health	✓			
Utsāha Proper enthusiasm, eagerness	✓			
Upachaya Proper growth and nourishment	✓			
Prabhā Proper glow, complexion, brightness	✓			
Ojas Natural immunity, resilience	✓			
Tejas Spark, drive, transformation	✓			
Agnaya Proper functioning of all other agnis	✓			
Prāṇa Proper intake of all life-supporting requirements	✓			

Cira jīva Long, full, complete life	√			
Anāmaya Absence of disease	√			

Viṣhamāgni Assessment

Viṣhamāgni lakṣhaṇas are described in Cha. Chi. 15/50, Cha. Vi. 6/12, Su. Sū. 35/26 and AH Śhā. 3/73-76. These describe the improper functions of *agni* when it is in an abnormal state due to vāta.

Viṣhamāgni Outcomes of dysfunctional digestion caused by *Vāta*	Cha. Chi. 15/50	Cha. Vi. 6/12	Su. Sū. 35/26	AH Śhā. 3/73-76
Dhātu-vaiṣhamya Abnormal state of *dhātus*	√			
Viṣhama pachan Irregular digestion (cooking)	√			
Sama-lakṣhaṇa-viparīta-lakṣhaṇa Presents with features opposite to *samāgni*		√		
Kadācit samyak pachati Digests (cooks) food properly sometimes			√	
Kadācit – ādhmāna Sometimes produces distension			√	
Kadācit – śhūla Sometimes produces colic pain			√	
Kadācit – udāvarta Sometimes produces upward movement of *vāta*			√	
Kadācit – atisāra Sometimes produces diarrhea			√	
Kadācit – jaṭhara gaurava Sometimes produces heaviness in the abdomen			√	
Kadācit – āntra kūjana Sometimes produces borborygmus			√	
Kadācit – pravāhaṇi Sometimes produces tenesmus			√	

Samyak-āśhu samyak-chirā pachet Sometimes fast or slow to digest				√

Tīkṣhṇāgni Assessment

Tīkṣhṇāgni lakṣhaṇas are described in Cha. Chi. 15/50, Cha. Vi. 6/12, Su. Sū. 35/26 and AH Śhā. 3/73-76. These describe the improper functions of *agni* when it is in an abnormal state due to pitta.

Tīkṣhṇāgni Outcomes of dysfunctional digestion caused by *Pitta*	Cha. Chi. 15/50	Cha. Vi. 6/12	Su. Sū. 35/26	AH Śhā. 3/73-76
Dhātu-viśhoṣhana with *manda-indhana* Depletion with insufficient fuel or nutrition	√			
Sarva-apachāra-saha Overcomes all improper habits		√		
Āśhu pachati of prabhūta anna Quickly digests too much food			√	
Śhighra-pachet of samyak, etc. *bhojana* Fast digestion of proper food (meals)				√

Mandāgni Assessment

Mandāgni lakṣhaṇas are described in Cha. Chi. 15/51, Cha. Vi. 6/12, Su. Sū. 35/26 and AH Śhā. 3/73-76. These describe the improper functions of *agni* when it is in an abnormal state due to kapha.

Mandāgni Outcomes of dysfunctional digestion caused by *Kapha*	Cha. Chi. 15/51	Cha. Vi. 6/12	Su. Sū. 35/26	AH Śhā. 3/73-76
Vidahati-anna Incompletely digested meals	√			
Chirāt-pahcet of samyak, upayukta anna Slow digestion of proper food (meals)				√
Na sarva-apachāra-saha Does not tolerate inconsistent meals		√		
Mahatā kālena pachati of alpa yukta Long time to digest small meals			√	

Udara and śhiro-gaurava Heaviness in the abdomen and head			✓	
Kāsa Cough			✓	
Śhvāsa Difficulty breathing on exertion			✓	
Praseka Salivation			✓	
Chhardi Regurgitation or vomiting			✓	
Gātra-sadana Fatigue, exhaustion of the limbs			✓	
Asya-śhoṣha Dry mouth				✓
Āṭopa Bloating				✓
Āntra kūjana Borborygmus				✓
Ādhmāna Abdominal distension				✓
Gaurava Heaviness				✓

Assessing koṣhṭha

Recall from Volume 2, Chapters 5 and 18, that the *koṣhṭha* is the pathway from mouth to anus which encompasses all of the components and activities of *jaṭharāgni*. It can be considered as the gastrointestinal tract or alimentary canal.

The three types of *koṣhṭha* represent various predominant states of the *doṣhas* or a general state of *svastha*. The predominant *doṣhas* in each state are found in specific types of *koṣhṭha*.

Koṣhṭha	Cha. Sū. 13/69	Su. Chi. 33/21	AH Sū. 18/34
Krūra	*Vāta*	*Vāta* and *kapha*	*Vāta*
Mṛdu	*Pitta*	*Pitta*	*Pitta*
Madhyama	not specified	*Sama doṣha*	not specified

Krūra koṣhṭha purges and passes bowel movements with difficulty because of the increased presence of *vāta*. Suśhruta adds that *kapha* is involved in this presentation.

Mṛdu koṣhṭha passes bowels and purges easily because of the increased presence of *pitta*.

Madhyama koṣhṭha is that which is experienced in a state of *sama doṣha* marked by normal, healthy *doṣhas* in equilibrium.

While an individual's *koṣhṭha* is often related to their baseline *prakṛti*, there are cases where the two may be different. In some situations, this difference might be due to *svabhāva*, or nature of the individual. In other cases, there may be variations in the presentation of *koṣhṭha* due to other factors especially long-term habits and behaviors. Variations among congruent states of components are often found in the stages of *vikṛti*, or pathological development.

For example, repeated habits of certain types of foods having specific *guṇas* that influence the *doṣhas* can gradually mask the presentation of an individual's normal *koṣhṭha* over a long period of time. These types of scenarios must be considered while assessing the *koṣhṭha* as they can directly impact management protocols.

To assess an individual's *koṣhṭha* type, Charaka provides a method called *koṣhṭha parīkṣha*.

गुडमिक्षुरसं मस्तु क्षीरमुल्लोडितं दधि |
पायसं कृशरां सर्पिः काश्मर्यत्रिफलारसम् || ६६
द्राक्षारसं पीलुरसं जलमुष्णमथापि वा |
मद्यं वा तरुणं पीत्वा मृदुकोष्ठो विरिच्यते || ६७
विरेचयन्ति नैतानि क्रूरकोष्ठं कदाचन |
भवति क्रूरकोष्ठस्य ग्रहण्यत्युल्बणानिला || ६८
उदीर्णपित्ताऽल्पकफा ग्रहणी मन्दमारुता |
मृदुकोष्ठस्य तस्मात् स सुविरेच्यो नरः स्मृतः || ६९

च. सू. १३।६६-६९

Guḍam, ikṣhu-rasaṁ, mastu, kṣhīram, ulloḍitaṁ dadhi |
Pāyasaṁ, kṛśharāṁ, sarpiḥ, kāśhmarya, triphalā-rasam || 66
Drākṣhā-rasaṁ, pīlu-rasaṁ jalam-uṣhṇam-athāpi vā |
Madyaṁ vā taruṇaṁ pītvā mṛdu-koṣhṭho virichyate || 67
Virechayanti naitāni krūra-koṣhṭhaṁ kadāchana |
Bhavati krūra-koṣhṭhasya grahaṇyaty-ulbaṇānilā || 68
Udīrṇa-pittā ' lpa-kaphā grahaṇī manda-mārutā |
Mṛdu-koṣhṭhasya tasmāt sa suvirechyo naraḥ smṛtaḥ || 69

Cha. Sū. 13/66-69

Guḍam (Jaggery,) ikṣhu-rasaṁ (sugarcane juice,) mastu (whey,) kṣhīram (milk,) ulloḍitaṁ dadhi (water produced when homemade yogurt is prepared,) pāyasaṁ (desserts prepared with cooked milk,) kṛśharāṁ (rice cooked with various pulses,) sarpiḥ (ghee [of cow],) kāśhmarya (juice or decoction of *kāśhmarya* [*Gmelina arborea*],) triphalā-rasam (juice or decoction of *triphala* [*Terminalia chebula*, *Terminalia bellirica* and *Emblica officinalis*],) drākṣhā-rasaṁ (juice or decoction of grape [*Vitis vinifera*],) pīlu-rasaṁ (juice or decoction of *Salvadora persica*,) jalam-uṣhṇam-(hot water) athāpi vā (or) madyaṁ (alcohol, especially fresh wine;) vā (any of these) taruṇaṁ pītvā (drunk in their fresh state) mṛdu-koṣhṭho virichyate (will produce purgations in individuals having *mṛdu koṣhṭha*).

Virechayanti naitāni ([However], purgations) krūra-koṣhṭhaṁ (in individuals having *krūra koṣhṭha*) kadāchana bhavati (are never produced [with these same *dravya*]) krūra-koṣhṭhasya (due to the hardness of the *koṣhṭha*) grahaṇyaty-ulbaṇānilā (because of increased presence of *vāta* in the *grahaṇi*).

Udīrṇa-pittā (Increased *pitta*) alpa-kaphā (and less *kapha*) grahaṇī (in the *grahaṇī*, or primary location of *pāchaka pitta*) manda-mārutā (along with slowness [reduced, diminished response] of *vāta*) mṛdu-koṣhṭhasya (in an individual having *mṛdu koṣhṭha*) tasmāt sa suvirechyo naraḥ smṛtaḥ (are always known to cause easy, comfortable purgations in people).

This explanation provides important underlying principles of the basic roles of the three *doṣhas* to produce easy bowel movements. The terms related to *vireka* used above literally mean to throw out of the body. The actual production of bowel movements may occur in lower or higher degrees of looseness which can also be considered within the context of the *doṣhas* involved.

The purpose of *koṣhṭha parīkṣha* is to provide a simple method of testing any individual for their current state of *koṣhṭha*. Consumption of any of the *dravyas* mentioned produces a corresponding result which can be assessed for the involvement of *doṣhas* and any additional concurrent factors. A historical assessment can also be made based on eliciting a proper, thorough history of relevant factors. This may or may not be indicative of the individual's state of baseline *koṣhṭha*.

Koṣhṭha parīkṣha dravya	Nearest English equivalent
Guḍam	Jaggery
Ikṣhu-rasaṁ	Sugarcane juice
Mastu	Whey
Kṣhīram	Milk
Ulloḍitaṁ dadhi	Water produced when homemade yogurt is made
Pāyasaṁ	Desserts prepared with cooked milk
Kṛśharāṁ	Rice cooked with various pulses
Sarpiḥ	Ghee (of cow)
Kāśhmarya	Juice (decoction) of *kāśhmarya* (*Gmelina arborea*)
Triphalā-rasam	Juice (decoction) of *triphala* (*Terminalia chebula*, *Terminalia bellirica* and *Emblica officinalis*)
Drākṣhā-rasaṁ	Juice or decoction of grape (*Vitis vinifera*)
Pīlu-rasaṁ	Juice or decoction of *Salvadora persica*
Jalam-uṣhṇam	Hot water
Madyaṁ	Alcohol, especially fresh wine

Assessing āhāra śhakti (intake)

Assessment of an individual's *āhāra śhakti* intends to measure their capacity for consumption, digestion and assimilation of food. This parameter is included in Charaka's *daśhavidha parīkṣha*.

आहारशक्तितश्चेति आहारशक्तिरभ्यवहरणशक्त्याजरणशक्त या च परीक्ष्या; बलायुषी ह्याहारायत्ते || १२०

च. वि. ८।१२०

Āhāraśhaktitaśhcheti āhāraśhaktirabhyavaharaṇaśhaktyā jaraṇaśhaktayā cha parīkṣhyā; balāyuṣhī hyāhārāyatte || 120

Cha. Vi. 8/120

Āhāra-śhaktita-śhcheti (One's ability [strength, power, capacity] to consume, digest and assimilate food) parīkṣhyā (must be examined or assessed) āhāra-śhaktir (as the actual power of food consumption, digestion and assimilation) abhyavaharaṇa-śhaktyā (in terms of *abhyavaharaṇa*, or ingestion) jaraṇa-śhaktayā cha (and *jaraṇa*, or output;) bala ([one's] strength) āyuṣhī (and life, quality of life or lifespan) hyāhārāyatte (depend on food and diet).

The purpose of understaing *āhāra śhakti* is to gain insight into an individual's current ability to intake food and drink and effectively convert it into useful outputs that support strength and life.

Like many factors in *daśhavidha parīkṣha*, *āhāra śhakti* is measured in three levels, *hīna*, *madhyama* and *uttama*. Both the healthy, baseline state and the current state should be determined. These two points are compared to each other to better understand deviation and the current state.

Mātra as the primary factor

When assessing *āhāra śhakti*, the main factor that must be considered is the *āhāra mātra*, or quantity of consumed food. Charaka states this very clearly in Cha. Sū. 5/3.

मात्राशी स्यात् | आहारमात्रा पुनरग्निबलापेक्षिणी || ३

च. सू. ५।३

Mātrāśhī syāt | Āhāramātrā punaragnibalāpekṣhiṇī || 3

Cha. Sū. 5/3

Mātrāśhī syāt (One should eat the proper quantity [of food]). Āhāra-mātrā (The correct quantity of food) punar-agni-balāpekṣhiṇī (is always dependent on the strength of *agni*).

Chakrapāṇi fully supports this position and elaborates on its specifics when applying the principle in practice. He recognizes that factors including *vyāyāma*, *kāla*, *ṛtu*, *vaya*, and others influence an individual's *āhāra śhakti*. However, the quantity consumed is ultimately the most significant determining factor.

Chakrapāṇi adds that in order to properly measure an individual's *āhāra śhakti*, a large meal must be consumed.

Charaka further describes the benefits of consuming the proper quantity of food according to the individual's requirements.

मात्रावद्ध्यशनमशितमनुपहत्य प्रकृतिं बलवर्णसुखायुषा योजयत्युपयोक्तारमवश्यमिति ||८||

च. सू. ५।८

Mātrāvaddhyaśhanamaśhitam anupahatya prakṛtiṁ bala varṇa sukhāyuṣhāyojayaty-upayoktāramavaśhyamiti ||8||

Cha. Sū. 5/8

Consuming the proper quantity of food according to the individual's requirements promotes *bala* (strength), *varṇa* (complexion), *sukha* (healthy contentment), and *āyuṣhā* (longevity). This supports the individual's *prakṛti* (normal baseline).

Mātrāvat: Proper quantity

Considering *āhāra mātra* as the primary tool for assessing *āhāra śhakti*, Charaka further specifies in Cha. Vi. 2/ that *āhāra mātra* may be proper or improper. When improper, it can be further classified as insufficient or excessive quantity.

He states that the purpose of chapter two in *Vimānasthāna* is to understand how to measure proper and improper quantity for any given individual. There are many aspects to consider in the complete measurement, or assessment, of a meal.

तत्रायं तावदाहारराशिमधिकृत्य
मात्रामात्राफलविनिश्चयार्थः प्रकृतः |
एतावानेव ह्याहारराशिविधिविकल्पो
यावन्मात्रावत्त्वममात्रावत्त्वं च || ५

च. वि. २।५

Tatrāyaṁ tāvadāhārarāśhimadhikṛtya mātrāmātrāphalaviniśhchayārthaḥ prakṛtaḥ | Etāvāneva hyāhārarāśhividhivikalpo yāvanmātrāvattvamamātrāvattvaṁ cha || 5

Cha. Vi. 2/5

Tatrāyaṁ tāvad (And so) āhāra-rāśhim (the specifications of measurements of food) adhikṛtya (in regards to its) mātra-amātrā (proper or improper quantity) phala-viniśhchaya-arthaḥ prakṛtaḥ (is the primary topic of the instructions in this chapter). Etāvāneva hi (Such) āhāra-rāśhi (quantity of food) vidhi-vikalpo (and its specifications and measurements are) yāvan (the determining factors) mātrāvat tvam (that produce the correct amount) amātrāvat tvaṁ cha (or the incorrect amount).

This explanation implies that the assessment of *āhāra śhakti* begins with careful analysis of *āhāra mātra*. Then, additional factors can be considered secondarily within this context.

Both proper and improper quantities of consumed food are capable of producing specific *lakṣhaṇas* to guide clinical assessment. Review these in the following tables.

तत्र मात्रावत्त्वं पूर्वमुद्दिष्टं कुक्ष्यंशविभागेन,
तद्भूयो विस्तरेणानुव्याख्यास्यामः | तद्यथा
- कुक्षेरप्रणीडनमाहारेण, हृदयस्यानवरोधः,
पार्श्वयोरविपाटनम्, अनतिगौरवमुदरस्य,
प्रीणनमिन्द्रियाणां, क्षुत्पिपासोपरमः
स्थानासनशयनगमनोच्छ्वासप्रश्वास -
हास्यसङ्कथासु सुखानुवृत्तिः, सायं प्रातश्च
सुखेन परिणमनं; बलवर्णोपचयकरत्वं च;
इति मात्रावतो लक्षणमाहारस्य भवति || ६

च. वि. २।६

Tatra mātrāvattvaṁ pūrvamuddiṣhṭaṁ kukṣhyaṁśhavibhāgena, tadbhūyo vistareṇānuvyākhyāsyāmaḥ | Tadyathā – kukṣherapraṇīḍanamāhāreṇa, hṛdayasyānavarodhaḥ, pārśhvayoravipāṭanam, anatigauravamudarasya, prīṇanamindriyāṇāṁ, kṣhutpipāsoparamaḥ, sthānāsanaśhayanagamanochchhvāsap raśhvāsahāsyasaṅkathāsu sukhānuvṛttiḥ, sāyaṁ prātaśhcha sukhenapariṇamanaṁ; balavarṇopachayakaratvaṁ cha; iti mātrāvato lakṣhaṇamāhārasya bhavati || 6

Cha. Vi. 2/6

Tatra (And so,) mātrāvat-tvaṁ (determining the correct quantity [of food]) pūrvam-uddiṣhṭaṁ (as previously discussed) kukṣhyaṁśha (is based on the portions of the belly, abdomen or stomach) vibhāgena (being divided into three parts); tadbhūyo (these same topics) vistareṇānu vyākhyāsyāmaḥ (are being discussed here in more detail). Tadyathā (Such that) – kukṣher (within the stomach) apraṇīḍanam (there is no exertion or pressure) āhāreṇa (due to the food), hṛdayasya-anavarodhaḥ (the heart and its functions are not obstructed by covering or a sensation of blockage), pārśhvaya ura-vipāṭanam (the flanks and sides of the thorax do not experience a splitting type of pain), anati (there is not too much) gauravam (heaviness) udarasya (throughout the abdominal cavity), prīṇanam (a feeling of satiation and nourishment) indriyāṇāṁ (is recognized through the senses), kṣhut (hunger) pipāsa (and thirst) uparamaḥ (are quelled), sthānāsanaśhaya (standing, sitting) na gamana (walking) uchchhvāsa-praśhvāsaha (inhaling and exhaling) āsya-saṅkathāsu (laughing and talking) sukhānuvṛttiḥ (are easy and comfortable), sāyaṁ (when taken in the evening) prātaśhcha (and morning) sukhena (it easily and comfortably) pariṇamanaṁ (undergoes transformation [digestion, metabolism, assimilation]); bala (strength), varṇa (complexion) upachaya (and proper nourishment and growth) karatvaṁ cha (are produced); iti (thus), mātrāvato lakṣhaṇam (the characteristics of proper quantity) āhārasya (of food) bhavati (are as described).

Charaka identifies several key indicators that must be assessed to determine whether food has been consumed in the proper quantity. These include:

1. Consuming two meals per day, one in the morning (before noon) and one in the evening (around sunset)
2. The quantity of food consumed at both times is digested, metabolized and assimilated before the next meal
3. This quantity produces the *lakṣhaṇas* described as immediate and long-term outcomes

The assessment and analysis of each of these lakṣhaṇas provides valuable insight into the possible causes for improper digestion. Review each in the following table and consider its assessment methodology. The presence of any lakṣhaṇa may indicate a wide variety of causative factors depending on the individual's unique circumstances.

Mātrāvat lakṣhaṇas Indicators of proper food quantity consumed	Cha. Vi. 2/6			
Kukṣher apraṇīḍanam āhāreṇa No exertion or pressure in the abdomen due to the consumed food	✓			
Hṛdayasya-anavarodhaḥ The heart and its functions feel unobstructed	✓			
Pārśhvaya ura-vipāṭanam The flanks and sides of the thorax do not experience a splitting type of pain	✓			

Prīṇanam indriyāṇāṁ Satiation and nourishment recognized in the sense organs and perception	√			
Kṣhut pipāsa uparamaḥ Hunger and thirst are quelled	√			
Sthānāsanaśhaya na gamana uchchhvāsa-praśhvāsaha āsya-saṅkathāsu sukhānuvṛttiḥ Standing (sitting), walking, inhaling and exhaling, laughing and talking are easy and comfortable	√			
Sāyaṁ prātaśhcha sukhena pariṇamanaṁ When taken in the evening and morning, it easily and comfortably undergoes transformation [digestion, metabolism, assimilation]	√			
Bala Physical strength	√			
Varṇa Complexion	√			
Upachaya Proper nourishment, growth and development	√			

***Amātrāvat*: Insufficient quantity**

Consuming food in improper quantity is similarly described in Cha. Vi. 2/ as either insufficient or excessive. Charaka clearly states this classification.

अमात्रावत्त्वं पुनर्द्विविधमाचक्षते - हीनम्,
अधिकं च | ...

च. वि. २/७

Amātrāvattvaṁ punardvividhamāchakṣhate - hīnam, adhikaṁ cha |

Cha. Vi. 2/7

Amātrāvat-tvaṁ (Improper quantity of food) punar (is again) dvividham (divided into two types) āchakṣhate (explained as) – hīnam (insufficient), adhikaṁ cha (and excessive).

These two opposite scenarios have distinct causes and presentations. Both are described with their specific lakṣhaṇas.

... तत्र हीनमात्रमाहारराशिं
बलवर्णोपचयक्षयकरमतृप्तिकरमुदावर्तक
रमनायुष्यवृष्यमनौजस्यं
शरीरमनोबुद्धीन्द्रियोपघातकरं
सारविधमनमलक्ष्म्यावहमशीतेश्च
वातविकाराणामायतनमाचक्षते, ...

च. वि. २/७

... Tatra hīnamātramāhārarāśhiṁbalavarṇopachayakṣhayakaramatṛptikaramudāvartakaramanāyuṣhyavṛṣhyamanaujasyaṁśharīramanobuddhīndriyopaghātakaraṁ sāravidhamanamalakṣhmyāvahamaśhīteśhchavātavikārāṇāmāyatanamāchakṣhate, ...

Cha. Vi. 2/7

Tatra (And so), hīna-mātram (an insufficient quantity) āhāra-rāśhiṁ (of consumed food produces) bala-varṇa-upachaya kṣhaya karam (a reduction in overall strength, complexion and proper nourishment, growth and development), atṛpti karam (absence of the sense of satiation or satisfaction), udāvarta karam (upward movement of *vāta*), anāyuṣhya-vṛṣhyam-anaujasyaṁ-śharīram-anobuddh-īndriya-upaghāta karaṁ (damage to life and life span, fertility and virility, *ojas*, the physical body, *buddhi*, and the senses), sāra-vidham ([damage to] the various types of *sāra*), anam-alakṣhmyāvaham-aśhīteśh-cha (reduction or absence of affluence, prosperity), vāta-vikārāṇām-āyatanam (and many varieties of diseases of *vāta*) āchakṣhate (manifest).

Any of these *lakṣhaṇas* may be seen singly or in conjunction when food is consumed in insufficient quantity over time. *Lakṣhaṇas* may present immediately or progressively with reduced consumption. These *lakṣhaṇas* are listed next.

Amātrāvat Assessment

Amātrāvat lakṣhaṇas Indicators of insufficient food quantity consumed	Cha. Vi. 2/7			
Bala, varṇa, upachaya kṣhaya karam Reduction of strength, complexion and proper nourishment and growth	√			
Atṛpti karam Absence of the sense of satiation or satisfaction	√			
Udāvarta karam Upward movement of *vāta*	√			
Anāyuṣhya, vṛṣhyam, anaujasyaṁ, śharīram, anobuddh, īndriya upaghāta karaṁ sāra-vidham Damage to life and life span, fertility and virility, *ojas*, the physical body, *buddhi*, and the senses; damage to the various types of *sāra*	√			
Anam-alakṣhmyāvaham-aśhīteśhcha Reduction or absence of affluence, prosperity, wealth	√			
Vāta vikārāṇāmāyatanam Many types *vāta* disorders	√			

Atimātrāvat: Excessive quantity

Charaka then describes the outcomes of excessive intake of food. This process increases formation of *doṣhas*. It often is associated with the production of *āma* and then *sāma doṣhas*.

... अतिमात्रं पुनः सर्वदोषप्रकोपणमिच्छन्ति कुशलाः| यो हि मूर्तानामाहारजातानां सौहित्यं गत्वा द्रवैस्तृप्तिमापद्यते भूयस्तस्यामाशयगता वातपित्तश्लेष्माणोऽभ्यवहारेणातिमात्रेणाति प्रपीड्यमानाः सर्वे युगपत् प्रकोपमापद्यन्ते, ते प्रकुपितास्तमेवाहारराशिमपरिणतमाविश्य कुक्ष्येकदेशमन्नाश्रिता विष्टम्भयन्तः सहसा वाऽप्युत्तराधराभ्यां मार्गाभ्यां प्रच्यावयन्तः पृथक् पृथगिमान् विकारानभिनिर्वर्तयन्त्यतिमात्रभोक्तुः | ...

च. वि. २।७

Atimātraṁ punaḥ sarvadoṣhaprakopaṇamichchhanti kuśhalāḥ | Yo hi mūrtānāmāhārajātānāṁ sauhityaṁ gatvā dravaistṛptimāpadyate bhūyastasyāmāśhayagatāvātapittaśhleṣhmāṇo ' bhyavahāreṇātimātreṇātiprapīḍyamānāḥ sarve yugapat prakopamāpadyante, teprakupitāstamevāhārarāśhimapariṇatamāviśhya kukṣhyekadeśhamannāśhritā viṣhṭambhayantaḥ sahasāvā ' pyuttarādharābhyāṁ mārgābhyāṁ prachyāvayantaḥ pṛthak pṛthagimānvikārānabhinirvartayantyatimātrabhoktuḥ |

Cha. Vi. 2/7

Ati-mātraṁ (Excessive quantity) punaḥ (as discussed previously) sarva doṣha prakopaṇam ichchhanti (produces immediate aggravation of all the *doṣhas*) kuśhalāḥ (from their otherwise normal, healthy state). Yo hi mūrtānām (When a substantial) āhāra-jātānāṁ (quantity of food is consumed) sauhityaṁ gatvā (that is overly satisfying) dravais-tṛptim āpadyate (along with liquid to produce excess satiation [like a food coma]), bhūyas-tasyām (this excessive combination is sufficient to) āśhaya-gatā vāta pitta śhleṣhmāṇo (cause the *vāta*, *pitta* and *kapha* which are moving in their places in the organs [like *āmāśhaya*]) abhyavahāreṇa (due to eating) ati-mātreṇa (too much quantity of food) ati-prapīḍya (to create excessive pressure or squeezing) mānāḥ sarve yugapat prakopam āpadyante (causing all of them [the *doṣhas*] to undergo aggravation from their normal state). Te (The *doṣhas*) prakupitāstam (in their aggravated state) eva (due to) āhāra-rāśhim (the quantity of) apariṇatam āviśhya (food in an incomplete state of conversion, form completely into a conglomerated mass), kukṣhyeka-deśham (find a location inside the belly or stomach), annāśhritā (residing within the food), viṣhṭambhayantaḥ (obstruct and restrain) sahasāvā (with great strength) apy-uttarādharābhyāṁ mārgābhyāṁ (or go in either the upward or downward pathways) prachyāvayantaḥ pṛthak (being suddenly unrestrained [ejected, expelled]), pṛthak imān-vikārān-abhinirvarta-yanty (and they suddenly produce disorders as a result) ati-mātra bhoktuḥ (of eating an excessive quantity).

The *lakṣhaṇas* of excess food consumption are listed in the next table.

Atimātrāvat lakṣhaṇas Indicators of excessive food quantity consumed	Cha. Vi. 2/7			
Sarva doṣha prakopaṇam ichchhanti kuśhalāḥ Immediate aggravation of all doṣhas from their otherwise normal, healthy state	✓			

Assessing *jarana śhakti* (output)

Assessment of an individual's *jaraṇa śhakti* intends to measure their ability to output the waste products of consumed food. This parameter is included in Charaka's *daśhavidha parīkṣha*.

आहारशक्तितश्चेति आहारशक्तिरभ्यवहरणशक्त्याजरणशक्त या च परीक्ष्या; बलायुषी ह्याहारायत्ते || १२०
च. वि. ८।१२०

Āhāraśhaktitaśhcheti āhāraśhaktirabhyavaharaṇaśhaktyā jaraṇaśhaktayā cha parīkṣhyā; balāyuṣhī hyāhārāyatte || 120
Cha. Vi. 8/120

Āhāra-śhaktita-śhcheti (One's ability [strength, power, capacity] to consume, digest and assimilate food) parīkṣhyā (must be examined or assessed) āhāra-śhaktir (as the actual power of food consumption, digestion and assimilation) abhyavaharaṇa-śhaktyā (in terms of *abhyavaharaṇa*, or ingestion) jaraṇa-śhaktayā cha (and *jaraṇa*, or output;) bala ([one's] strength) āyuṣhī (and life, quality of life or lifespan) hyāhārāyatte (depend on food and diet).

The purpose of understaing *jaraṇa śhakti* is to gain insight into an individual's current ability to process and excrete waste products of consumed food and drink. This assessment is often performed in conjunction with *koṣhṭha parīkṣha*. The individual's current state and their baseline should both be considered as components of this assessment.

Like many factors in *daśhavidha parīkṣha*, *jaraṇa śhakti* is measured in three levels, *hīna*, *madhyama* and *uttama*. Both the healthy, baseline state and the current state should be determined. These two points may be compared to each other to better understand the current state.

The key components of this assessment are determined primarily by enquiring about the patient's exretion habits, quantity, frequency and related characteristics. Each of these must be considered in the context of their time of presentation.

Assessing jīrna āhāra lakṣhanas

The *jīrṇa āhāra lakṣhaṇas* assess key parameters that indicate the completeness of digestion of the previous meal over a period of time. These *lakṣhaṇas* generally appear over the course of 1 to 6 hours after an individual consumes a meal. In abnormal circumstances, these *lakṣhaṇas* may appear up to 24 hours after the meal or they may not appear at all.

Their appearance should be considered normal within the range of 4 to 6 hours after the proper quantity of food has been consumed. Each *lakṣhaṇa* can be measured individually and independently. When more *lakṣhaṇas* appear towards the end of the assessment period (approximately 6 hours), the meal should be considered completely digested.

In many cases, all *lakṣhaṇas* will not manifest. This may be due to a number of factors including *vikṛti*, *kāla*, *ṛtu*, *vaya*, *nidrā* and others. The absence or incomplete manifestation of any of these *lakṣhaṇas* should be identified and investigated as an important indicator of underlying *agni vaiṣhamya*. Further examination should be performed to determine the cause, duration, triggering and relieving factors, typical presentation and any additional, important details.

The *jīrṇa āhāra lakṣhaṇas* first appear in the *Laghu Trayī* through Mādhava Nidāna (MN 6/24) and Bhāva Prakāśha (BP Pū. 5/109).

उद्गारशुद्धिरुत्साहो वेगोत्सर्गो यथोछितः ।

लघुता क्षुत्पिपासा च जीर्णाहारस्य लक्षणम् ॥

भा. प्र. पू. ५।१०९

Udgāraśhuddhirutsāho vegotsargo yathochitaḥ |
Laghutā kṣhutpipāsā cha jīrṇāhārasya lakṣhaṇam ||

BP Pū. 5/109

Udgāra-śhuddhir (Clean, clear, pure belching), utsāho (enthusiasm), vegotsargo (proper release of *vegas*) yathochitaḥ (in the downward direction), laghutā (lightness), kṣhut-pipāsā cha (hunger and thirst) jīrṇāhārasya lakṣhaṇam (are the signs of proper, complete transformation [digestion] of food).

Review each of these *lakṣhaṇas* in the following tables.

Jīrṇa āhāra lakṣhaṇas Indicators of correct outcomes of digestion				BP Pū. 5/109
Udgāra śhuddhir Clean, clear, pure belching				✓
Utsāho Enthusiasm				✓
Vegotsargo yathochitaḥ Proper release of *vegas* in the downward direction				✓
Laghutā Lightness				✓
Kṣhut-pipāsā cha Manifestation of hunger and thirst				✓

Āma

The presence of *āma* is indicated by potential causative factors in addition to known *lakṣhaṇas*. Charaka states that the process of *āma* formation initiates when an individual consumes food in excessive quantity.

Nidāna (Causative Factors)

As described in Cha. Vi. 2/7, the increased pressure of the excessive food compresses all three *doṣhas* in their locations of the GIT organs. These *doṣhas* are immediately aggravated, then mix with the consumed food and become lodged in their location(s). They can either create obstruction in the channels or the urge to be expelled through upward or downward tracts.

In this state the aggravated *doṣhas* should be considered as improperly formed waste products. These constitute *āma*.

In addition to excessive intake of food as the primary causative factor for *āma*, Charaka mentions factors about the qualities of the food, the individual's state of mind and their immediate environment. He explains the direct, causative factors for the production of *āma* in Cha. Vi. 2/8.

न च खलु केवलमतिमात्रमेवाहारराशिमामप्रदोषकरमिच्छन्ति अपि तु खलु गुरुरूक्षशीतशुष्कद्विष्टविष्टम्भिविदाह्यशुचि विरुद्धानामकाले चान्नपानानामुपसेवनं, कामक्रोधलोभमोहेर्ष्याह्रीशोकमानोद्वेगभयोपतप्तमनसा वा यदन्नपानमुपयुज्यते, तदप्याममेव प्रदूषयति || ८

च. वि. २।८

Na cha khalu kevalamatimātramevāhārarāśhimāmapradoṣhakaramichchhanti api tu khalugururūkṣhaśhītaśhuṣhkadviṣhṭaviṣhṭambhividāhyaśhuchiviruddhānāmakāle chānnapānānāmupasevanaṁ, kāmakrodhalobhamoherṣhyāhrīśhokamānodvegabhayopataptamanasā vā yadannapānamupayujyate, tadapyāmameva pradūṣhayati || 8

Cha. Vi. 2/8

Na cha khalu kevalam (It is not only) ati-mātram (the use of excessive quantity) eva āhāra-rāśhim (of food portions) āma-pradoṣha karam-ichchhanti (that produce conditions of *āma-pradoṣha* [waste-product *doṣhas*]), api tu khalu (but also food which is) guru (heavy), rūkṣha (dry), śhīta (cold), śhuṣhka (dried up, shrivelled, desiccated), dviṣhṭa (disliked), viṣhṭambhi (causing obstruction of the channels), vidāhy (producing burning sensation because of incomplete, sour digestion), aśhuchi (unclean, polluted), viruddhānām (having improper food combinations), akāle cha (or improper timing) anna-pānānām (of food and drinks) upasevanaṁ (on a regular basis); kāma (desire), krodha (anger), lobha (greed), moha (delusion), irṣhyā (jealousy), hrī (shame), śhoka (sorrow, grief), mānod-vega (disorders of the mind due to emotional disturbance), bhaya (fear), upatapta-manasā vā (or overheating of the mind) yad anna-pānam (while consuming food and drink) upayujyate (also produce the same [*āma-pradoṣha*, or waste-product *doṣhas*]); tad-apyāmameva pradūṣhayati (all of these [specific causes] can produce vitiation).

This comprehensive list of causative factors for production of *āma* make it clear that many factors are involved. Realistically, it is very difficult for anyone to fully control each of these factors at every meal. The more likely outcome is that every person will experience the formation of *āma* in varying degrees every time they consume food or drink.

When *āma* forms, it may be produced in varying quantities. This can create immediately noticeable signs and symptoms, or ones which are delayed. Normally, some amount of discomfort or disturbance is recognizable. If this occurs, and the causative factors for production of *āma* continue, the quantity and presentation generally increase in severity and frequency.

The state of manas, rajas and tamas influence digestion and the production of *āma*. This mental state creates *āma* on physical level, not "mental *āma*."

भवति चात्र- मात्रयाऽप्यभ्यवहृतं पथ्यं चान्नं न जीर्यति|
चिन्ताशोकभयक्रोधदुःखशय्याप्रजागरैः ||९||

च. वि. २।९

Bhavati chātra – mātrayā ' pyabhyava hṛtaṁ pathyaṁ chānnaṁ na jīryati |
Chintāśhokabhayakrodhaduḥkhaśhayyā prajāgaraiḥ ||9||

Cha. Vi. 2/9

And so, even wholesome food in proper quantity is not digested when anxiety, grief, fear, anger, discontent or sleeplessness interfere with an individual's mental state.

Āma nidāna Causative factors that produce metabolic waste	Cha. Vi. 2/7	Cha. Vi. 2/8		
Ati-mātraṁ Excessive quantity (of food)	✓			
Āhāra-jātānāṁ sauhityaṁ gatvā dravais-tṛptim āpadyate When a substantial quantity of food is consumed that is overly satisfying along with liquid to produce excess satiation (like a food coma)	✓			
Guru Heaviness		✓		
Rūkṣha Dry		✓		
Śhīta Coldness		✓		
Śhuṣhka Dried up, shrivelled, desiccated		✓		
Dviṣhṭa Disliked		✓		
Viṣhṭambhi Causing obstruction of the channels		✓		
Vidāhi Producing burning sensation because of incomplete, sour digestion		✓		
Aśhuci Unclean, impure, polluted		✓		
Viruddhānām Improper food combinations		✓		
Akāle cha anna-pānānām upasevanaṁ Improper timing of food and drinks on a regular basis		✓		
Kāma Desire		✓		
Krodha Anger		✓		
Lobha Greed		✓		
Moha		✓		

Delusion				
Irṣhyā Jealousy		✓		
Hrī Shame		✓		
Śhoka Sorrow, grief		✓		
Mānod-vega Disorders of the mind due to emotional disturbance		✓		
Bhaya Fear		✓		
Upatapta-manasā vā yad anna-pānam Overheating or overworking of the mind while consuming food and drink		✓		

Sāmānya āma lakṣhaṇas

When waste-product *doṣhas* remain lodged inside the body, they will continue in an aggravated state and can eventually produce a variety of disorders. They may present in a generalized state of abnormality or they may physically associate with one or more of the *doṣhas*.

The generalized state of presentation may be referred to as *āma*, *āma lakṣhaṇas*, or *sāmānya āma lakṣhaṇas*. When associated with *doṣhas*, each type is referred to as *sāma vāta*, *sāma pitta* or *sāma kapha*, depending on the presentation.

The *āma lakṣhaṇas* described by Vāgbhaṭa provide a thorough and detailed assessment methodology for determining the presence and duration of generalized *āma* in an individual.

स्रोतोरोधबलभ्रंशगौरवानिलमूढताः ॥ २३
आलस्यापक्तिनिष्ठीवमलसङ्गारुचिक्लमाः ।
लिङ्गं मलानां सामानां, निरामाणां विपर्ययः
॥ २४

अ. हृ. सू. १३।२३-२४

Srotorodhabalabhraṁśhagauravānilamū ḍhatāḥ || 23
Ālasyāpaktiniṣhṭīvamalasaṅgāruchiklam āḥ |
Liṅgaṁ malānāṁ sāmānāṁ, nirāmāṇāṁ viparyayaḥ ||

AH Sū. 13/23-24

Sroto-rodha (Obstruction of the *srotases*), bala-bhraṁśha (loss of strength), gaurava (heaviness), ānila-mūḍhatāḥ ("death," stoppage or stagnancy of *vāta* [obstipation]), ālasya (fatigue), apakti (loss of power of conversion, digestion, transformation), niṣhṭīva (increased expectoration, mucus, phlegm), mala-saṅga (accumulation of waste materials), aruchi (lack of appetite), klamāḥ (and exhaustion) liṅgaṁ (are the signs and symptoms) malānāṁ sāmānāṁ (of the presence of *āma*); nirāmāṇāṁ (the absence of *āma*) viparyayaḥ (is known by the opposite of these).

Sāmānya āma lakṣhaṇas Causative factors that produce metabolic waste			AH Sū. 13/23-24	
Sroto-rodha Obstruction of the *srotases*			✓	
Bala-bhraṁśha Loss of strength			✓	
Gaurava Heaviness			✓	
Ānila mūḍhatāḥ "Death," stoppage or stagnancy of *vāta* [obstipation]			✓	
Ālasya Fatigue			✓	
Apakti Loss of power of conversion, digestion, transformation			✓	
Niṣhṭīva Increased expectoration, mucus, phlegm			✓	
Mala saṅga Accumulation of waste materials			✓	
Aruchi Lack of appetite			✓	
Klamāḥ Exhaustion			✓	

Sāma lakṣhaṇas

Charaka also explains the concept of *sāma doṣha lakṣhaṇas* as a result of generated *āma* mixing with aggravated *doṣhas* in Cha. Vi. 2/7. This explanation immediately follows the description of the formation of *āma* due to the consumption of an excessive quantity of food.

The term *sāma* is formed by the prefix "*sa*-" appended to "*āma*." It literally means "with *āma*" and refers to the *doṣha* associated with the generated *āma*.

Review the *sāma doṣha lakṣhaṇas* stated by Charaka below along with their clinical descriptions and assessment methods at the end of this section.

तत्र वातः
शूलानाहाङ्गमर्दमुखशोषमूर्च्छाभ्रमाग्निवैष
म्यपार्श्वपृष्ठकटिग्रहसिराकुञ्चनस्तम्भनानि
करोति, पित्तं
पुनर्ज्वरातीसारान्तर्दाहतृष्णामदभ्रमप्रलप
नानि, श्लेष्मा तु
छर्द्यरोचकाविपाकशीतज्वरालस्यगात्रगौर
वाणि || ७

च. वि. २।७

Tatra vātaḥ śhūlānāhāṅgamardamukhaśhoṣhamūrchchhābhramāgnivaiṣhamyapārśhvapṛṣhṭhakaṭigrahasirākuñchanastambhanāni karoti, pittaṁ punarjvarātīsārāntardāhatṛṣhṇāmadabhramapralapanāni, śhleṣhmā tu chhardyarochakāvipākaśhītajvarālasyagātragauravāṇi ||

Cha. Vi. 2/7

Tatra (And so), vātaḥ (*vāta* is [known by the *sāma vāta lakṣhaṇas* of]) śhūla (abdominal pain, discomfort), ānāha (abdominal distention, bloating), aṅgamarda (squeezing pain in the bodily limbs), mukhaśhoṣha (dryness of the mouth and oral cavity), mūrchchhā (fainting), bhrama (dizziness), āgnivaiṣhamya (abnormal state of *agni*), pārśhva-pṛṣhṭha-kaṭi-graha (tightness, limited mobility of the sides of the waist, back and spine and hips), sirā-kuñchana (contraction of the veins), stambhanāni (and stiffness) karoti (being produced); pittaṁ (*pitta* is [known by the *sāma pitta lakṣhaṇas* of]) punarjvara (recurrent fever), ātīsāra (diarrhea), āntardāha (internal burning sensation), tṛṣhṇā (thirst), mada (behavior similar to intoxication), bhrama (dizziness), pralapanāni (and excessive, irrelevant talking); śhleṣhmā tu (*kapha* is [known by the *sāma kapha lakṣhaṇas* of]) chhardi (vomiting), arochakā (loss of the normal sense of taste), vipāka (improper or abnormal final outputs of digestion), śhītajvara (cold fever), ālasya (complete lack of enthusiasm or motivation), gātra-gauravāṇi (and heaviness in the limbs).

Sāma vāta lakṣhaṇas Causative factors that produce metabolic waste	Cha. Vi. 2/7			
Sroto-rodha Obstruction of the *srotases*	✓			
Śhūla Abdominal pain, discomfort	✓			
Ānāha Abdominal distention, bloating	✓			
Aṅgamarda Squeezing pain in the bodily limbs	✓			
Mukhaśhoṣha Dryness of the mouth and oral cavity	✓			
Mūrchchhā Fainting	✓			
Bhrama Dizziness	✓			
Agnivaiṣhamya Abnormal state of *agni*	✓			

Pārśhva, pṛṣhṭha, kaṭi graha Tightness, limited mobility, of the sides of the waist, back and spine and hips	✓			
Sirā-kuñchana Contraction of the veins	✓			
Stambhanāni Stiffness	✓			

Sāma pitta lakṣhaṇas Causative factors that produce metabolic waste	Cha. Vi. 2/7			
Punarjvara Recurrent fever	✓			
Atīsāra Diarrhea	✓			
Antardāha Internal burning sensation	✓			
Tṛṣhṇā Thirst	✓			
Mada Behavior similar to intoxication	✓			
Bhrama Dizziness	✓			
Pralapanāni Excessive, irrelevant talk	✓			

Sāma kapha lakṣhaṇas Causative factors that produce metabolic waste	Cha. Vi. 2/7			
Chhardi Vomiting	✓			
Arochakā Loss of the normal sense of taste	✓			
Vipāka Improper or abnormal final outputs of digestion	✓			
Śhītajvara Cold fever	✓			

Ālasya Complete lack of enthusiasm or motivation	✓			
Gātra-gauravāṇi Heaviness in the limbs	✓			

Āhāra

Everything which is consumed on a physical level by the human body can contribute or detract from svastha and ultimately āyu. While the guṇa and karma of the āhāra are critically important to this outcome, they are not the only factors. The external environment, season, routines, mental state and *agni* of the individual contribute dramatically to how the consumed food is processed and assimilated.

This section on āhāra and its role in contributing to svastha will review major classical perspectives on food and its modulations. Processing methods and food combinations are essential to properly understanding the final effect on any individual.

In the Charaka Saṁhitā, the teacher Punarvasu Ātreya recognizes the importance of food to overall lifespan and quality of life.

प्राणाःप्राणभृतामन्नमन्नंलोकोऽभिधावति ।
वर्णःप्रसादःसौस्वर्यंजीवितंप्रतिभासुखम् ॥

च. सू. २७।३४९

Prāṇāḥ prāṇabhṛtāmannamannaṁ loko ' bhidhāvati |
Varṇaḥ prasādaḥ sausvaryaṁ jīvitaṁ pratibhā sukham ||

Cha. Sū. 27/349

Prāṇāḥ (Continuity of life) prāṇabhṛtām (and all living beings) annam (is [possible because of] food) annaṁ loko ' bhidhāvati (and the entire world is dependent upon food). Varṇaḥ (Healthy complexion), prasādaḥ (clear, unimpeded energetic output), sausvaryaṁ (proper vocal expression and voice), jīvitaṁ (full quality of life), pratibhā (proper understanding and comprehension) sukham (and contentment [are all dependent on food]).

Food is a critical component to experiencing the highest potential of life. The conversion of consumed food into bodily tissues is equally important.

बलमारोग्यमायुश्चप्राणाश्चाग्नौप्रतिष्ठिताः।
अन्नपानेन्धनैश्चाग्निर्ज्वलतिव्येतिचान्यथा ॥

च. सू. २७।३४२

Balamārogyamāyuśhcha prāṇāśhchāgnau pratiṣhṭhitāḥ |
Annapānendhanaiśhchāgnirjvalati vyeti chānyathā ||

Cha. Sū. 27/342

Balam (Physical strength and resilience), ārogyam (complete absence of disease), āyuśhcha (life, lifespan, vitality) prāṇāśhcha (and continuity of life) agnau pratiṣhṭhitāḥ (are all depending on *agni*, which is a function of both) anna (food) pāna (and drink) indhanaiśhcha (as the fuel) agnirjvalati (which sustains it [*agni*, the digestive power]) vyeti chānyathā (or diminishes it, otherwise [in the absence of food and drink]).

Agni is responsible for the conversion of all consumed food and drink. This is the starting point for understanding the creation of human life and health.

In some spheres of New Age Āyurveda, it has been proposed that the "mind digests thoughts and emotions" in a way that is similar to the processes of āhāra and agni. This hypothesis has no basis in Classical Āyurveda and should be questioned to demonstrate its logical functioning. The processing of information and emotions are described classically through their own framework beginning in Cha. Sū. 11/.

Through direct interaction, study and testing of foods and drinks, traditional Āyurvedic scholars and clinicians understood their complex mechanics. They developed the framework of Āyurveda on the multifactorial approach which allows seemingly disparate concepts to relate and function inter-dependently.

इष्टवर्णगन्धरसस्पर्शंविधिविहितमन्नपानंप्रा
णिनांप्राणिसञ्ज्ञकानांप्राणमाचक्षतेकुशलाः,
प्रत्यक्षफलदर्शनात्;
तदिन्धनाह्यन्तरग्नेःस्थितिः; तत्सत्त्वमूर्जयति,
तच्छरीरधातुव्यूहबलवर्णेन्द्रियप्रसादकरंय
थोक्तमुपसेव्यमानं,
विपरीतमहितायसम्पद्यते ॥

च. सू. २७।३

Iṣhṭavarṇagandharasasparśhaṁ vidhivihitamannapānaṁ prāṇināṁ prāṇisañjñakānāṁ prāṇamāchakṣhate kuśhalāḥ, pratyakṣhaphaladarśhanāt; tadindhanā hyantaragneḥsthitiḥ; tat sattvamūrjayati, tachcharīradhātuvyūhabalavarṇendriyap rasādakaraṁ yathoktamupasevyamānaṁ, viparītamahitāya sampadyate ||

Cha. Sū. 27/3

Iṣhṭa (Desirable [proper, correct]) varṇa (color), gandha (smell), rasa (taste), sparśhaṁ (and feel) vidhivi (in the correct proportions and manners [of season, growth period, etc]) hitam ([produce] healthy) anna (food) pānaṁ (and drinks) prāṇināṁ (for all living beings) prāṇi sañjñakānāṁ prāṇam āchakṣhate kuśhalāḥ (according to the wise and learned experts). Pratyakṣha (Direct observation and methodical study) phala darśhanāt (provided these results). Tad indhanā (This fuel [ie, proper food and drink]) hyantaragneḥsthitiḥ (is responsible for the stable functioning of *agni*); tat (it also) sattvamūrjayati (invigorates and strengthens *sattva*), tac (it also) karaṁ (increases) charīra-dhātuvyūha (encourages proper development of the bodily tissues), bala (physical strength and resilience), varṇa (complexion and skin tone), indriyaprasāda (clear, unimpeded functioning of the sense organs). Yatha (These) uktam-upasevyamānaṁ (are all possible when the correct measurements area applied meticulously); viparītamahitāya (otherwise, the opposite) sampadyate (results).

When food and drink are used judiciously throughout an individual's life, the expectation is that, barring other uncontrollable factors, they will experience longevity in quantity and quality.

षड्त्रिंशतंसहस्राणिरात्रीणांहितभोजनः।
जीवत्यनातुरोजन्तुर्जितात्मासम्मतःसताम्

च. सू. २७।३४८

Ṣhaḍtriṁśhataṁ sahasrāṇi rātrīṇāṁ hitabhojanaḥ |
Jīvatyanāturo janturjitātmā sammataḥ satām ||

Cha. Sū. 27/348

Ṣhaḍtriṁśhataṁ sahasrāṇi rātrīṇāṁ (Achieving [accomplishing, or successfully living through] 36,000 nights) hita-bhojanaḥ (is due to proper eating habits). Jīvatyanāturo (It promotes a life free from disease), janturjitātmā (supports spiritual development) sammataḥ satām (and encourages respect from all).

Adaptability and sustainability

The use of foods and drinks to support and

promote health today is significantly different from what would have been typical several centuries ago. With modern transportation systems, industrial farming and increasing popularity of marketable concepts like superfoods, the food landscape is flooded with choices.

Making exotic foods available to people globally comes at a cost which is much higher than what the consumer pays. At the expense of habitat destruction, pollution and climate change, food demands are pushing the limits of the earth's environment.

Classically, Āyurveda was meant to be practiced on a local scale using readily available materials. It is likely that this approach may have evolved from over-exploitation of natural resources several thousand years ago .

A significant number of dravya mentioned in the older texts, including the Charaka Saṁhitā and Suśhruta Saṁhita, are unidentifiable today. Bhāvamiśhra recognizes this and states in Bhāva Prakāśha that when specific dravya are no longer available, they should be replaced with their nearest equivalent that is readily available. This indicates the probable over-harvesting of medicinal resources.

Additionally, Charaka supports the use of locally available dravya in different regions. His reference states this indirectly, likely because of the limitations of transportation of goods at the time of writing.

Today, it is imperative that cultures globablly focus on creating and maintaining sustainable resources. To properly apply Āyurveda outside of the Indian subcontinent, it must be adapted to the needs of the local culture and place. Appropriate dravya and protocols must be researched and developed to support its adaptations.

Export of dravya and medicinal formulations from India creates an unsustainable market for Āyurveda which will burst as every other capitalistic bubble does. It also allows the over-exploitation of people and natural resources to continue in a country that was under foreign rule for hundreds of years.

When considering the information in this chapter and its application outside of India, keep these implications in mind. The true practice of Āyurveda should produce a sustainable, holistic health care system.

अन्नपानैकदेशोऽयमुक्तःप्रायोपयोगिकः ।
द्रव्याणिनहिनिर्देष्टुंशक्यंकात्स्न्येननामभिः ॥ ३२९
यथानानौषधंकिञ्चिद्देशजानांवचोयथा ।
द्रव्यंतत्तत्थावाच्यमनुक्तमिहयद्भवेत् ॥ ३३०

च. सू. २७।३२९-३३०

Annapānaikadeśho'yamuktaḥ prāyopayogikaḥ |
Dravyāṇi na hi nirdeṣhṭuṁ śhakyaṁ kārtsnyena nāmabhiḥ || 329
Yathā nānauṣhadhaṁ kiñciddeśhajānāṁ vacho yathā |
Dravyaṁ tattattathā vāchyamanuktamiha yadbhavet || 330

Cha. Sū. 27/329-330

Anna (The foods) pāna (and drinks) eka-deśho (described here [in this chapter]) ' yamuktaḥ (are only one source) prāyopayogikaḥ (for the application of this science). Dravyāṇi na hi nirdeṣhṭuṁ (It is not possible to enumerate all of the dravya in existence) śhakyaṁ kārtsnyena nāmabhiḥ (with their names, details and properties). Yathā nānauṣhadhaṁ (Ultimately, everything can be used medicinally) kiñcid-deśhajānāṁ (according to the location and people) vacho (who are able to convey that knowledge). Yathā dravyaṁ (And so those dravya) tattattathā (can be utilized [in the framework of Āyurveda]) vāchyam {through the experts of their use) anuktamiha yadbhavet (when they have not been mentioned here).

Additionally, the terms *hita* and *ahita* are regularly used in the context of *āhāra*. These two terms refer to the healthy or unhealthy implications of any food. Depending on the context of usage, this may apply to a single individual or more than one person.

It is commonly seen in practice that certain individuals respond very well or very poorly to specific *dravya* or certain food combinations. Likewise, a group of people, such as a family or ethnic subpopulation, may respond in similar ways. *Hita* and *ahita* can be used to describe these responses in both individual and group scenarios.

हिताहारोपयोग एकएव पुरुषवृद्धिकरो भवति,

च. सू. २५।३१

Hitāhāropayoga ekaeva puruṣhavṛddhikaro bhavati,

Cha. Sū. 25/31

Hita āhāra upayoga (Wholesome food when regularly consumed) ekaeva bhavati (is the primary factor for) puruṣha vṛddhi karo (causing growth in human beings).

Hita āhāra is that which is wholesome when used regularly. Wholesome can be determined by the outcome of proper growth and development of the individual.

अहिताहारोपयोगः पुनर्व्याधिनिमित्तमिति ॥

च. सू. २५।३१

Ahitāhāropayogaḥ punarvyādhinimittamiti ||

Cha. Sū. 25/31

Ahita āhāra upayogaḥ (Unwholesome food when regularly consumed) punar-vyādhi nimittam iti (as mentioned earlier, is the cause for disease).

Ahita āhāra is that which consistently causes disease when used regularly.

Determination of healthy food

Differentiating between *hita* and *ahita āhāra* is essentially the determination between healthy and unhealthy, or wholesome and unwholesome food.

While many things exist that can be considered universally harmful, clinical practice of healthy diet requires an individual approach. The parameters to make this determination must be assessed against the individual using themselves as the baseline for measurement.

This approach also impacts the perception that certain foods are always healthy while others may not be. This simplistic perception obstructs the clinician's ability to understand the scale of impact that food can have on an individual.

Depending on the state of the individual in various factors, tolerance to certain foods can change over time. Therefore, it is possible that any given food (or combination) can cause health or disease depending on the state of the individual.

येषामेव हि भावानां सम्पत् सञ्जनयेन्नरम् ।
तेषामेव विपद्व्याधीन्विविधान्समुदीरयेत् ॥

च. सू. २५।२९

Yeṣhāmeva hi bhāvānāṁ sampat sañjanayennaram |
Teṣhāmeva vipadvyādhīnvividhānsamudīrayet ||

Cha. Sū. 25/29

Yeṣhāmeva (Those very same foods) hi bhāvānāṁ (which are) sampat sañjanayennaram (properly utilized as food) teṣhāmeva (can also be) vipad-vyādhīn (the cause of disease) vividhān samudīrayet (when applied incorrectly).

The question then arises as to how to determine the proper or improper application of food for an individual. Charaka provides general guidance for this through the scientific application of Āyurveda using specifics of Dravya-guṇa Śhāstra. Suśhruta elaborates on this in chapters 41/ through 46/ in sūtrasthāna.

... लघूनि हि द्रव्याणि वाय्वग्निगुणबहुलानि भवन्ति;
पृथ्वीसोमगुणबहुलानीतराणि,तस्मात् स्वगुणादपि
लघून्यग्निसन्धुक्षणस्वभावान्यल्पदोषाणि
चोच्यन्तेऽपि सौहित्योपयुक्तानि,
गुरूणिपुनर्नाग्निसन्धुक्षणस्वभावान्यसामा न्यात्, अतश्चातिमात्रं दोषवन्ति
सौहित्योपयुक्तान्यन्यत्र व्यायामाग्निबलात्;
सैषाभवत्यग्निबलापेक्षिणी मात्रा ||

च. सू. ५।६

... gurulāghavamakāraṇaṁ manyeta,
laghūni hi dravyāṇi
vāyvagniguṇabahulānibhavanti;
pṛthvīsomaguṇabahulānītarāṇi, tasmāt
svaguṇādapilaghūnyagnisandhukṣhaṇa
svabhāvānyalpadoṣhāṇi chohcyante'pi
sauhityopayuktāni,
gurūṇipunarnāgnisandhukṣhaṇasvabhāv
ānyasāmānyāt, ataśhchātimātraṁ
doṣhavanti
sauhityopayuktānyanyatravyāyāmāgnib
alāt; saiṣhā bhavatyagnibalāpekṣhiṇī
mātrā || 6

Cha. Sū. 5/6

Laghūni hi dravyāṇi (*Dravya* which are inherently *laghu*) vāyv-agni guṇa bahulāni bhavanti (are predominant in *guṇas* related to *vāyu* and *agni*). Pṛthvī soma guṇa bahulānītarāṇi (Likewise, [*dravya* which are inherently *guru*] are predominant in *guṇas* related to *pṛthvī* and *soma* [*ap*, or *jala*]). Tasmāt (Therefore), sva-guṇād-api (by their own similar *guṇas*), laghūni (those *dravya* which are *laghu*) agni sandhu (are similar to *agni*) kṣhaṇa svabhāvāni (by their very nature) alpa-doṣhāṇi chochyante (and thus produce minimal *doṣhas*). Api (And so), sauhitya (they are still less harmful) upayuktāni (even if they are used excessively). Gurūṇi (*Dravya* which are *guru*) punar na-agni sandhu (are dissimilar to *agni*) kṣhaṇa svabhāvāni (by their very nature) asāmānyāt (based on their opposite qualities). Ataśhcha (Therefore), atimātraṁ (excessive use [of *guru dravya*]) doṣhavanti (increases the *doṣhas*). Sauhitya (They can still be less harmful) upayuktāni (even if they are used excessively) anyatra (and the individual) vyāyāma (performs sufficient vyāyāma, or physical training) agnibalāt (to promote the strength of agni). Saiṣhā bhavati agni-bala (And so ultimately, it is the state of *agni*) āpekṣhiṇī (which determines) mātrā (the proper quantity of food).

Multifactorial perspective

In the determination of healthy versus unhealthy food, the main factors to take into consideration are

- *mātra*
- *agni bala*

Once these have been determined, several additional factors should be assessed as required.

These additional factors are found in several references classically. However, there does not seem to be a definitive, final conclusion on which factors must always be assessed. This indicates that the clinician is responsible to apply whichever are required for each patient.

Agniveśha asks his teacher, Punarvasu Ātreya for guidance on understanding this multifactorial approach.

एवंवादिनं भगवन्तमात्रेयमग्निवेश उवाच - कथमिह भगवन् !
हिताहितानामाहारजातानां लक्षणमनपवादमभिजानीमहे;
हितसमाख्यातानामाहारजातानामहितसमाख्यातानां च मात्राकालक्रियाभूमिदेहदोषपुरुषावस्थान्तरेषुविपरीतकारित्वमुपलभामह इति ||
च. सू. २५।३२

Evaṁvādinaṁ bhagavantamātreyamagniveśha uvācha - kathamiha Bhagavan!
Hitāhitānāmāhārajātānāṁlakṣhaṇamanapavādamabhijānīmahe;
hitasamākhyātānāmāhārajātānāmahitasamākhyātānāṁ chamātrākālakriyābhūmidehadoṣhapuruṣhāvasthāntareṣhu viparītakāritvamupalabhāmaha iti ||
Cha. Sū. 25/32

Evaṁvādinaṁ (And so, after listening to what was stated) bhagavantam ātreyam (by his teacher, Bhagavan Ātreya), agniveśha (Agniveśha) uvācha (asked) - kathamiha (Then, what do we do,) Bhagavan (Sir)?

Hita ([Sometimes], wholesome) ahitānām (and unwholesome) āhāra (food or diet) jātānāṁ lakṣhaṇam (having known properties and actions) anapavādam abhijānīmahe (do not produce expected results). Hita samākhyātānām āhāra (Instead, that food which is known to be wholesome) jātānām (produces) ahita (unwholesome) samākhyātānāṁ cha (results, and vice versa, due to) mātrā (quantity), kāla (time), kriyā (processing or preparation methods), bhūmi (location), deha (the physical body [of the individual]), doṣha (*doṣha*[s]) puruṣha avastha (and the stage of development of the individual [age, disease, etc]). Antareṣhu viparīta kāritvam upalabhāmaha iti (How are these two oppositions possible)?

Here, Agniveśha begins to identify the multiple factors that influence the determination of *hita* or *ahita āhāra*. He includes:

- mātrā
- kāla
- kriyā
- bhūmi
- deha
- doṣha
- puruṣha avastha

These factors had been previously identified in Cha. Sū. 25/46.

मात्राकालक्रियाभूमिदेहदोषगुणान्तरम् |
प्राप्य तत्तद्धि दृश्यन्ते ते ते भावास्तथा तथा ||
च. सू. २५।४६

Mātrākālakriyābhūmidehadoṣhaguṇāntaram |
Prāpya tattaddhi dṛśhyante te te bhāvāstathā tathā ||
Cha. Sū. 25/46

Mātrā (Quantity), kāla (time), kriyā (processing or preparation methods), bhūmi (location), deha (the physical body), doṣha (the doṣhas) guṇāntaram (and all of their related *guṇas*) prāpya tattaddhi dṛśhyante (contribute as determinant factors) te te bhāvāstathā tathā (to the variety of outcomes).

Charaka specifically identifies the factors which are responsible for producing viruddha āhāra, incompatible food combinations. These will be discussed later in this section.

Viruddha āhāra is *ahita* and produces detrimental effects on human health. To avoid these food combinations, the following factors should always be considered so that food maintains natural homeostasis.

यच्चापि
देशकालाग्निमात्रासात्म्यानिलादिभिः |
संस्कारतो वीर्यतश्च कोष्ठावस्थाक्रमैरपि ||
च. सू. २६।८६

Yachchāpi
deśhakālāgnimātrāsātmyānilādibhiḥ
Saṁskārato vīryataśhcha
koṣhṭhāvasthākramairapi ||
Cha. Sū. 26/86

Yachchāpi (And so, the) deśha (location), kāla (time), agni (state and power of agni), mātrā (quantity), sātmya (state of *sātmya*) anilādibhiḥ (*vāta*, and the other *doṣhas*), saṁskārato (all processing and preparation methods), vīryataśhcha (potency and effects), koṣhṭha (type of digestive system), avasthā (and all related stages) kramairapi (must always be considered).

Here, the key factors are more extensive, and presented in a different order.

- deśha
- kāla
- agni
- mātrā
- sātmya
- anilādibhiḥ
- saṁskāra
- vīryataśhcha
- koṣhṭha
- avasthā

In the context of clinical assessment, Punarvasu Ātreya provides an explicit list which includes assessment of food. In the context of the current review of *āhāra*, these should be considered related factors.

इह खलु व्याधीनां
निमित्तपूर्वरूपरूपोपशयसङ्ख्याप्राधान्य
विधिविकल्प
बलकालविशेषाननुप्रविश्यानन्तरं
दोषभेषजदेशकालबलशरीरसाराहारसा
त्म्यसत्त्वप्रकृतिवयसां मानमवहितमनसा
यथावज्ज्ञेयं भवति भिषजा,
दोषादिमानज्ञानायत्तत्वात् क्रियायाः |
न ह्यमानज्ञो दोषादीनां भिषग्
व्याधिनिग्रहसमर्थो भवति |
तस्माद्दोषादिमानज्ञानार्थं
विमानस्थानमुपदेक्ष्यामोऽग्निवेश! || ३
च. वि. १।३

Iha khalu vyādhīnāṁ
nimittapūrvarūparūpopaśhayasaṅkhyāpr
ādhānyavidhivikalpa
balakālaviśheṣhānanupraviśhyānantara
ṁ
doṣhabheṣhajadeśhakālabalaśharīrasār
āhārasātmyasattvaprakr̥tivayasāṁ
mānamavahitamanasā yathāvajjñeyaṁ
bhavati bhiṣhajā,
doṣhādimānajñānāyattatvāt kriyāyāḥ |
Na hyamānajño doṣhādīnāṁ bhiṣhag
vyādhinigrahasamartho bhavati |
Tasmāddoṣhādimānajñānārthaṁ
vimānasthānamupadekṣhyāmo '
gniveśha! || 3
Cha. Vi. 1/3

The key factors include:

- *doṣha*
- *bheṣhaja*
- *deśha*
- *kāla*
- *bala*
- *śharīra*
- *sāra*
- *āhāra sātmya*
- *sattva*

- *prakṛti*
- *vayasāṁ*

A similar and more elaborate explanation is given in Cha. Sū. 28/7 to reiterate the importance of thorough clinical assessment in practice.

How these factors determine any outcome in a given individual depends entirely on that person's unique situation. In some cases, certain factors will contribute greater weight or priority. This can be calculated and estimated by investigating causative factors.

Charaka provides a general rule for calculating outcomes within a multifactorial approach. Because of the infinitely variable number of possible inputs, it is impossible to arrive at a single calculation method to derive predictable outcomes.

संसर्गविकल्पविस्तरो ह्येषामपरिसङ्ख्येयो भवति, विकल्पभेदापरिसङ्ख्येयत्वात् ||
च. वि. १|८

Saṁsargavikalpavistaro hyeṣhāmaparisaṅkhyeyo bhavati, vikalpabhedāparisaṅkhyeyatvāt ||
Cha. Vi. 1/8

Saṁsarga (The number of possible combinations [as presentations]) vikalpa-vistaro (based on permutations of inputs) hyeṣhām aparisaṅkhyeyo bhavati (cannot be enumerated because) vikalpa bhed (the number of combinations) āpari-saṅkhyeyatvāt (is infinite).

The reason for inifite combinations and permutations spans through each of the factors in this framework. This variability means that no study of human health can be completely controlled. This applies to all systems of medicine in various ways, depending on their paradigm and systematic methods for measuring indicators and calculating outcomes.

Most notably, the factor of *kāla*, or time, can never be controlled in any experiment or study.

When assessing food, the factors which relate to the *dravya* are of primary significance.

तत्र खल्वनेकरसेषु द्रव्येष्वनेकदोषात्मकेषु च विकारेषु
रसदोषप्रभावमेकैकश्येनाभिसमीक्ष्य ततो द्रव्यविकारयोः प्रभावतत्त्वं व्यवस्येत् ||
च. वि. १|९

Tatra khalvanekaraseṣhu dravyeṣhvanekadoṣhātmakeṣhu cha vikāreṣhu rasadoṣhaprabhāvamekaikaśhyenābhis amīkṣhya tato dravyavikārayoḥ prabhāvatattvaṁ vyavasyet || 9
Cha. Vi. 1/9

Tatra khalvan (In any situation, whether it be) eka-raseṣhu dravyeṣhu (a *dravya* having a single, primary *rasa*) aneka-doṣhātmakeṣhu cha vikāreṣhu (or a complex pathology presenting with multiple *doṣhas*), rasa (the *rasa*) doṣha (and the *doṣha*) prabhāvam (and their own special effects) ekaikaśhyena abhisamīkṣhya (must be critically analyzed individually, first). Tato (Then), dravya-vikārayoḥ prabhāva (the special effect of the dravya to counteract the disease) tattvaṁ vyavasyet (can be determined).

When assessing appropriate and inappropriate *āhāra*, the same methodology should be followed.

In the following line (Cha. Vi. 1/10), however, Charaka clarifies that in complex presentations and disorders, this general approach is insufficient.

This provides baseline guidance to demarcate the practice of clinical Āyurveda at various professional levels.

न त्वेवं खलु सर्वत्र ।
न हि विकृतिविषमसमवेतानां नानात्मकानां परस्परेण चोपहतानामन्यैश्च विकल्पनैर्विकल्पितानामवयवप्रभावानुमाने नैव समुदायप्रभावतत्त्वमध्यवसातुं शक्यम् ॥

च. वि. १।१०

Na tvevaṁ khalu sarvatra |
Na hi vikr̥tiviṣhamasamavetānāṁ nānātmakānāṁ paraspareṇa chopahatānāmanyaiśhcha vikalpanairvikalpitānāmavayavaprabhāvānumānenaiva samudāyaprabhāvatattvamadhyavasātuṁ śhakyam ||

Cha. Vi. 1/10

But this rule is not applicable universally because in case of complex disorders (and dravyas) where the effect is not exactly in accordance with the cause due to multiple causative factors operating, with differing (often conflicting) modes of operation, it is not possible to determine the effect of the dravya or the disease on the basis of the effect of individual rasas or doshas. [10]

At all levels of practice, the total outcome over time can also provide insight into the effect of continuous use of specific *āhāra*.

तथायुक्ते हि समुदये समुदायप्रभावतत्त्वमेवमेवोपलभ्य ततो द्रव्यविकारप्रभावतत्त्वं व्यवस्येत् ॥

च. वि. १।११

Tathāyukte hi samudaye samudāyaprabhāvatattvamevamevopalabhya tato dravyavikāraprabhāvatattvaṁ vyavasyet ||

Cha. Vi. 1/11

In such cases, the effect of the dravya or the disease is ascertained on the basis of their cumulative action.

And so the presentation of information in the Charaka Saṁhitā is organized to focus on rasa through its input *dravya* and *doṣha* as the outcome effect.

तस्माद्रसप्रभावतश्च द्रव्यप्रभावतश्च दोषप्रभावतश्च विकारप्रभावतश्च तत्त्वमुपदेक्ष्यामः ॥

च. वि. १।१२

Tasmādrasaprabhāvataśhcha dravyaprabhāvataśhcha doṣhaprabhāvataśhcha vikāraprabhāvataśhcha tattvamupadekṣhyāmaḥ ||

Cha. Vi. 1/12

Therefore, we shall describe the concept according to the effect of *rasa* (individual) and *dravya* (total) on one side and *doṣha* (individual) and disease (total) on the other.

Charaka discusses examples of improper application of the multifactorial approach in Cha. Sū. 26/86-101. Review the original text for that discussion.

Dual-factor perspective (guru and laghu)

When assessing *āhāra*, the two primary factors to consider are the total effect in terms of *guru* and *laghu*. These *guṇas* are ultimately responsible for the quantity of food consumed and the *agni* required to digest and assimilate it properly.

The determination of heaviness or lightness of a food or meal will also depend on the quantity consumed and the individual's current state of *agni*. A proportionate relationship should therefore exist among these.

अल्पादानेगुरूणांचलघूनांचातिसेवने ।

मात्राकारणमुद्दिष्टंद्रव्याणांगुरुलाघवे ॥
३४०
गुरूणामल्पमादेयंलघूनांतृप्तिरिष्यते ।
मात्रांद्रव्याण्यपेक्षन्ते मात्राचाग्निमपेक्षते ॥
३४१

च. सू. २७।३४०-३४१

Alpādāne gurūṇāṁ cha laghūnāṁ cātisevane |
Mātrā kāraṇamuddiṣhṭaṁ dravyāṇāṁ gurulāghave || 340
Gurūṇāmalpamādeyaṁ laghūnāṁ tṛptiriṣhyate |
Mātrāṁ dravyāṇyapekṣhante mātrā cāgnimapekṣhate || 341

Cha. Sū. 27/340-341

Heavy articles should be consumed in small measures and light ones in large quantities.

Food articles should thus be consumed in proper measure and the proper measure should be in accordance with the strength of the individual's *agni*.

When considering how heaviness and lightness may impact an individual's digestive capacity and function, their current state and energetic demand must also be considered.

Those who are less active, suffering from disease, generally weak or accustomed to an easy life should consider heaviness and lightness of food as a priority.

गुरुलाघवचिन्तेयंप्रायेणाल्पबलान्प्रति ।
मन्दक्रियाननारोग्यान्सुकुमारान्सुखोचितान्
॥

च. सू. २७।३४३

Gurulāghavacinteyaṁ prāyeṇālpabalān prati |
Mandakriyānanārogyān sukumārānsukhocitān ||

Cha. Sū. 27/343

The consideration of heaviness and lightness of food articles is particularly important for those who are generally weak, indolent, unhealthy, fragile or in a delicate condition of health, and those given to luxury.

Consideration of heaviness and lightness is most important for the following:

- *Manda kriya*
- *Ananārogyān*
- *Sukumāra*
- *Ansukhocitān*

Classically, the examples of common foods demonstrate the application of lightness and heaviness. Note that these foods were common at the time of writing and many are still in regular use today in various parts of India.

तत्र
शालिषष्टिकमुद्गलावकपिञ्जलैणशशशरभ
शम्बरादीन्याहारद्रव्याणि प्रकृतिलघून्यपि
मात्रापेक्षीणि भवन्ति |
तथा
पिष्टेक्षुक्षीरविकृतितिलमाषानूपौदकपिशिता
दीन्याहारद्रव्याणि प्रकृतिगुरूण्यपि
मात्रामेवापेक्षन्ते || ५

च. सू. ५।५

Tatra śhāliṣhaṣhṭikamudgalāvakapiñjalaiṇaśhaśhaśharabhaśhambarādīnyāhāradravyāṇi prakṛtilaghūnyapimātrāpekṣhīṇi bhavanti |
Tathā piṣhṭekṣhukṣhīravikṛtitilamāṣhānūpaudakapiśhitādīnyāhāradravyāṇi prakṛtigurūṇyapimātrāmevāpekṣhante || 5

Cha. Sū. 5/5

Thus, shali rice (Oryza sativum), shashtika rice (variety of Oryza sativum), mudga (Vigna radiata green gram), common quail, gray partridge, antelope, rabbit, wapiti, Indian sambar deer, and such other food-articles, though light to digest by their inherent properties, depends on the proper quantity. Similarly, preparations of flour (pastry), sugar-cane juice and sugar preparations, milk and milk preparations, til (Sesamum indicum-sesame), masha (Vigna mungo-black gram), flesh of aquatic animals, marshy land animals are inherently heavy to digest foods.

Certain individuals will not be affected by the heaviness or lightness of food primarily due to their baseline constitution and influenced by their energetic demand. People who have a strong *agni*, or used to hard-to-digest foods, or do physically demanding work daily, or have a high capacity for consumption and digestion, are generally unaffected.

दीप्ताग्नयःखराहाराःकर्मनित्यामहोदराः ।
येनराःप्रतितांश्चिन्त्यंनावश्यंगुरुलाघवम् ॥

च. सू. २७।३४४

Dīptāgnayaḥ kharāhārāḥ karmanityā mahodarāḥ |
Ye narāḥ prati tāṁśhcintyaṁ nāvaśhyaṁ gurulāghavam ||

Cha. Sū. 27/344

For those whose *agni* is strong, are accustomed to tough-to-digest food articles, are accustomed to hard labor and have a large capacity for consumption and digestion of food, the consideration of heavy and light food is not necessary.

Consideration of heaviness and lightness generally does not affect the following:

- *Dīptāgnayaḥ*
- *kharāhārāḥ*
- *karmanityā*
- *mahodarāḥ*

To determine heaviness or lightness of any dravya, Charaka provides several examples in the context of animal meat. Using the various parts of the body for consumption, specific guṇas can be connected to understand the effect on the physical body.

These examples demonstrate the underlying principles of *Sāmānya-Viśheṣha*, *Samavāya-Samavāyi* and *Vṛddhi-Kṣhaya*. The function together to transmute the *guṇas* of the consumed *āhāra* by the animal into its constituent parts. When consumed by humans, these *guṇas* are again converted into the corresponding tissues and components. See Cha. Sū. 27-331-338 for examples.

Proper outcomes and benefits

Judicious use of food over the course of life is stated to promote āyu and positive health outcomes. This allows one to fully be present in their life and accomplish desired goals.

आहिताग्निःसदापथ्यान्यन्तरग्नौजुहोतियः ।
दिवसेदिवसेब्रह्मजपत्यथददातिच ॥ ३४६
नरंनिःश्रेयसेयुक्तंसात्म्यज्ञंपानभोजने ।
भजन्तेनामयाःकेचिद्भाविनोऽप्यन्तराद्दते ॥ ३४७

च. सू. २७।३४६-३४७

Āhitāgniḥ sadā pathyānyantaragnau juhoti yaḥ |
Divase divase brahma japatyatha dadāti cha || 346
Naraṁ niḥśhreyase yuktaṁ sātmyajñaṁ pānabhojane |
Bhajante nāmayāḥ kecidbhāvino'pyantarādṛte || 347

Cha. Sū. 27/346-347

The man whose agni is well tended, who feeds it duly with wholesome diet, who does daily meditation, charity and the pursuit of spiritual salvation, and who takes food and drinks that are wholesome to him, will not fall to approaching diseases except for special reasons.

Consumed food has a direct effect on the *doṣhas*. Recall that the *doṣhas* function to promote health or produce disease, depending on their state.

दोषाः पुनस्त्रयो वातपित्तश्लेष्माणः |
ते प्रकृतिभूताः शरीरोपकारका भवन्ति,
विकृतिमापन्नास्तु खलु नानाविधैर्विकारैः
शरीरमुपतापयन्ति || ५

च. वि. १।५

Doṣhāḥ punastrayo vātapittaśhleṣhmāṇaḥ |
Te prakṛtibhūtāḥ śharīropakārakā bhavanti, vikṛtimāpannāstu khalu nānāvidhairvikāraiḥ śharīramupatāpayanti || 5

Cha. Vi. 1/5

The three *doṣhas* are *vāta*, *pitta* and *śhleṣhma* (*kapha*). In their normal state, they support and sustain the body. In an abnormal state, they are the causes of various disorders in the body.

General guidelines for food consumption

To promote *svastha*, Charaka clearly states that one should adhere to daily regimens that are wholesome. This also prevents the onset of disease.

तच्च नित्यं प्रयुञ्जीत स्वास्थ्यं येनानुवर्तते |
अजातानां विकाराणामनुत्पत्तिकरं च यत् ||

च. सू. ५।१३

Tacca nityaṁ prayuñjīta svāsthyaṁ yenānuvartate |
Ajātānāṁ vikārāṇāmanutpattikaraṁ cha yat ||

Cha. Sū. 5/13

One should maintain a daily regimen that supports health and prevents the onset of diseases.

Recommendations and restrictions

Food in classical Āyurveda consists of extensive documentation on the qualitites, actions and special effects of single *dravya*. *Dravya* are classified into 12 groups used for regular consumption. These categories will be discussed in the following section.

Several lists of recommendations are also provided for general use. The should be considered for every individual, and in the context of the intended audience of India at the time of writing.

The most wholesome and unwholesome foods are listed in Cha. Sū. 25/38-40. Review the tables in Chapter 1 of this volume for an explanation.

Additionally, Charaka describes specific foods that should always be avoided in Cha. Sū. 5/10-11. Following that, foods that should be consumed regularly are provided in Cha. Sū. 5/12 and Cha. Sū. 27/4.

Certain dravya are restricted for regular use, or in their quantity. Three special dravya are significant because they are highly medicinal and are likely reserved for therapeutic effect. These are discussed in Cha. Vi. 1/16-18.

If any of the restricted dravya are used

excessively, they should be identified and controlled appropriately. The schedule for removing asātmya and okasātmya dravya can be followed here.

तस्मात्तेषां तत्सात्म्यतः क्रमेणापगमनं श्रेयः | सात्म्यमपि हि क्रमेणोपनिवर्त्यमानमदोषमल्पदोषं वा भवति || १९

च. वि. १।१९

Tasmātteṣhāṁ tatsātmyataḥ krameṇāpagamanaṁ śhreyaḥ |
Sātmyamapi hi krameṇopanivartyamānamadoṣhamalpa doṣhaṁ vā bhavati ||

Cha. Vi. 1/19

It is always beneficial to gradually eliminate the use of these substances. Habituated usage can be adjusted gradually and cause little or no harm.

Classification methods

There are numerous classification methods for *āhāra*. Each serves a purpose by providing a perspective on food or diet that may be applicable to individual clinical scenarios.

Single type

As a single type, all food can be consumed.

आहारत्वमाहारस्यैकविधमर्थाभेदात्;

च. सू. २५।३६

Āhāratvamāhārasyaikavidhamarthābhedāt;

Cha. Sū. 25/36

Food is all of one kind in the view of eatability as a common feature.

Dual type (vegetarian, non-vegetarian)

Based on the source or type of food, it can be classified as vegetarian or non-vegetarian. Eggs are considered non-vegetarian, but other animal products, including milk and its derivatives, fall under a separate sub-classification.

स पुनर्द्वियोनिः, स्थावरजङ्गमात्मकत्वात्;

च. सू. २५।३६

Sa punardviyoniḥ, sthāvarajaṅgamātmakatvāt;

Cha. Sū. 25/36

According to the source, food articles are of two types – those based on vegetable sources and those that are based on animal products.

Dual type (wholesome, unwholesome)

Food can be classified as *hita* or *ahita*, depending on its effect for the individual. This classification is commonly used in the context of regular, daily application for health maintenance.

द्विविधप्रभावः,हिताहितोदर्कविशेषात्;

च. सू. २५।३६

Dvividhaprabhāvaḥ, hitāhitodarkaviśheṣhāt;

Cha. Sū. 25/36

It is also of two types based on specific action: actions that have a positive effect and actions that have an unhealthy, unwholesome, or negative effect.

Three types based on effect

Food can also be considered as having an effect for therapeutic outcome.

किंचिद्दोषप्रशमनं किंचिद्धातुप्रदूषणम् ।
स्वस्थवृत्तौ मतं किंचित्त्रिविधं द्रव्यमुच्यते ॥

च. सू. १।६७

Kiñciddoṣhapraśhamanaṁ kiñciddhātupradūṣhaṇam |
Svasthavṛttau mataṁ kiñcittrividhaṁ dravyamucyate ||

Cha. Sū. 1/67

See also AH Sū. 1/16.

Trividhaṁ dravyam ucyate (These three types of *dravya* are explained as):

Kiñcid doṣha praśhamanaṁ

Some types (of *dravya*) have the purpose or effect of doṣha praśhamanaṁ, or returning *doṣha*(s) to their normal state

Kiñcid dhātu pradūṣhaṇam

Some types (of *dravya*) have the purpose or effect of *dhātu pradūṣhaṇam*, or vitiating (aggravating, dirtying, ruining) the *dhātus*

Svasthavṛttau mataṁ kiñcit

Some types (of *dravya*) have the purpose or effect of *svastha-vṛtta*, or maintaining health

Four types based on density

Based on the way the food is consumed, it is classified in four ways. This classification can apply to single *dravya* but it is more commonly used with prepared food, meals and drinks.

विविधमशितं पीतं लीढं खादितं

च. सू. २८।३

Vividhamaśhitaṁ pītaṁ līḍhaṁ khāditaṁ

Cha. Sū. 28/3

Different types of wholesome foods ingested in the form of eatables, drinkables, lickables and masticables

The four types are:

1. aśhita – eatables (soft meals)
2. pīta – drinkables
3. līḍha – lickables
4. khādita – chewables (hard food)

A variant of this classification includes:

चतुर्विधोपयोगः,
पानाशनभक्ष्यलेह्योपयोगात्; षडास्वादः,

च. सू. २५।३६

Caturvidhopayogaḥ,
pānāśhanabhakṣhyalehyopayogāt;ṣhaḍ āsvādaḥ,

Cha. Sū. 25/36

Food can also be classified into four groups by the way it is ingested: drinkables, eatables, chewables, and linctuses.

The four types are:

1. pānā – drinkables
2. āśhana – eatables
3. bhakṣhya – chewables (meals)
4. lehya – lickables

Six types based on rasa

The six *rasas* create a classification method for food based on its predominant *rasa*. Because each *rasa* has its own specifications of expected characteristics and effects, this is a very practical way to predict a generalized outcome for unfamiliar *dravya*.

रसभेदतः षड्विधत्वात्;

च. सू. २५।३६

Rasabhedataḥ ṣhaḍvidhatvāt;

Cha. Sū. 25/36

Another method of classification categorizes food by taste – and these are six categories.

The six *rasas* include:

1. Madhura
2. Amla
3. Lavaṇa
4. Kaṭu
5. Tikta
6. Kaṣhaya

Twenty types based on guṇa

Dravya and food can also be classified based on their predominant *guṇa*. Like *rasa*, this provides an effective practical approach to understanding new dravya in the context of classical Āyurveda.

विंशतिगुणः,गुरुलघुशीतोष्णस्निग्धरूक्षमन्द तीक्ष्णस्थिरसरमृदुकठिन - विशदपिच्छिलश्लक्ष्णखरसूक्ष्मस्थूलसान्द्रद्र वानुगमात्;

च. सू. २५।३६

Viṁśhatiguṇaḥ,gurulaghuśhītoṣhṇasnig dha rūkṣhamandatīkṣhṇasthirasaramṛdu kaṭhina viśhadapicchhilaśhlakṣhṇakhara sūkṣhmasthūlasāndradravānugamāt;

Cha. Sū. 25/36

Considering the characteristics and properties of food, they can be classified according to their twenty *guṇas*: heavy, light, cold, hot, unctuous, dry, slow, sharp, stable, fluid, soft, hard, clear, viscid, smooth, rough, subtle, gross, dense and liquid.

Infinite types

Ultimately, the classification of *dravya* and food is infinite.

अपरिसङ्ख्येयविकल्पः, द्रव्यसंयोगकरणबाहुल्यात् ||

च. सू. २५।३६

Aparisaṅkhyeyavikalpaḥ,dravyasaṁyog akaraṇabāhulyāt ||

Cha. Sū. 25/36

Classifications of food can be unlimited based on the variety and variability of ingredients, combinations and preparation methods.

Types of foods

The classification system of dietary food items and their detailed descriptions of qualities, actions and special effects is found in Cha. Sū. 27/. This is one of the largest chapters in the entire *saṁhitā*.

Foods are classified into 12 major groups. Similar systems are found throughout classical literature, most notably in Su. Su. 46/ and AH Sū. 5/.

The 12 food groups include:

- Śhūka-dhānya – corns
- Śhamī-dhānya – pulses
- Māṁsa – meats
- Śhāka –green leafy vegetables
- Phala – fruit
- Harita – vegetables, salad
- Madya – alcohol
- Ambu – water
- Gorasa – milk products
- Ikṣhu-vikārikān – sugarcane and its products
- Kṛtānna – prepared foods, meals
- Āhārayogin – condiments and accessories

Meal practices

Charaka describes specific practices for meals to promote optimal digestion and assimilation. See Cha. Vi. 1/ and 2/ for the complete discussion.

Chapter 7: Review

ADDITIONAL READING

Read and review the references listed below to expand your understanding of the concepts in this chapter. Write down the date that you complete your reading for each. Remember that consistent repetition is the best way to learn. Plan to read each reference at least once now and expect to read it again as you continue your studies.

References marked with (skim) can be read quickly and do not require commentary review.

CLASSICS		1st read	2nd read
Charaka	Cha. Sū. 5/, 27/, 28/ Cha. Vi. 1/, 2/		
Suśhruta	Su. Sū. 45/, 46/		
Aṣhṭāṅga Hṛdaya	AH Sū. 5/, 6/, 7/13-44, 8/		
Bhāva Prakāśha	BP Pū. 5/		

JOURNALS & CURRENT RESOURCES

Studies on the physicochemical characteristics of heated honey, honey mixed with ghee and their food consumption pattern by rats
https://www.ncbi.nlm.nih.gov/pmc/articles/PMC3215355/

https://highline.huffingtonpost.com/articles/en/everything-you-know-about-obesity-is-wrong/

QUESTIONS & ANSWERS

Record your questions for this chapter here for further research and discussion.

Question:

Answer:

Question:

Answer:

Question:

Answer:

SELF-ASSESSMENT

1. Which is not an outcome of normal digestion?
   a. *bala* (strength)
   b. *sama doṣha*
   c. *utsāha* (proper enthusiasm, eagerness)
   d. *varṇa* (proper skin tone and complexion)
   e. *vyādhi* (disease)
2. Which type of *agni* takes a long time to digest small meals?
   a. *mandāgni*
   b. *samāgni*
   c. *tīkṣhnāgni*
   d. *visamāgni*
   e. *visamāgni and mandāgni*
3. A *mṛdu koṣhṭha* purges and passes bowels easily. *Mṛdu koṣhṭha* is associated with which *doṣha*?
   a. *pitta*
   b. *sama doṣha*
   c. *sannipāta doṣha*
   d. *vāta*
   e. *vāta and kapha*
4. What is the primary tool for assessing *āhāra śhakti*?
   a. *āhāra mātra*
   b. *drākṣha-rasaṁ (juice of grapes)*
   c. *koṣhṭha parīkṣha*
   d. *varṇa*
   e. *vyāyāma*
5. *Āma* can be produced by all of the following factors: excessive quantity of food, food which is heavy, dry or cold, food which is disliked, food which is unclean and improper food combinations.
   a. True
   b. False
6. *Āma* mixed with aggravated *doṣhas* is called *sāma doṣha nidāna*.
   a. True
   b. False
7. Which is not a *sāma vāta lakṣhana*?
   a. *aṅgamarda* (squeezing pain in the limbs)
   b. *chhardi* (vomiting)
   c. *mukhaśhoṣha* (dryness of the mouth)
   d. *parśhva*, *pṛṣhṭha*, *kaṭi graha* (tightness of the sides of the waist, back, spine, hips)
   e. *śhūla* (abdominal pain or discomfort)
8. *Dravya* which are *laghu* produce minimal *doṣha* because they are similar to *agni*.
   a. True
   b. False
9. Which of the following are classification methods for food?
   a. animal and vegetable
   b. *guṇa*
   c. *hīta* and *ahīta*
   d. *rasa*
   e. All of the above
10. Which of the following meal practices does Charaka recommend in Cha. Vi. 1/ and 2/?
   a. don't eat in a hurry
   b. don't eat too slowly
   c. eat food in a proper quantity
   d. eat without talking and laughing
   e. All of the above

CRITICAL THINKING

1. Explain in your own words why a study of human health cannot be completely controlled.

2. Imagine a scenario that demonstrates when the effect of a *dravya* is ascertained on the basis of cumulative action. Describe that scenario to demonstrate your understanding.

References

Chapter 8 : Bala

KEY TERMS

aṅguli pramāṇa
añjali pramāṇa
bala
ojas
pramāṇa
saṁhanana
svastha
vyādhi kṣhamatva
vyāyāma
vyāyāma śhakti

CLASSICAL REVIEW

Bala is classically considered in two significant contexts:

Bala can be:	Bala can be assessed through:
Physical strength or capacity	Deha, saṁhanana and vyāyāma śhakti
Ability to resist disease	Ojas

This chapter covers the breadth and depth of classical knowledge of bala in both contexts using the major references. The information available for each topic is presented at the beginning of its own section. It is followed by the assessment methodologies used to measure the related components.

Bala as physical strength

When considered as physical strength, or the capacity to perform physical activity or work, bala is created through *vyāyāma*, the practice of physical training to improve capacity, endurance and stamina. In order to fully understand the assessment methodologies related to *vyāyāma*, a critical review of complete topic is required.

<u>Factors that promote *bala*</u>

While specific factors can improve the state of *bala* for any individual, each person also has certain limitations, or a range in which they can feasibly operate. Every person cannot become incredibly strong or weak because each one has a natural tendency towards a certain state. This state can be enhanced or impeded depending on how it is manipulated through the major factors of *sātmya* such as *āhāra*, *nidrā*, *vyāyāma*, *sattva*, etc.

The factors that promote *bala* described by Charaka can have a direct effect on the individual's natural tendency, or range of *bala*, as well as their capacity to manipulate it. The major factors include:

कार्त्स्न्येन शरीरवृद्धिकरास्त्विमे भावा भवन्ति; तद्यथ - कालयोगः, स्वभावसंसिद्धि, आहारसौष्ठवम्, अविघातश्चेति ॥

च. शा. ६।१२

Kārtsryena śharīravṛddhikarāstvime bhāvā bhavanti; tadyatha - kālayogaḥ, svabhāvasaṁsiddhi, āhārasauṣhṭavam, avighātaśhceti ||

Cha. Śhā. 6/12

Bhāvā bhavanti (These specific factors are) kārtsryena (the causes or reasons) śharīra-vṛddhi-karāstvime (for making the body grow); tadyatha (they are) - kālayogaḥ (opportune time), svabhāva-saṁsiddhi (one's own properly manifested nature), āhārasauṣhṭavam (excellent food and nourishment), avighātaśhceti (absence of inhibiting factors).

The first two factors should be considered to influence the potential range, while the second two directly affect the level of *bala* that can be achieved. Consider them as follows.

Factor influencing *bala*	Affects	Practical examples
Kāla-yoga Opportune time	Potential *bala*	*Bāla* (the period of youth) is the ideal time for physical growth.
Svabhāva-saṁsiddhi One's properly manifested nature	Potential *bala*	The unique nature of an individual's *prakṛti*, *karma*, etc. creates or enhance or impede the potential for physical growth.
Āhārasauṣhṭavam Excellent food and nourishment	Manifested *bala*	Excellent qualities of food and nourishment directly increase physical growth by providing available building blocks.
Avighāta Absence of inhibiting factors	Manifested *bala*	Avoidance of activities which impede physical growth, like indulgence in sexual intercourse or stress.

Examples of how these factors manifest can be practically demonstrated as explained in the following *śhloka*:

बलवृद्धिकरास्त्वमे भाव भवन्ति । तद्यथा - बलवत्पुरुषे देशे जन्म बलवत्पुरुषे काले च, सुखश्च कालयोगः, बीजक्षेत्रगुणसंपच्च, आहारसंपच्च, शरीरसंपच्च, सात्म्य संपच्च, सत्त्व संपच्च, स्वभाव संसिद्धिश्च, यौवनं च, कर्म च, संहर्षश्चेति ॥

च. शा. ६।१३

Balavṛddhikarāsvame bhāva bhavanti | Tadyathā - balavatpuruṣhe deśhe janma balavatpuruṣhe kāle cha, sukhaśhcha kālayogaḥ, bījakṣhetraguṇasaṁpacca, āhārasaṁpacca, śharīrasaṁpacca, sātmya saṁpacca, sattva saṁpacca, svabhāva saṁsiddhiśhcha, yauvanaṁ cha, karma cha, saṁharṣhaśhceti ||

Cha. Śhā. 6/13

Bhāvā (The specific factors) bala-vṛddhi-karāsvame (responsible for the increase in *bala*) bhavanti (are as follows):

Bala vṛddhi kara bhāva	Factors responsible for the increase in *bala*
Balavat-puruṣhe deśhe janma	Birth in a *deśha* (location) where people tend to be strong
Balavat-puruṣhe kāle	Birth during a *kāla* (time period) which naturally imparts strength to the environment and living beings
Sukha kālayoga	Pleasant and opportune time period
Bīja kṣhetra guṇa saṁpat	Proper features, characteristics and functions of the seed and field for healthy conception
Āhāra saṁpat	Proper diet and food
Śharīra saṁpat	Proper physical body
Sātmya saṁpat	Proper wholesomeness of all influential factors utilized as *sātmya*
Sattva saṁpat	Proper mental disposition
Svabhāva saṁsiddhi	Perfect natural disposition
Yauvana	Youth
Karma	Actions (past and present) and all activities
Saṁharṣha	Proper excitement for life and contentment

The factors listed above include those things which are set by choices and actions of the parents as well as the individual. This results in some being fixed and unchangeable, while others may be manipulated to improve the state of *bala*. The single most influential factor which can be controlled by every individual is *vyāyāma*, discussed in detail below.

Vyāyāma, the main cause for bala

The term *vyāyāma* is defined in the Monier-Williams dictionary as:

1. Dragging different ways, contest, strife, struggle
2. Exertion, manly effort, athletic or gymnastic exercise
3. Right exercise or training
4. Drawing out, extending

It is created from two component terms:

Vy (Vi) Intensity, distinction, peculiarity, specificity

Āyāma → Stretching, extending, expanding, lengthening (either in space or time)

Vyāyāma is the practice of specifically stretching or extending one's limits of physical capacity, endurance and stamina to increase the ability to perform physical work. While *vyāyāma* is often translated as exercise, it may be more appropriately considered physical training.

The Merriam Webster dictionary defines exercise within this context as:

1. Regular or repeated use of a faculty or bodily organ
    a. Bodily exertion for the sake of developing and maintaining physical fitness
    b. Example: Trying to get more exercise
2. Something performed or practiced in order to develop, improve, or display a specific capability or skill arithmetic exercises vocal exercises
3. Performance or activity having a strongly marked secondary or ulterior aspect
    a. Party politics has always been an exercise in compromise - H. S. Ashmore
4. A maneuver, operation, or drill carried out for training and discipline naval exercises
    a. Exercises (plural): a program including speeches, announcements of awards and honors, and various traditional practices of secular or religious character
    b. Example: commencement exercises

The term exercise may refer to activities that maintain physical capacity to perform work as well as extend or improve them, while *vyāyāma* indicates the extension of capacity. The concept of exercise for physical maintenance is not specifically mentioned in the classics. That level of activity was likely a normal part of daily life and not considered to be an additional requirement for health maintenance as it is in modern, sedentary lifestyles.

If the term *vyāyāma* is used today to indicate a wide range of physical activity, it must be remembered that in order to truly qualify as *vyāyāma*, the activities must push the individual to their limit for an appropriate period of time. This is an area which requires some research and focus to develop standardized terms and criteria for measuring *vyāyāma*, its range and effects on individuals.

Charaka defines *vyāyāma* as:

शरीरचेष्टा या चेष्टा स्थैर्यार्था बलवर्धिनी |
देहव्यायामसङ्ख्याता मात्रया तां समाचरेत् ||

च. सू. ७।३१

Śharīracheṣhṭā yā cheṣhṭā sthairyārthā balavardhinī |
Dehavyāyāmasaṅkhyātā mātrayā tāṁ samācaret ||

Cha. Sū. 7/31

The physical actions (movements, activities) of the body which improve overall stability and increase strength are called *vyāyāma*. The methods of practice and duration must be carefully monitored (and performed appropriately for the individual).

शरीरायासजननं कर्म व्यायामसंज्ञितम् ॥

सु. चि. २४।३७

Śharīrāyāsajananaṁ karma vyāyāmasaṁjñitam

Su. Chi. 24/37

Śharīra-āyāsa-jananaṁ (Exertion of the physical body by) karma (work or effort) vyāyāma-saṁjñitam (is known as *vyāyāma*).

Additional explanations of *vyāyāma* can be found in Su. Chi. 24/38-50, AH Sū. 2/10-14, and BP Pū. 5/47-55.

When performed correctly, *vyāyāma* produces the following benefits:

लाघवं कर्मसामर्थ्यं स्थैर्यं दुःखसहिष्णुता |
दोषक्षयोऽग्निवृद्धिश्च व्यायामादुपजायते ||

च. सू. ७।३२

Lāghavaṁ karmasāmarthyaṁ sthairyaṁ duḥkhasahiṣhṇutā |

Doṣhakṣhayo ' gnivṛddhiśhcha vyāyāmādupajāyate || 32

Cha. Sū. 7/32

Lāghavaṁ (Lightness), karma-sāmarthyaṁ (the ability to perform physical work and activities), sthairyaṁ (stability), duḥkha-sahiṣhṇutā (the ability to bear discomfort and stress), doṣha-kṣhayo (reduction of the *doṣhas* [especially of *kapha*]), agni-vṛddhiśhcha (and an increase of the power of digestion, metabolism and assimilation) vyāyāmād-upajāyate (are the results of [proper] exercise).

However, when performed excessively, *vyāyāma* can cause:

श्रमः क्लमः क्षयस्तृष्णा रक्तपित्तं प्रतामकः
| अतिव्यायामतः कासो ज्वरश्छर्दिश्च
जायते ||

च. सू. ७।३३

Śhramaḥ klamaḥ kṣhayastṛṣhṇā raktapittaṁ pratāmakaḥ |

Ativyāyāmataḥ kāso jvaraśhchardiśhcha jāyate ||

Cha. Sū. 7/33

Ati-vyāyāma (Excessive practice of vyāyāma) jāyate (gives rise to symptoms and disorders including) śhrama (exhaustion), klama (fatigue), kṣhaya (emaciation, wasting), tṛṣhṇā (thirst), raktapitta (a named disorder characterized by bleeding from different parts of the body), pratāmaka (a named sub-disorder, a type of śhvāsa, characterized by dyspnea with fainting), kāsa (cough, as a symptom or disorder), jvara (fever) and chardi (vomiting).

Vyāyāma should be practiced for a duration that allows one to expend energy up to half of their physical capacity, and then it should be stopped.

(स्वेदागमः श्वासवृद्धिर्गात्राणां लाघवं तथा |
हृदयाद्युपरोधश्च इति व्यायामलक्षणम् || १
)

च. सू. ७।३३ (१)

(Svedāgamaḥ śhvāsavṛddhirgātrāṇāṁ lāghavaṁ tathā |

hṛdayāduparodhaśhcha iti vyāyāmalakṣhaṇam ||)

Cha. Sū. 7/33 (1)

Iti vyāyāma-lakṣhaṇam (And so, the features and characteristics of properly practiced vyāyāma are) svedā-gamaḥ (the appearance of perspiration), śhvāsa-vṛddhi gātrāṇāṁ (increase in respiration), lāghavaṁ (a feeling of lightness), hṛdayād-uparodha (a feeling of the heart reaching its comfortable maximum capacity, bordering on overfilling).

When this stage is reached and the individual recognizes the appearance of these *lakṣhaṇas*, they should stop practicing *vyāyāma* intensely.

Compare the effects of *vyāyāma* when it is performed too little, at the proper level or too much:

Effects of vyāyāma			
	Too little	Correct amount	Too much
Respiration	Remains normal	Increased comfortably / borderline	Uncomfortably increased
Heart rate	Remains normal	Increased comfortably / borderline	Uncomfortably increased
Perspiration	None or little	Moderate or profuse	Profuse
Energy levels	Less or same	Increased	Depleted
Doṣhas	No effect or may increase any	Normalizes all especially *kapha*	Increases *vāta* Decrease *kapha*, *pitta*
Agni	No effect or slight increase	Increased	Overly increased or extinguished

Excessive practice of *vyāyāma* can lead to a number of varied health issues. Because general perceptions of exercise often fall in the "more is better" category, individuals with that belief may become more prone to disregarding or ignoring the negative effects of too much activity.

The signs and symptoms can vary from insidious to acute onset, and if they are ignored the issues can become deeply set and chronic. For that reason, Charaka states that individuals who are accustomed to certain activities in excess should make a concerted effort to change this negative habit.

व्यायामहास्यभाष्याध्वग्राम्यधर्मप्रजागरान् |
नोचितानपि सेवेत बुद्धिमानतिमात्रया ||

च. सू. ७।३४

Vyāyāmahāsyabhāṣhyādhvagrāmyadharmaprajāgarān |

Nochitānapi seveta buddhimānatimātrayā ||

Cha. Sū. 7/34

Vyāyāma (physical training), hāsya (laughing) bhāṣhyā (speaking), dhva (walking), grāmyadharma (sexual activities) prajāgarān (and staying awake during the night) na-uchitānapi (should not be practiced) seveta (regularly) buddhimān (by one who is aware of their health) atimātrayā (even if these activities have become habitual).

The recommendations to avoid these activties stem from the understanding that they can cause overexertion of vāta. By limiting these, one will better reserve their energy for maintenance of physiological activities that promote robust health.

Charaka provides an important simile that demonstrates the potential negative outcomes of over exertion.

एतानेवंविधांश्चान्यान् योऽतिमात्रं निषेवते |
गजं सिंह इवाकर्षन् सहसा स विनश्यति |

च. सू. ७।३५

Etānevaṁvidhāṁśhchānyān yo ' timātraṁ niṣhevate |
Gajaṁ siṁha ivākarṣhan sahasā sa vinaśhyati ||

Cha. Sū. 7/35

One who indulges in these and such other activities in excess, suddenly perishes like a lion trying to drag an (huge) elephant. [35]

Etānevaṁ vidhāṁśhchānyān (These and similar activities) yo atimātraṁ niṣhevate (that require one to over exert themselves) gajaṁ siṁha ivākarṣhan sahasā sa vinaśhyati (cause one to perish suddenly just like a lion who attacks an elephant).

Suśhruta provides another important explanation of sitting versus walking in Su. Chi. 24/80. And Bhāva Prakāśha includes similar descriptions in BP Pū. 5/221-222.

Assessing deha

In Su. Sū. 35/33-36, Suśhruta explains the methods of assessing *deha*.

देहः स्थूलः, कृशो, मध्य, इति प्रागुपदिष्टः ।
३३
कर्शयेद् बृंहयेच्चापि सदा स्थूलकृशौ नरौ ।
रक्षणं चैव मध्यस्य कुर्वीत सततं भिषक् ॥
३४
बलमभिहितगुणं; दौर्बल्यं तु
स्वभावदोषजरादिभिरवेक्षितव्यम् ।
यस्माद्बलवतः सर्वक्रियाप्रवृत्तिस्तस्माद्बलमेव
प्रधानमधिकरणानम् ॥

सु. सू. ३५।३५

Dehaḥ sthūlaḥ, kṛśho, madhya, iti prāgupatiṣhṭaḥ || 33
Karśhayed bṛṁhatechchāpi sadā sthūlakṛśho naro | Rakṣhaṇaṁ chaiva madhyasya kurchīta satataṁ bhiṣhak || 34
Balamabhihitaguṇaṁ; daurbalyaṁ tu svabhāvadoṣhajarādibhiravekṣhitavyam | Yasmādbalavataḥ sarvakriyāpravṛttistasmādbalameva pradhānamadhikaraṇānam ||

Su. Sū. 35/35

Assessing saṁhanana

The assessment of *saṁhanana* is explained by Charaka as a separate component of *daśhavidha parīkṣha*. In the consolidated Clinical Svastha Assessment, it is organized within the context of *bala* because of its direct impact.

While *saṁhanana* can change to some degree for an individual depending on their *sātmya*, *vyāyāma* and efforts toward building the physical body, there is a normal range in which any individual naturally operates. There are always limitations to how much an individual can change their physical structure due to their innate nature and constitution.

The purpose of assessing *saṁhanana* is to better understand an individual's baseline state and current presentation of health.

Saṁhati and *saṁyojana* are synonyms for *saṁhanana*.

संहननतश्चेति संहननं, संहतिः,
संयोजनमित्येकोऽर्थः | तत्र
समसुविभक्तास्थि, सुबद्धसन्धि,
सुनिविष्टमांसशोणितं, सुसंहतं
शरीरमित्युच्यते | तत्र सुसंहतशरीराः पुरुषा
बलवन्तः, विपर्ययेणाल्पबलाः, मध्यत्वात्
संहननस्य मध्यबला भवन्ति ||

च. वि. ८।११६

Saṁhananataśhcheti saṁhananaṁ, saṁhatiḥ, saṁyojanamityeko ' rthaḥ | Tatra samasuvibhaktāsthi, subaddhasandhi, suniviṣhṭamāṁsaśhoṇitaṁ, susaṁhataṁ śharīramityuchyate | Tatra susaṁhataśharīrāḥ puruṣhā balavantaḥ, viparyayeṇālpabalāḥ, madhyatvāt saṁhananasya madhyabalā bhavanti ||
Cha. Vi. 8/116

Saṁhananataśhcheti (And so *saṁhanana* is assessed [considering the context of the previous *śhloka*'s descriptions of *sāra*) ityeko ' rthaḥ ([and it] is also known by one of the following synonyms) saṁhananaṁ (*saṁhanana*), saṁhatiḥ (*saṁhati*), saṁyojanam (*saṁyojana*). Tatra (And so) ityuchyate (it is said to be) sama (normal, complete) suvibhaktāsthi (well-divided, symmetrical skeletal structure and bones), subaddha (well-bound) sandhi (joints), suniviṣhṭa (well-developed, properly situated) māṁsa (muscular structures and muscle) śhōṇitaṁ ([and] blood, vascular system, supportive system to *māṁsa*), susaṁhataṁ (properly compacted, well-developed) śharīram (body [overall]). Tatra (And so) susaṁhata (a properly compacted, well-developed) śharīrāḥ (physical body) puruṣhā (in human beings) balavantaḥ ([results in] increased strength), viparyayeṇa (the opposite [results in]) alpa [less, reduced) balāḥ (strength), madhyatvāt ([and] a moderate amount) saṁhananasya (of *saṁhanana* [results in]) madhya (a medium amount) balā (of strength) bhavanti (is how it is explained).

Lakṣhaṇas Assessment criteria	Assessment methods
Sama suvibhakta asthi Properly proportioned, symmetrical and well-divided bones	Visual inspection and manual palpation of the skeletal structure and bones, cartilage and tendons.
Subaddha sandhi Well-bound joints	Inspection and palpation of various joints, and investigation of history of accidents, fractures, injuries.
Suniviṣhṭa māṁsa śhoṇita Well-bound muscle tissue and blood (vascular system)	Inspection and palpation of the muscular system and muscles. Investigation of the vascular system.
Susaṁhata śharīra Properly compact physical body	Assessment of symmetry, form, proportion

Pramāṇa

The assessment of *pramāṇa* is covered in the major classical texts and includes measurement of *aṅguli pramāṇa* (length and other dimensions) and *añjali pramāṇa* (volumetric measurement). The information provided in the classical references lists measurable aspects of the human body and their ideal values which indicate proper proportion.

While these lists of measurements are interesting, they do not provide reliable data that can be utilized today without further research, testing and large-scale analysis. It is important to recognize the value that this type of information can provide to professional Āyurvedic practice, and consider how these methodologies might be applicable today.

Use the chart below to review the classical references for assessing *pramāṇa*.

	Charaka	Suśhruta	Vāgbhaṭa
Aṅguli pramāṇa	Cha. Vi. 8/117	Su. Sū. 35/12	
Añjali pramāṇa	Cha. Śhā. 7/15		

Assessing vyāyāma śhakti

A primary method of assessing *vyāyāma* is the determination of an individual's capacity to perform physical work or activity.

Prior to assessing *vyāyāma śhakti*, Suśhruta mentions that an individual's physique may not always indicate their capacity for physical work. This must be taken into account when performing the assessment, and a thorough investigation should elicit indicators of capacity through type of work, duration, and other specific characteristics.

केचित् कृशाः प्राणवन्तः स्थूलाश्चाल्पबला नराः । तस्मात् स्थिरत्वं व्यायामैर्बलं वैद्यः प्रतर्कयेत् ॥

सु. सू. ३५।३६

Kechit kṛśhāḥ prāṇvantaḥ sthūlāśhchālpabalā narāḥ |
Tasmāt sthiratvaṁ vyāyāmairbalaṁ vaidyaḥ pratarkayet ||

Su. Sū. 35/36

Kechit (Some who) kṛśhāḥ (are thin) prāṇvantaḥ (are actually strong), sthūlāśhchālpabalā narāḥ (and some who are large are actually weak). Tasmāt (Accordingly) sthiratvaṁ ([one's] stability) vyāyāmairbalaṁ ([as a function] of physical strength) vaidyaḥ pratarkayet (must be properly assessed by the *vaidya*).

External appearance is not sufficient to draw conclusions about one's *vyāyāma śhakti.*

Charaka further explains the grades of assessment for *vyāyāma śhakti* as low, medium and high.

व्यायामशक्तितश्चेति व्यायामशक्तिरपि कर्मशक्त्या परीक्ष्या । कर्मशक्त्याह्यनुमीयतेबलत्रैविध्यम् ॥

च. वि. ८।१२१

Vyāyāmaśhaktitaśhcheti vyāyāmaśhaktirapi karmaśhaktyā parīkṣhyā | Karmaśhaktyā hyanumīyate balatraividhyam ||

Cha. Vi. 8/121

Vyāyāmaśhaktitaśhcheti (Proper assessments of one's capacity to perform physical work) vyāyāmaśhaktirapi (must be done by actually assessing one's capacity) karmaśhaktyā (through the performance of physical work) parīkṣhyā (and its measured outcomes). Karmaśhaktyā (The performance of physical work) hyanumīyate (is practically seen in) balatraividhyam (three categories [low, medium, high]).

Practical assessment of *vyāyāma śhakti* requires knowing the baseline for comparison. Classically, an individual can be assessed against the expected behavior for their *prakṛti* for a general comparison. More specifically, the individual can also be assessed against their own *prākṛta* state of *doṣhas* that is unique to them only.

Chapter 8: Review

ADDITIONAL READING

Read and review the references listed below to expand your understanding of the concepts in this chapter. Write down the date that you complete your reading for each. Remember that consistent repetition is the best way to learn. Plan to read each reference at least once now and expect to read it again as you continue your studies.

References marked with (skim) can be read quickly and do not require commentary review.

CLASSICS	1st read	2nd read
Charaka		
Suśhruta		
Aṣhṭāṅga Hṛdaya		
Bhāva Prakāśha		

JOURNALS & CURRENT RESOURCES

https://archive.org/details/Mallapurana/page/n39

QUESTIONS & ANSWERS

Record your questions for this chapter here for further research and discussion.

Question:

Answer:

Question:

Answer:

Question:

Answer:

SELF-ASSESSMENT

1. Which factor(s) are responsible for the increase of *bala*?
   a. Adaptability
   b. *Amātrāvat*
   c. Proper mental disposition
   d. Youth
   e. Both C and D

2. Which definition for *vyāyāma* is the most accurate?
   a. Drawing out, extending
   b. Proper physical body
   c. The practice of promoting all aspects of health
   d. All of the above
   e. None of the above

3. What do *vy*(*vi*)- and *āyāma* translate to?
   a. Distinction and extending
   b. Intensity and stretching
   c. Peculiarity and expanding
   d. All of the above
   e. None of the above

4. What type of effect does a physical activity have to possess in order to qualify as *vyāyāma*?
   a. The activity must be able to be performed at a consistent, long duration.
   b. The activity must be performed at a high intensity.
   c. The activity must maintain physical capacity to perform work.
   d. The activity must push the individual to their limit for an appropriate period of time.
   e. Both C and D

5. What is an effect of too little *vyāyāma*?
   a. Depleted energy levels
   b. Increased energy levels
   c. Normalized *doṣhas* especially *kapha*
   d. Profuse perspiration
   e. Respiration remains normal

6. What is an effect of the correct amount of *vyāyāma*?
   a. Increased *agni*
   b. Increased energy levels
   c. Moderate or profuse perspiration
   d. All of the above
   e. None of the above

7. What is an effect of too much *vyāyāma*?
   a. Increased *agni*
   b. Increased *vāta* and decreased *kapha* and *pitta*
   c. No effect or slight increase in *agni*
   d. None or little perspiration
   e. None of the above

8. What is a *lakṣhaṇa* of proper *saṁhanana*?
   a. Properly compact physical body
   b. Properly proportioned, symmetrical and well divided bones
   c. Well-bound joints
   d. Well-bound muscle tissue and blood (vascular system)
   e. All of the above

9. *Aṅguli* and *añjali pramāṇa* refer to
   a. Direct measurement and indirect measurement
   b. Indirect measurement and direct measurement
   c. Length/other dimensions and volumetric measurement
   d. Volumetric measurement and length/other dimensions
   e. None of the above

10. *Subaddha sandhi* refers to
   a. Properly proportioned, symmetrical and well divided bones
   b. Well-bound joints
   c. Well-bound muscle tissue and blood
   d. All of the above
   a. None of the above

CRITICAL THINKING

1.

2.

3.

4.

5.

References

Chapter 9 : Sattva

KEY TERMS

āchāra	dhāraṇīya vega	prajñāparādha	smṛti
āchāra rasāyana	dhī	pravara	svastha
ahaṅkāra	dhṛti	puruṣhārtha	tamas
asātmyendriyārtha saṁyoga	indriya	rajas	tisra eṣhaṇā
avara	madhyama	sadvṛtta	tri āyatana
buddhi	manas	sattva	tri-guṇa
	mānasika prakṛti		

CLASSICAL REVIEW

Assessment of *sattva* and *manas* play significant roles in the clinical practice of Āyurveda. Not only do they guide the clinician in determining appropriate treatment protocols, they also provide vast opportunities for the patient to improve their state of health and quality of life through interconnected guidance and supervision.

Classical literature provides a well-structured framework for assessment of *manas* and *sattva*. These methods primarily refer to the overall assessment as *sattva* rather than *manas*. This is a key point to note as it provides insight into the classical train of thought. Recall from Volume 2, Chapters 18, 23, 24 and 26 that *sattva* operates on a larger scale than *manas* as it flows through *ātma* to its final effects in human life.

On the other hand, *manas* is contained to more functional roles as a processor of information and delegator of actions. In Western psychology, it may be comparable to executive function. *Manas*' role includes management of the *indriyas*, calculating and analyzing information and sending that information along the chain of decision-making. It communicates with *ahaṅkāra*, *buddhi*, *smṛti* and *dhṛti* in addition to the *indriyas*.

Sattva, *rajas* and *tamas* can be considered to influence the lines of communication between all of these components. Therefore, in assessing the state of an individual from this perspective, it is the *sattva* that ultimately has the most influence.

The influence of an individual's states of *sattva*, *rajas* and *tamas* can be effectively observed and assessed through their *mati* (mental faculties), *vacha* (speech) and *karma* (activities). Charaka explains the importance of applying these properly to promote *svastha* and avoid disease.

मतिर्वचः कर्म सुखानुबन्धं सत्त्वं विधेयं
विशदा च बुद्धिः| ज्ञानं तपस्तत्परता च योगे
यस्यास्ति तं नानुपतन्ति [३२] रोगाः || ४७
च. शा. २।४७

Matirvachaḥ karma sukhānubandhaṁ sattvaṁ vidheyaṁ viśhadā cha buddhiḥ | Jñānaṁ tapastatparatā cha yoge yasyāsti taṁ nānupatanti rogāḥ || 47
Cha. Śhā. 2/47

Matir (Mental faculties), vachaḥ (speech), karma (and [right] action, which are) sukha-anubandhaṁ (comfortably or naturally present or bound) sattvaṁ (to one's *sattva*) vidheyaṁ (and readily compliant), viśhadā (clear, clean, pure), cha buddhiḥ (capable of innate intelligence) jñānaṁ (and knowledge), tapastatparatā cha yoge (aid one who regularly engages in the practice of *yoga*) yasyāsti taṁ nānupatanti rogāḥ (so that he never becomes afflicted by disease).

Similar to many of the other factors within the *daśhavidha parīkṣha*, *sattva* may be assessed from both a baseline perspective as well as a current perspective. Behaviors, actions and responses of an individual that occur naturally should be considered as their baseline state. With sufficient training and determination, modifications may be possible to any of these behaviors or actions. These learned behaviors should be considered as the individual's current state which may shift from their baseline over the course of their life.

Considering this, one of the most pressing questions that comes up in mental health might be able to be addressed through the practice of Āyurveda. To what degree are mental state and mental health a choice? What are the roles and responsibilities of the individual in determining their own state of mental health?

These questions are especially relelvant today. Using the classical frameworks for *sattva* assessment and management through Svastha Vṛtta, Āyurveda offers ample methods and approaches to improving mental health for anyone who is ready to utilize the tools and apply them.

Sattva assessment

Classical literature recognizes two types of *sattva* assessment. First, the type of *sattva*, also called *mānasika prakṛti*, reviews the presence of the *tri-guṇas* in the individual to determine a predominance of *sattva*, *rajas* or *tamas*. Second, the quantum of *sattva* present in an individual is measured using a simple scale to help determine the individual's capacity and tolerance for therapeutic interventions.

To determine *sattva* in terms of *mānasika prakṛti*, Charaka provides the following instructions.

यद्गुणं चाभीक्ष्णं पुरुषमनुवर्तते सत्त्वं
तत्सत्त्वमेवोपदिशन्ति मुनयो
बाहुल्यानुशयात् || ६

च. सू. ८|६

Yadguṇaṁ chābhīkṣhṇaṁ
puruṣhamanuvartate sattvaṁ
tatsattvamevopadiśhanti munayo
bāhulyānuśhayāt || 6

Cha. Sū. 8/6

Yad-guṇaṁ (That *guṇa*, or characteristic) cha-abhīkṣhṇaṁ (which is constantly, repeatedly) puruṣham-anuvartate (demonstrated or present in the individual's) sattvaṁ (*sattva* [ie, *mānasika prakṛti*]) tat-sattvam-eva-upadiśhanti (is said to be that type of *sattva*) munayo bāhulyānuśhayāt (which is predominant in him, according to the experts).

Assessing *sattva* as *mānasika prakṛti* requires careful analysis and determination of the *guṇas* and *lakṣhaṇas* that are normally and regularly present for the individual. These can again be differentiated as the baseline and current presentations.

Sattva type: Mānasika prakṛti

Charaka and Suśhruta provide two methods for assessing *sattva* as *mānasika prakṛti*. Suśhruta uses a generalized method that describes each of the *tri-guṇas* in detail while Charaka expands each of these three into a total of 16 minor types.

Charaka describes seven types of *sattva*-predominant *mānasika prakṛti*, six types of *rājasa*-predominant *mānasika prakṛti* and 3 types of *tāmasa*-predominant *mānasika prakṛti*. He reiterates the purpose of assessing these so that the patient can be provided with the most appropriate type of treatment according to what they can tolerate.

कथं च यथासत्त्वमुपचारः स्यादिति || ४०
च. शा. ४।४०

Kathaṁ cha yathāsattvamupachāraḥ syāditi || 40
Cha. Śhā. 4/40

Kathaṁ (In this manner), cha yathā-sattvam (all of these types of *sattva* [ie, *mānasika prakṛti*] have been explained) upachāraḥ syād iti (in order to determine the appropriate type of care, treatment, management [for the patient]).

When referring to the assessment of an individual's *sattva*, they may be considered to have a predominance of either *sattva*, *rajas* or *tamas*. Even when the outcome is a *rājasa* or *tāmasa* type, it is referred to as *rājasasya sattva* or *tāmasasya sattva*.

Both methodolgies are described here to allow the clinician to assess the range of classical parameters.

Review the specific *lakṣhaṇas* described for each type in the following tables. Assessment methodologies are generally most effective when that *lakṣhaṇa* is observed in the patient through *darśhana*. Attempting to elicit a truthful, accurate understanding through *praśhna* is often challenging and unproductive, except in the case of patients having *sattva sāra*, which is uncommon.

See also Su. Śhā. 4/81-98, AH Śhā. 3/7.

General sattva lakṣhaṇas Indicators of *sattva*-predominant characteristics	Cha. Śhā. 4/36	Su. Śhā. 1/18		
Adoṣham-ākhyātaṁ kalyāṇāṁśhatvāt Said to be free of *doṣha* due to its high proportion of benevolence	✓			
Ānṛśhaṁsya Kind, benevolent, compassionate		✓		
Saṁvibhāga-ruchitā Mindfully aware of how they share and proportion the things which they like		✓		
Titikṣhā Patient		✓		
Satya Truthful		✓		
Dharma Committed to their responsibilities		✓		
Āstikya Believers in a higher power		✓		
Jñāna Knowledgable		✓		

Buddhi Well-connected to their innate intelligence and able to discriminate and act accordingly		✓		
Medhā Wise		✓		
Smṛti Having a strong memory		✓		
Dhṛti Courageous, self-controlled		✓		
Anabhiṣhaṅga Free from attachments		✓		

General rajas lakṣhaṇas Indicators of *rajas*-predominant characteristics	Cha. Śhā. 4/36	Su. Śhā. 1/18		
Sadoṣham-ākhyātaṁ roṣhāṁśhatvāt Said to be associated with doṣha due to its high proportion of anger, rage, wrath, passion and fury	✓			
Duḥkha-bahulatā Very discontent, always dissatisfied		✓		
Aṭana-śhīlatā Having the character trait of always wanting to move around		✓		
Adhṛti ahaṅkāra Unsteady, unable to control their sense of individuality		✓		
Ānṛtikatva Addicted to lying, being untruthful, or misrepresenting the truth		✓		
Akāruṇya Harsh, cruel		✓		
Dambho Fraudulent, deceitful, hypocritical		✓		
Mano harṣhaḥ Always seeking ways to please their mind		✓		
Kāmaḥ Lustful, passionate, sensual		✓		
Krodha Angry, wrathful		✓		

General tamas lakṣhaṇas Indicators of *tamas*-predominant characteristics	Cha. Śhā. 4/36	Su. Śhā. 1/18		
Sadoṣham-ākhyātaṁ mohāṁśhatvāt Said to be associated with *doṣha* due to its high proportion of confusion, delusion, foolishness, inability to discriminate and error	✓			
Viṣhāditva Full of grief or despair, despondent		✓		
Nāstikya Atheists		✓		
Adharma-śhīlatā Having the character trait of always avoiding their responsibilities		✓		
Buddher-nirodho Blocking their innate intelligence		✓		
Ajñāna Prone to ignorance		✓		
Durmedhastva Prone to lack of wisdom		✓		
Akarma-śhīlatā Having the character trait of laziness, avoiding work and activities		✓		
Nidrālutva Always sleepy or drowsy		✓		

<u>Sattva capacity: Daśhavidha parīkṣha</u>

The capacity of one's *sattva* can be considered as the quantum of *sattva* naturally available to them. This is generally assessed as *pravara*, *madhyama* and *avara*.

Charaka describes this assesment in context of the *daśhavidha parīkṣha* as a tool for planning current management and treatment. Based on the individual's *sattva* capacity, certain therapeutic interventions and treatment protocols may be too extreme or harsh and thus contraindicated.

सत्त्वतश्चेतिसत्त्वमुच्यतेमनः |
तच्छरीरस्यतन्त्रकमात्मसंयोगात् |
तत्त्रिविधंबलभेदेन- प्रवरं, मध्यम्,
अवरंचेति;
अतश्चप्रवरमध्यावरसत्त्वाःपुरुषाभवन्ति |
तत्रप्रवरसत्त्वाःसत्त्वसारास्तेसारेषूपदिष्टाः,
स्वल्पशरीराह्यपितेनिजागन्तुनिमित्तासुमह
तीष्वपिपीडास्वव्यथा
दृश्यन्तेसत्त्वगुणवैशेष्यात्;
मध्यसत्त्वास्त्वपरानात्मन्युपनिधाय
संस्तम्भयन्त्यात्मनाऽऽत्मानंपरैर्वाऽपिसंस्त
भ्यन्ते;
हीनसत्त्वास्तुनात्मनानापिपरैःसत्त्वबलंप्रति
शक्यन्तेउपस्तम्भयितुं,
महाशरीराह्यपितेस्वल्पानामपिवेदनानामस
हादृश्यन्ते,
सन्निहितभयशोकलोभमोहमानारौद्रभैरवद्वि
ष्टबीभत्सविकृतसङ्कथास्वपिचपशुपुरुषमांस
शोणितानिचावेक्ष्यविषादवैवर्ण्यमूर्च्छोन्माद
भ्रमप्रपतनानामन्यतममाप्नुवन्त्यथवामरण
मिति || ११९

च. वि. ८।११९

Sattvataśhcheti sattvamuchyate manaḥ | Tachchharīrasya tantrakamātmasaṁyogāt | Tat trividhaṁ balabhedena - pravaraṁ, madhyam, avaraṁ cheti; ataśhcha pravaramadhyāvarasattvāḥ purușhā bhavanti | Tatra pravarasattvāḥ sattvasārāste sāreṣhūpadiṣhṭāḥ, svalpaśharīrā hyapi te nijāgantunimittāsu mahatīṣhvapi pīḍāsvavyathā dṛśhyante sattvaguṇavaiśheṣhyāt; madhyasattvāstvaparānātmanyupanidhāya saṁstambhayantyātmanātmānaṁ parairvā ' pi saṁstabhyante; hīnasattvāstu nātmanā nāpi paraiḥ sattvabalaṁ prati śhakyante upastambhayituṁ, mahāśharīrā hyapi te svalpānāmapi vedanānāmasahā dṛśhyante, sannihitabhayaśhokalobhamohamānā raudrabhairavadviṣhṭabībhatsavikṛtasaṅkathāsvapi cha paśhupuruṣhamāṁsaśhoṇitāni chāvekṣhya viṣhādavaivarṇyamūrchchhonmādabhramaprapatanānāmanyatamamāpnuvanty athavā maraṇamiti || 119

Cha. Vi. 8/119

Sattvataś-cheti (And the capacity of sattva) sattvam-uchyate manaḥ (is also considered in the context of sattva and manas). Tat (That [*sattva*]) tantrakam (is known in this science as) ātma-saṁyogāt (that which connects, associates or conjoins the *ātma*) śharīrasya (with the physical body). Tat (That [*sattva*]) trividhaṁ (is of three types) balabhedena (of strength, or capacity) - pravaraṁ (*pravara*, the highest), madhyam (*madhyama*, moderate), avaraṁ cheti (or *avara*, the lowest); ataśhcha (based on this), pravara (*pravara*), madhya (*madhyama*), avara (and *avara*) sattvāḥ (*sattva*) puruṣhā bhavanti (present as such in humans).

Tatra (And so), pravara-sattvāḥ (*pravara sattva*) sattva-sāra-āste (is found in those having *sattva sāra*), sāreṣhūpadiṣhṭāḥ (which has just been detailed in [the previous section on] *sāra*); svalpa-śharīrā hyapi te (though they have a small body), nija (disorders due to internal causes), āgantu nimittāsu (and disorders due to external causes) mahatīṣhvapi (even though they produce severe) pīḍāsvavyathā (pain and discomfort) dṛśhyante (are seen) sattva-guṇa vaiśheṣhyāt (to be handled unusually well in those having a predominance of sattva guṇa);

Madhya sattvā (*Madhyama sattva*) stvaparān-ātmany-upanidhāya (resorts to putting themselves in the position of) saṁstambhayanti (being supported [mentally and emotionally]) ātman-ātmānaṁ (by others) parairvā api saṁstabhyante (or completely through others);

Hīna sattvāstu (With *Hīna* or *avara sattva,*) nātmanā nāpi paraiḥ (the individual on their own nor with help of others) sattvabalaṁ prati śhakyante upastambhayituṁ (can maintain the strength of their *sattva*); mahā-śharīrā hyapi te (even though they have a large physical body) svalpānāmapi (they have a very low) vedanānām-asahā (tolerance to pain); dṛśhyante (just by seeing) sannihita (they are bound to be) bhaya (fearful), śhoka (sad), lobha (greedy), moha (confused, delusional), mānā (and arrogant, conceited, prideful); raudra (violent), bhairava (frightful), dviṣhṭa (hateful, hostile), bībhatsa (revolted, disgusted) vikṛta (or twisted, wronged) saṅkathāsvapi (or by discussions and talks about) cha paśhu (animals), puruṣha (people), māṁsa (flesh), śhoṇitāni (blood and gory things) chāvekṣhya (do they experience) viṣhāda (clearness, vacuity), vaivarṇya (discoloration of normal complexion), mūrchchha (fainting), unmāda (madness [a group of mental disorders]), bhrama (dizziness), prapatana (falling down on the floor), anāmanyat amamāpnuvantyathavā maraṇamiti (and even death).

These descriptions clearly delineate the characteristics and behaviors of *pravara*, *madhyama* and *avara sattva*. Again, both the baseline and current perspectives should be considered in these assessments.

सत्त्वं तु
व्यसनाभ्युदयक्रियादिस्थानेष्वविक्लवकरम्
॥ ३७
सत्त्ववान् सहते सर्वं संस्तभ्यात्मानमात्मना
। राजसः स्तभ्यमानोऽन्यैः सहते नैव
तामसः ॥ ३८

सु. सू. ३५।३७-३८

Sattvaṁ tu
vyasanābhyudayakriyādisthāneṣhvavikl
avakaram || 37
Sattvavān sahate sarvaṁ
saṁstabhyamāno ‘ nyaiḥ sahate naiva
tāmasaḥ || 38

Su. Sū. 35/37-38

Sattvaṁ tu (*Sattva* is) vyasana (even in times of adversity) abhyudaya (increased) kriyādi (in all activities), sthāna (places), iṣhva (and desires) viklava karam (even when the individual is unsteady or exhausted). Sattvavān (One predominant in *sattva*) sahate (overcomes) sarvaṁ (everything) saṁstabhyamāno (by taking courage) anyaiḥ (from himself) sahate (to overcome) naiva (any situation) tāmasaḥ (in a calm, subdued manner).

Review the *lakṣhaṇas* of each type in the following tables.

Pravara sattva lakṣhaṇas Indicators of the highest level of *sattva*	Cha. Vi. 8/119	Su. Sū. 35/37-38		
Svalpa-śharīrā A small body	√			
Nijāgantunimittāsu mahatīṣhvapi pīḍāsvavyathā Handles high levels of pain well due to internal and external disorders		√		
Vyasana-ābhyudaya-kriya ādisthāna-iṣhva viklava-karam Able to handle stress in all activities, places and desires even when exhausted		√		
Sarvaṁ saṁstabhyamāno anyaiḥ sahate naiva tāmasaḥ Overcomes all [challenges] by taking courage from himself and maintains a calm demeanor		√		

Madhyama sattva lakṣhaṇas Indicators of the medium level of *sattva*	Cha. Vi. 8/119	Su. Sū. 35/37-38		
Astvaparānātmanyupanidhāya saṁstambhayantyātmanātmānaṁ parairvā api saṁstabhyante Resorts to putting themselves in a position where they require [mental and emotional] support from others	√			

Avara sattva lakṣhaṇas Indicators of the lowest level of *sattva*	Cha. Vi. 8/119	Su. Sū. 35/37-38		
Nātmanā nāpi paraiḥ sattvabalaṁ prati śhakyante upastambhayituṁ mahāśharīrā hyapi te svalpānāmapi vedanānāmasahā The strength of their *sattva* cannot be supported by themselves or by others, even though they have a large physical body	√			
Dṛśhyante, sannihitabhayaśhokalobhamohamānā raudrabhairavadviṣhṭabībhatsavikṛta Just by seeing [something disturbing] they become fearful, sad, greedy, delusional, arrogant, violent, frightful, hostile, disgusted, or twisted		√		
Saṅkathāsvapi cha paśhupuruṣhamāṁsaśhoṇitāni chāvekṣhya viṣhādavaivarṇyamūrchchhonmādabhramaprapatanā		√		

nāmanyatamamāpnuvantyathavā maraṇamiti By talking about animals, people, flesh, or blood they experience loss of complexion, fainting, loss of mental stability, dizziness, falling down on the floor, and even death				

Managing sattva

In order to successfully integrate *sattva* in a clinical therapeutics, the factors which influence *sattva* and its functioning must be understood. *Sattva* is strongly connected to an individual's base desires, emotions and life goals.

This section covers a comprehensive review of these concepts as they relate to *sattva*, *manas* and ultimately *svastha*.

Puruṣhārthas and tisra eṣhaṇā

The four *puruṣhārthas* address the major goals and accomplishments that guide individuals to achieving satisfaction in their life. Charaka identifies these at the beginning of the text to set the context of the greater purpose of Āyurveda.

They include:

Puruṣhārtha	Life goal
Dharma	Efforts toward achieving or accomplishing one's life work or goals
Artha	The material gains, results or benefits
Kāma	The resulting satisfaction, pleasure, enjoyment
Mokṣha	Detachment, release, freedom

Each of these becomes a primary focus at various stages of life. By properly identifying each during the appropriate period of life, an individual can better understand their immediate and long-term goals. This promotes a sense of purpose.

In India, family and society typically play a major role in setting expectations for one's *puruṣhārthas*. In Western cultures, especialy in the US, the extreme opposite tends to be common where individuals are responsible for determining their life purpose. Different approaches and degrees of guidance or freedom are appropriate on an individual basis. However, both options should always be available.

धर्मार्थकाममोक्षाणामारोग्यं मूलमुत्तमम् || १५
रोगास्तस्यापहर्तारः श्रेयसो जीवितस्य च |

च. सू. १।१५

Dharmārthakāmamokṣhāṇāmārogyaṁ mūlamuttamam || 15
Rogāstasyāpahartārah ṡhreyaso jīvitasya cha |

Cha. Sū. 1/15

Health is the foundation for achieving *dharma*, *artha*, *kāma*, *mokṣha*. Disease destroys the chance for any of these and takes away life.

In order to achieve *mokṣha*, one must eliminate the *doṣhas* of *rajas* and *tamas*.

न चानतिवृत्तसत्त्वदोषाणामदोषैरपुनर्भवो धर्मद्वारेषूपदिश्यते||२८||

च. सू. ११।२८

Na chānativṛttasattvadoṣhāṇām adoṣhairapunarbhavo dharmadvāreṣhūpadiśhyate || 28

Cha. Sū. 11/28

Those who have not been able to free themselves from the *doṣhas* of *rajas* and *tamas* are said to be unable to achieve *dharma*, etc.

Chakrapāṇi elaborates on the meaning of each of these in the commentary.

Punarbhavo mokṣhaḥ, dharmadvāreṣhu dharmaśhāstreṣhu, adoṣhaiḥ nirmanodoṣhairmaharṣhibhiḥ, upadiśhyate na, iti sambandhaḥ

Tisra eṣhaṇā

The *tisra eṣhaṇā*, or the three basic desires in life, provide guidance on achieving purpose and satisfaction in life. These three are fundamental requirements for life, and should be normally found in healthy individuals.

Tisra eṣhaṇā	Three basic desires
Prāṇa eṣhaṇā	Desire for a long life
Dhana eṣhaṇā	Desire for money, wealth
Paraloka eṣhaṇā	Desire for happiness beyond the physical world

इह खलु पुरुषेणानुपहतसत्त्वबुद्धिपौरुषपराक्रमेण हितमिह चामुष्मिंश्च लोके समनुपश्यता तिस्र एषणाः पर्येष्टव्या भवन्ति | तद्यथा - प्राणैषणा, धनैषणा, परलोकैषणेति || ३

च. सू. ११।३

Iha khalu puruṣheṇānupahatasattvabuddhipauruṣhaparākrameṇa hitamiha chāmuṣhmiṁśhcha lokesamanupaśhyatā tisra eṣhaṇāḥ paryeṣhṭavyā bhavanti | Tadyathā - prāṇaiṣhaṇā, dhanaiṣhaṇā, paralokaiṣhaṇeti || 3

Cha. Sū. 11/3

A person with properly functioning *sattva*, *buddhi*, and *pauruṣha* (strength, physically and psychologically), and with the desire for achievement in the material world and beyond, should make efforts to fulfill three innate desires. These are - prāṇaiṣhaṇā (desire for a long, fulfilling life), dhanaiṣhaṇā (desire for financial independence), paralokaiṣhaṇ (and desire for satisfaction beyond the present life).

Dhāraṇīya vegas

The *dhāraṇīya vegas* are those urges which should be controlled. These are categorized into three main areas of thoughts, speech and action.

इमांस्तु धारयेद्वेगान् हितार्थी प्रेत्य चेह च | साहसानामशस्तानां मनोवाक्कायकर्मणाम् || २६

च. सू. ७।२६

Imāṁstu dhārayedvegān hitārthī pretya cheha cha | Sāhasānāmaśhastānāṁ manovākkāyakarmaṇām || 26

Cha. Sū. 7/26

A person who desires to be well in the present life and beyond should properly manage any impulses to engage in dangerous or inappropriate activities of thought, speech and action.

For each of these three, one should control their behavior so that it is not sāhasānām (exceeding their limit) or aśhastānāṁ (to be read as apraśhasta, inappropriate, or that which should be generally avoided).

When engaging in any thought, speech or action, these two criteria should always be considered. The cover perspectives from the individual and society.

From an individual perspective, one should always be aware of their limitations in thoughts, speech and action. Proper effort should be made to control these so that they do not exceed their limitations. This is most easily evident with physical actions.

From a larger, societal perspective, thoughts, speech and actions must also be considered based on their effects on others. This includes anything which is generally shunned upon or considered that which should be avoided.

Mānasika vegas

The *mānasika vegas* are the urges or desires of the mind which should be restricted or withheld. These are nearly identical to the causative factors for mental dysfunction due to *rajas* and *tamas*.

लोभशोकभयक्रोधमानवेगान् विधारयेत् |
नैर्लज्ज्येर्ष्यातिरागाणामभिध्यायाश्च बुद्धिमान् || २७

च. सू. ७।२७

Lobhaśhokabhayakrodhamānavegān vidhārayet |
Nairlajjyerṣhyātirāgāṇāmabhidhyāyāśhcha buddhimān || 27

Cha. Sū. 7/27

A wise person should refrain from acting upon any emotions of greed, grief, fear, anger, egoism, shamelessness, jealousy, excessiveness, and desire for others' property.

Mānasika vega	Controllable urges of the mind
Lobha	Greed
Śhoka	Grief, sadness
Bhaya	Fear
Krodha	Anger
māna	Arrogance, self-importance
Nairlajjya	Shamelessness
Irṣhya	Envy, jealousy, spite, malice
Ati-rāgāṇām	Excessive indulgence in any feeling or passion
Abhidhyāyā	Desire to aquire someone's wealth

Chakrapāṇi elaborates on the meaning of each of these in the commentary.

Aśhastaṁ manasaḥ karma darśhayati - lobhetyādi | lobhaḥ viṣhaye'nucitā prārthanā, śhokaḥ putrādivināśhajaṁ dainyam, bhayam apakārakānusandhānajaṁ dainyam, krodhaḥ pradveṣho yena prajvalitamivātmānaṁ manyate, mānaḥ sadasadguṇādhyāropeṇātmanyutkarṣhapratyayaḥ| jugupsitagopanecchā lajjā, tadabhāvo nairlajjyaṁ; samāne dravye parasambandhapratiṣhedhecchā īrṣhyā; atirāga ucita eva viṣhaye punaḥ punaḥ pravartanecchā | abhidhyā manasā parābhidrohacintanaṁ, yadi vā paradravyaviṣhaye spṛhā || 27

Vāchika vegas

The vāchika vegas are the urges or desires of speech which should be restricted or withheld. These include mannerisms and behaviors in speech.

परुषस्यातिमात्रस्य सूचकस्यानृतस्य च |
वाक्यस्याकालयुक्तस्य धारयेद्वेगमुत्थितम् || २८

च. सू. ७।२८

Paruṣhasyātimātrasya sūchakasyānṛtasya cha |
Vākyasyākālayuktasya dhārayedvegamutthitam || 28

Cha. Sū. 7/28

Harsh speech, excessive talking, that which intends to harm others, lying and untimely speech should be restricted.

Vāchika vega	Controllable urges of speech
Paruṣha	Harsh words or speech
Atimātra	Excessive talking
Sūcaka	Harmful, piercing
Ānṛtasya	Lies
Akāla yukta	Improper or inappropriate timing of speech

Kāyika vega

The *kāyika vegas* are the urges or desires of the body which should be restricted or withheld.

देहप्रवृत्तिर्या काचिद्विद्यते परपीडया |
स्त्रीभोगस्तेयहिंसाद्या तस्यावेगान्विधारयेत् || २९

च. सू. ७।२९

Dehapravṛttiryā kāchidvidyate parapīḍayā | Strībhogasteyahiṁsādyā tasyāvegānvidhārayet || 29

Cha. Sū. 7/29

Physical actions intended to harm others; excessive indulgence in sex, stealing, violence, etc. should be restricted.

Kāyika vega	Controllable urges of action (or the body)
Parapīḍaya	Actions intended to cause stress to others
Strī- bhoga	Excessive indulgence in sex
Steya	Stealing
Hiṁsādyā	Causing harm, etc.

See AH Sū. 4/ for a similar explanation.

Sadvṛtta and āchāra

The terms *sadvṛtta* and *āchāra* refer to an individual's behavior, mannerisms, interactions and ethics as daily or regular practices.

Sadvṛtta is composed of two terms, *sad* which is an altered form of *sat*, and *vṛtta. Sat* indicates that which is true, good or real. *Vṛtta* is the cycle of life in this context. *Sadvṛtta* are the codes of conduct that promote a healthy life. It includes the behaviors of those considered to be good people.

Āchāra are codes of conduct that are considered as fundamental laws of society. They include traditional, customary practices that span generations.

Sadvṛtta are the codes of conduct seen in practice of a current generation, while *āchāra* are those which are timeless.

General recommendations

Charaka provides general recommendations to follow *āchāra* for *sukha* (satisfaction) throughout one's lifetime, and after death.

आहाराचारचेष्टासु सुखार्थी प्रेत्य चेह च |
परं प्रयत्नमातिष्ठेद्बुद्धिमान् हितसेवने || ६०
च. सू. ७|६०

Āhārāchāracheṣhṭāsu sukhārthī pretya cheha cha | Paraṁ prayatnamātiṣhṭhedbuddhimān hitasevane || 60

Cha. Sū. 7/60

Individuals who are aware of their health and development, and who desire satisfaction in the present life and beyond should make every possible effort to adhere to the correct routine of diet, personal conduct and action.

Additionally, it is recommended to follow *brahmacharya*. This should be understood within the context of the individual's span of life, and applied in the correct time period.

ब्रह्मचर्यज्ञानदानमैत्रीकारुण्यहर्षोपेक्षाप्रशम
परश्च स्यादिति || २९
च. सू. ८|२९

Brahmacharyajñānadānamaitrīkāruṇyah arṣhopekṣhāpraśhamaparaśhcha syāditi || 29

Cha. Sū. 8/29

One should adhere to a lifestyl of brahmacharya, knowledge, charity, friendship, compassion, cheerfulness, detachment and peace.

Āchāra	General recommendations
Hita sevana of *āhāra*	Regular aderence to a healthy diet of food and drinks
Hita sevana of *āchāra*	Regular adherence to a timeless code of conduct
Hita sevana of *cheṣhṭa*	Reguar adherence to healthy activities
Brahmacharya	Following a brahmacharya lifestyle when appropriate
Jñāna	Knowledge
Dāna	Charity
Maitrī	Friendship
Kāruṇya	Compassion
Harṣha upekṣha	Cheerfulness
Āpraśhamapara	Practicing detachment and calmness

Specific recommendations

Sadvṛtta is stated to be practiced in order to fulfill two main goals:

1. *ārogya* – complete absence of disease
2. *indriya-vijaya* – total control over the senses

तद्ध्यनुतिष्ठन् युगपत्
सम्पादयत्यर्थद्वयमारोग्यमिन्द्रियविजयं
चेति; तत् सद्वृत्तमखिलेनोपदेक्ष्यामो ...
च. सू. ८|१८

Taddhyanutiṣhṭhan yugapat sampādayatyarthadvayamārogyamindriy avijayaṁ ceti; tatsadvr̥ttamakhilenopadekṣhyāmo ...

Cha. Sū. 8/29

The practices (of *sadvṛtta*) fulfill two objectives when applied properly – they maintain optimal health and allow for control over sense organs.

Charaka provides extensive references on various aspects of *sadvṛtta*.

Reference	Instructions
Cha. Sū. 8/18	*Sadvṛtta* Codes of conduct of the prevalant times
Cha. Sū. 1/14c	*Upavasa* Control over all desires
Cha. Sū. 7/ and 8/	Relationships Individual, interpersonal, family, community, etc
Cha. Sū. 7/56-59	Company to avoid or prefer
Cha. Sū. 8/24	Guidelines for study and recitation
Cha. Sū. 8/22	Guidelines for intimate relationships
Cha. Sū. 5/104	Money, job
Cha. Sū. 8/35	Flexibility in recommending appropriate guidelines
Cha. Sū. 8/17-end	
Cha. Sū. 8/19	
Cha. Sū. 8/23	
Cha. Sū. 8/25-27	

Āchāra rasāyana

A specific practice of *āchāra* is explained to promote a *rasāyana* effect. This provides a restorative, rejuvenative effect on the individual who practices these codes of conduct regularly.

Additionally, these practices may be especially effective during a period of therapeutic *rasāyana*. As part of an overall treatment protocol, a *rasāyana* period may last for a few days to several months, depending on the methods.

Review Charaka's explanation of behaviors and codes of conduct to understand the expectations of *āchāra rasāyana* in Cha. Chi. 1(4)/30-35.

Causes of mental dysfunction

When *manas* and *sattva* are unable to maintain proper control over the *indriya*, *ahaṅkāra*, *rajas*, *tamas* and other components, the individual is prone to suffer from mental dysfunction. Presentations and outcomes can vary greatly depending on the components involved and the degree of dysfunction.

Charaka explain the outcomes due to *mānasika doṣhas* in Cha. Vi. 6/5-6. The disorders caused due to *rajas* and *tamas* are:

Disorder	Likely *doṣha*
Kāma Passion, lust, desire	*Rajas*
Krodha Anger	*Rajas*
Lobha Greed	*Tamas*
Moha Delusion, confusion, foolishness	*Tamas*
Irṣhyā Envy, jealousy, spite, malice	*Rajas*
Māna Arrogance, self-importance	*Rajas*
Mada Pride, lust, intoxication	*Rajas*

Śhoka Grief, sadness	*Tamas*
Cittodvega Anxiety neurosis	*Rajas*
Bhaya Fear	*Tamas*
Harṣhā Lust, desire, excitement (sexual)	*Rajas*

In each of these disorders, both *rajas* and *tamas* are involved in different ways and varying degrees. *Rajas* and *tamas* cannot act without the other. The likely *doṣha* listed in the previous table is that which is primarily involved. The other *doṣha* will always play a subordinate role in the disease process.

Tri āyatana and prajñāparādha

The *tri āyatana* explain three major causes of disease with psychological origins.

Origin	Occurs due to
Artha	Association of the senses with their objects
Karma	Thoughts, speech and action of the body
Kāla	Time and its effects

Each of these can produce disease in three ways, through:

1. *Ati-yoga* – excessive use
2. *Ayoga* – lack of use
3. *Mithya-yoga* – improper use

In total, there are nine possible causes of disease based on psychological origin.

Kāla, or time, may seem to be out of the purview of control for an individual. There are two ways to understand the effects of time.

In the classical Āyurvedic framework, the effects of time are considered to be under the influence of *daiva* and *puruṣhakāra*. Therefore, one who is living appropriately within their means would theoretically avoid untimely disease only. The normal effects of time, especially as timely ageing, decay and death, were unavoidable.

त्रीण्यायतनानीति - अर्थानां कर्मणः
कालस्य चातियोगायोगमिथ्यायोगाः ।

च. सू. ११।३७

Trīṇyāyatanānīti - arthānāṁ karmaṇaḥ
kālasya chātiyogāyogamithyāyogāḥ |

Cha. Sū. 11/37

Trīṇy-āyatanān-īti (The three causes of disease are -) arthānāṁ (association of the sense organs with their objects), karmaṇaḥ (actions [of the speech, mind and body]), kālasya (and time, along with its natural effects). Cha (And [these may be used]) atiyoga (too much), ayoga (too little) mithyāyogāḥ (or incorrectly, or improperly).

Vāgbhaṭa defines this as:

कालार्थकर्मणां योगो हीनमिथ्यातिमात्रकः
। सम्यग्योगश्च विज्ञेयो रोगारोग्यैककारणम्
॥

अ। हृ. सू. १।१९

Kālārthakarmaṇāṁ yogo
hīnamithyātimātrakaḥ |
Samyagyogaśhcha vijñeyo
rogārogyaikakāraṇam ||

AH Sū. 1/19

The complex topic of tri āyatana described in detail in Cha. Sū. 11/37-44 and AH Sū. 12/34-44. The authors include examples and additional subcategories to complete the explanation.

A major cause of disease is considered to the the inappropriate use of the sense organs to perceive their objects. Charaka states that this over-use, under-use or inappropriate acts as the initial cause for disease.

तदर्थातियोगायोगमिथ्यायोगात्
समनस्कमिन्द्रियं विकृतिमापद्यमानं
यथास्वं बुद्ध्युपघाताय सम्पद्यते,
सामर्थ्ययोगात् पुनः प्रकृतिमापद्यमानं
यथास्वं बुद्धिमाप्याययति || १५

च. सू. ८।१५

Tadarthātiyogāyogamithyāyogāt samanaskamindriyaṁ vikṛtimāpadyamānaṁ yathāsvaṁbuddhyupaghātāya sampadyate, sāmarthyayogāt punaḥ prakṛtimāpadyamānaṁ yathāsvaṁbuddhimāpyāyayati || 15

Cha. Sū. 8/15

The over-use, under-use and inappropriate use of the sense organs in perception of their objects leads to disease. The opposite produces normal health. These concepts are described in Cha. Sū. 8/15-16, 11/37-44 and AH Sū. 12/34-44.

The inappropriate application of the senses is stated to be prajñāparādha. This is a defect in proper application of wisdom, knowledge and understanding.

धीधृतिस्मृतिविभ्रष्टः कर्म यत्
कुरुतेऽशुभम्| प्रज्ञापराधं तं विद्यात्
सर्वदोषप्रकोपणम्||१०२||

Dhīdhṛtismṛtivibhraṣhṭaḥ karma yat kurute ' śhubham | Prajñāparādhaṁ taṁ vidyāt sarvadoṣhaprakopaṇam || 102

Cha. Śhā. 1/102

When comprehension, will power and memory are faulty, an individual acts in ways that allow all of the *doṣhas* to become aggravated.

बुद्ध्या विषमविज्ञानं विषमं च प्रवर्तनम् |
प्रज्ञापराधं जानीयान्मनसो गोचरं हि तत् ||
१०९

च. शा. १।१०९

Buddhyā viṣhamavijñānaṁ viṣhamaṁ cha pravartanam | Prajñāparādhaṁ jānīyānmanaso gocharaṁ hi tat || 109

Cha. Śhā. 1/109

Improperly functioning buddhi and jñāna which lead to innapropriate action are known as prajñāparādha. This results in perception of manas and indriya which is impaired.

Specific examples are described in Cha. Śhā. 1/103-108.

To overcome these defects in behavior and understanding, Charaka recommends promoting the power of smṛti (memory) and dhṛti (self control, restraint) to eliminate prajñāparādha. These are described in Cha. Śhā. 1/148-149, Cha. Śhā. 1/98, Cha. Śhā. 1/100 and Cha. Śhā. 1/102.

Chapter 9: Review

ADDITIONAL READING

Read and review the references listed below to expand your understanding of the concepts in this chapter. Write down the date that you complete your reading for each. Remember that consistent repetition is the best way to learn. Plan to read each reference at least once now and expect to read it again as you continue your studies.

References marked with (skim) can be read quickly and do not require commentary review.

CLASSICS	1st read	2nd read
Charaka		
Suśhruta		
Aṣhṭāṅga Hṛdaya		
Bhāva Prakāśha		

JOURNALS & CURRENT RESOURCES

QUESTIONS & ANSWERS

Record your questions for this chapter here for further research and discussion.

Question:

Answer:

Question:

Answer:

Question:

Answer:

SELF-ASSESSMENT

1. How many possible causes of disease are based on psychological orgin?
   a. innumberable
   b. 3
   c. 7
   d. 2
   e. None of the above

2. How many types of *sattva*-predominant *mānasika prakṛti* does Charaka describe?
   a. 3
   b. 14
   c. 16
   d. 12
   e. 7

3. Which is one of the *kāyika vegas*?
   a. *dāna*
   b. *akāla yukta*
   c. *lobha*
   d. *abhidhyāya*
   e. *strī-bhoga*

4. What are some the *lakṣhanas* of an *avara sattva* assessment?
   a. *raudra*
   b. *lobha*
   c. *unmāda*
   d. None of the above
   e. All the above

5. Why is assessing and managing *sattva* important?
   a. It can determine if you accept someone as a client.
   b. It will help determine appropriate treatment protocols.
   c. It ensures whether or not the client will maintain health protocols.
   d. None of the above
   e. All the above

6. What is one of the general recommendations provided by Charaka to follow *āchāra* for *sukha*?
   a. *dhṛti*
   b. *smṛti*
   c. *prajñāparādha*
   d. *jñāna*
   e. None of the above

7. What likely *doṣha*(s) is/are responsible for *harṣhā*?
   a. *pitta*
   b. *kapha*
   c. *rajas*
   d. *tamas*
   e. Both c and d

8. Which item below explains how disease can be produced as explained by *tri āyatana*?
   a. *doṣha*
   b. *tamas*
   c. *ati yoga*
   d. *rajas*
   e. All the above

9. Which is NOT a *rājasa*-predominant *mānasika prakṛti* described by Charka)? *Hint: Cha. Śā. 4/28*
   a. *gāndharva*
   b. *śhākuna*
   c. *sārpa*
   d. *rākṣhasa*
   e. *āsura*

10. What is one of the two types of *sattva* assessments?
    a. *tisra eṣhaṇā*
    b. *mānasika prakṛti*
    c. *pravara*
    d. *dhṛti*
    a. *dhana*

CRITICAL THINKING

1.

2.

3.

4.

5.

References

Chapter 10 : Vayas and āyu

KEY TERMS

āyu
bāla
madhyama
vayas
vṛddha

CLASSICAL REVIEW

Vayas

The classifications of age groups are significant in the context of assessing svastha for several reasons. The expectations of svastha and their practical implications can change greatly with each age group. Within each group, these can also change gradually through each subgroup. The methods of assessing various factors that influence svastha must also be modified accordingly for each age group, along with recommendations and management protocols.

Recall from Volume 2, Chapter 14, that Vāgbhaṭa roughly classifies the influence of the three *doṣhas* in the three major periods of life in AH Sū. 1/.

वयोहोरात्रिभुक्तानां तेऽन्तमध्याधिगाः क्रमात् ।

अ. हृ. सू. १।७.५

Vayohorātribhuktānāṁ te ' ntamadhyādhigāḥ kramāt |

AH Sū. 1/7.5

(In each stage of) vaya (lifespan), ahorātri (day and night) and bhuktānāṁ (stages of digestion after eating a meal), they (the doṣhas) undergo a cycle (of chaya, prakopa and praśhamā) in anta (the end), madhya (the middle) and ādhi (the beginning) of each.

Additionally, Suśhruta describes the lakṣhaṇas of each of these stages in Su. Sū. 35/29. These can be combined and understood as follows.

Period	Doṣha	Lakṣhaṇas
Bāla Childhood	Kapha	Kṣhīrapā, kṣhīrānnādā, annādā They drink milk only, drink milk and consume some solid food, or consume normal solid food
Madhyama Middle age	Pitta	Vṛddhi Growth (from 16-20 years)
		Yauvana Youthful energy and activity (from 20-30 years)
		Sarva dhātu-indriya-bala-vīrya sampūrṇatā All dhātus (supportive tissues), indriya (sense organs), bala (physical strength), and vīrya (potency) become fully manifested

		(from 30-40 years)
		Ūrdhvam-īṣhat parihāṇi Gradual decline and deterioration (from 40-70 years)
Vṛddha Old age	Vāta	Kṣhīyamāṇa dhātu, indriya, bala, vīrya, utsāha, mahanya hani Continuous general decline of dhātus (supportive tissues), indriya (sense organs), bala (physical strength), vīrya (potency) and utsāha (enthusiasm)
		Valī, palita, khālitya juṣhṭa Appearance of wrinkles (of the skin), grey hair, hair loss
		Kāsa, śhvāsa, prabhṛtibhirupadravairabhi bhūyamāna Cough, difficulty breathing, and other complications (of existing diseases) arise easily
		Sarvakriyāsvasamarthaṁ Unable to do any activities
		Jīrṇāgāramivābhivṛṣhṭamavasīdantaṁ Is like a worn-out house in the rain

Recall that different authors provide different ranges for ages in each of these groups. While Suśhruta considers bāla to end at 16 years old, Charaka states it to last until the age of 30.

The *lakṣhaṇas* provided by Suśhruta above can be applied in both classification methods because the specific age ranges are included in the descriptions.

By understanding what should be expected, or normal, for an individual within a specific age range, assessments, management protocols and expectations for results can be better estimated and planned.

Suśhruta states the practical application of this, and the underlying principles can be utilized and applied in other areas of health management. These principles will be discussed in the following section, Key principles.

Āyu

The assessment of āyu is explained by Suśhruta in Su. Sū. 35/3-11. This component is considered as the most important aspect of assessment from the clinician's perspective because it would provide insight into which patients would be less risky to treat.

Depending on the potential lifespan (long, medium or short), the patient could be managed in the way most appropriate to their situation. For those with a potentially long lifespan, the recommended action is to assess the remaining factors and then determine the line of treatment.

Suśhruta categorizes this assessment into general and specific *lakṣhaṇas*. When the general *lakṣhaṇas* appear in their full or complete presentation, the individual should be considered to have a long lifespan.

Medium or moderate presentations, and smaller or absent lakṣhaṇas are meant to indicate the reduced lifespan accordingly. This description is followed by the specific lakṣhaṇas for determining long, medium and short in more detail.

Each of these methods is reviewed next. Consider the assessment criteria and remember that in order to gauge an individual's assessed outcome, comparisons should be made against their immediate family members, extended family, or within their closest ethnic group.

While classically, this component may have been specified to be assessed first, it will be considered as the final, culminating component. This allows the professional to review all other significant components first and use their outcomes to contribute to assessing this factor. Basing this outcome on classical guidance is largely speculative today and confident future assessments require significant research and development.

General assessment of āyu

तत्र महापाणिपादपार्श्वपृष्ठस्तनाग्रदशनवदनस्कन्धललाटं दीर्घाङ्गुलिपर्वोच्छ्वासप्रेक्षणबाहुं, विस्तीर्णभ्रूस्तनान्तरोरस्कं, ह्रस्वजङ्गामेढ्रग्रीवं, गम्भीरसत्त्वस्वरनाभिम्, अनुच्चैर्बद्धस्तनम्, उपचितमहारोमशकर्णं, पश्चान्मस्तिष्कं, स्नातानुलिप्तं मूर्धानुपूर्व्या विशुष्यमाणशरीरं पश्चाच्च विशुष्यमाणहृदयं पुरुषं जानीयाद्दीर्घायुः खल्वयमिति । तमेकान्तेनोपक्रमेत् । एभिर्लक्षणैर्विपरीतैरल्पायुः; मिश्रैर्मध्यमायुरिति ॥

सु. सू. ३५।४

Tatra mahā-pāṇi-pāda-pārśhva-pṛṣhṭha-stanāgra-daśhana-vadana-skandha-lalāṭaṁ dīrgha-āṅguli-parvoccvāsa-prekṣhaṇa-bāhuṁ, vistīrṇabhrūstanāntaroraskaṁ, hrasva-jaṅgā-meḍhra-grīvaṁ, gambhīra-sattva-svara-nābhim, anuccairbaddhastanam, upachita -mahā-romaśha-karṇaṁ, paśhcān-mastiṣhkaṁ, snātān-uliptaṁ mūrdhānu-pūrvyā viśhuṣhyamāṇaśharīraṁ paśhcācca viśhuṣhyamāṇahṛdayaṁ puruṣhaṁ jānīyāddīrghāyuḥ khalvayamiti | Tamekāntenopakramet | Ebhirlakṣhaṇairviparītairalpāyuḥ, miśhrairmadhyamāyuriti ||

Su. Sū. 35/4

An individual having the following characteristics should be understood as having a long life span. For these types of individuals, treatment can be provided without hesitation. However, those with contrary (or opposite) characteristics should be understood as having a short lifespan. And those with moderate characteristics have a medium lifespan.

General āyu lakṣhaṇas Assessment criteria	Assessment methods
Mahā pāṇi, pāda, pārśhva, pṛṣhṭha, stanāgra, daśhana, vadana, skandha, lalāṭa Big hands, feet, sides (of the trunk of the body), back, nipples, teeth, face, shoulders and forehead	
Dīrgha āṅguli parva, uccvāsa, prekṣhaṇa, bāhu Long interphalangeal joints, breath (inhalation), eyes and arms	
Vistīrṇa bhrū, stanāntara, uras Broad eyebrows, space between the breasts, chest	
Hrasva jaṅgā, meḍhra, grīva Short legs, penis and neck	
Gambhīra sattva, svara, nābhi Deep (level of) sattva, voice, navel or umbilicus	
Anuccair-baddha stana Breasts are neither too prominent nor too firm	
Upachita mahā romaśha karṇa Thick, large, hairy ears	
Paśhcān mastiṣhka Well-developed posterior part of the brain	
Snātān uliptaṁ mūrdhānu pūrvyā viśhuṣhyamāṇa-śharīraṁ paśhcācca viśhuṣhyamāṇa-hṛdayaṁ After applying oil and taking a shower or bath, the person naturally dries first from the head, then the body and lastly the area around the heart	

Specific assessment for dīrgha āyu

गूढसन्धिसिरास्नायुः संहताङ्गः स्थिरेन्द्रियः ।
उत्तरोत्तरसुक्षेत्रो यः स दीर्घायुरुच्यते ॥ ५
गर्भात् प्रभृत्यरोगो यः शनैः समुपचीयते ।
शरीरज्ञानविज्ञानैः स दीर्घायुः समासतः ॥
सु. सू. ३५।६

Gūḍa-sandhi-sirā-snāyuḥ saṁhatāṅgaḥ sthirendriyaḥ |
Uttarottara-sukṣhetro yaḥ dīrghāyurucyate || 5
Garbhāt prabhṛtyarogo yaḥ śhanaiḥ samupacīyate |
Śharīrajñānavijñānaiḥ sa dīrghāyuḥ samāsataḥ ||

Su. Sū. 35/6

An individual with a long expected life span has the following characteristics:

Specific dīrgha āyu lakṣhaṇas Assessment criteria	Assessment methods
Gūḍa sandhi-sirā-snāyuḥ Joints, veins (vessels), and ligaments are well hidden (covered with well-developed bodily tissues)	
Saṁhatāṅgaḥ Bodily limbs are compact (strong, firm and well-built)	
Sthirendriyaḥ Stable (well-grounded) sense organs	
Uttarottara-sukṣhetro From below upwards (of the body), the bodily parts and features are better formed	
Garbhāt prabhṛtyarogo Absence of disease from conception onward	
Śhanaiḥ samupacīyate śharīra, jñāna, vijñānaiḥ The physical body, intellectual knowledge and scientific knowledge (application of thought) develop slowly and gradually	

Specific assessment for madhyama āyu

मध्यमस्यायुषो ज्ञानमत ऊर्ध्वं निबोध मे ।
अधस्तादक्षयोर्यस्य लेखाः स्युर्व्यक्तमायताः
॥ ७
द्वे वा तिस्रोऽधिका वाऽपि पादौ कर्णौ च
मांसलौ । नासाग्रमूर्ध्वं च भवेदूर्ध्वं लेखाश्च
पृष्ठतः ॥ ८
यस्य स्युस्तस्य परममायुर्भवति सप्ततिः ।

सु. सू. ३५।८.५

Madhyamasyāyuṣho jñānamata ūrdhvaṁ nibodha me |
Adhastādkṣhayoryasya lekhāḥ syurvyaktamāyatāḥ || 7
Dve vā tisro ‘ dhikā vā ‘ pi pādau karṇau cha māṁsalau |
Nāsāgramūrdhvaṁ cha bhavedūrdhvaṁ lekhāśhcha pṛṣhṭhataḥ || 8
Yasya syustasya paramamāyurbhavati saptatiḥ |

Su. Sū. 35/8.5

An individual with a medium (or moderate) expected life span has the following characteristics:

Specific madhyama āyu lakṣhaṇas Assessment criteria	Assessment methods
Adhastādkṣhayoryasya lekhāḥ syurvyaktamāyatāḥ dve vā tisro ' dhikā vā Two, three or more clear and long lines below the clavicle region	
Pādau karṇau cha māṁsalau Both hands and ears are fleshy	
Nāsāgramūrdhvaṁ Tip of the nose points upward	
Bhavedūrdhvaṁ lekhāśhcha pṛṣhṭhataḥ Vertical lines appear on the back	

Specific assessment for alpa āyu

जघन्यस्त्यायुषो ज्ञानमत ऊर्ध्वं निबोध मे ॥ ९
ह्रस्वानि यस्य पर्वाणि सुमहच्चापि मेहनम् ।
तथोरस्यवलीढानि न च स्यात्पृष्ठमायतम् ॥ १०
ऊर्ध्वं च श्रवणौ स्थानान्नासा चोच्चा शरीरिणः ।
हसतो जल्पतो वाऽपि दन्तमांसं प्रदृश्यते ।
प्रेक्षते यश्च विभ्रान्तं स जीवेत्पञ्चविंशतिम् ॥

सु. सू. ३५।११

Jaghanyastyāyuṣho jñānamata ūrdhvaṁ nibodha me |
Hrasvāni yasya parvāṇi sumahaccāpi mehanam |
Tathorasyavalīḍhāni na cha syātpṛṣhṭhamāyatam || 10
Ūrdhvaṁ cha śhravaṇau sthānānnāsā coccā śharīriṇaḥ |
Hasato jalpato vā ' pi dantamāṁsaṁ pradṛśhyate |
Prekṣhate yaśhcha vibhrāntaṁ sa jīvetpañchaviṁśhatim ||

Su. Sū. 35/11

An individual with a short expected life span has the following characteristics:

Specific alpa āyu lakṣhaṇas Assessment criteria	Assessment methods
Hrasvāni yasya parvāṇi Small joints of the fingers are short	
Sumahaccāpi mehanam The penis is very large	
Tatha urasya valīḍhāni na cha syātpṛṣhṭhamāyatam Chest has hairs that point in many different directions and spread to the back	

Ūrdhvaṁ cha śhravaṇau Both ears are placed higher on the head	
Sthānānnāsā cha uccā The position of the nose is placed higher	
Hasato jalpato vā ' pi dantamāṁsaṁ pradṛśhyate The gums become visible while speaking or laughing	
Prekṣhate yaśhcha vibhrāntaṁ Has a look of confusion, or wandering without purpose	

KEY PRINCIPLES

The following principles can be extracted from the classics and utilized to provide general guidance for current practice.

Principle #1: Age, predominant *doṣhas* and general restrictions

बाले विवर्धते श्लेष्मा मध्यमे पित्तमेव तु ।
भूयिष्ठं वर्धते वायुर्वृद्धे तद्वीक्ष्य योगयेत् ॥ ३१
अग्निक्षारविरेकैस्तु बालवृद्धौ विवर्जयेत् ।
तत्साध्येषु विकारेषु मृद्वीं कुर्यात् क्रियां शनैः ॥

सु. सू. ३५।३२

Bāle vivardhate śhleṣhmā madhyame pittameva tu |
Bhūyiṣhṭaṁ vardhate vāyurvṛddhe tadvīkṣhya yogayet || 31
Agnikṣhāravirekaistu bālavṛddhau vivarjayet |
Tatsādhyeṣhu vikāreṣhu mṛdvīṁ kuryāt kriyāṁ śhanaiḥ ||

Su. Sū. 35/32

In bāla (childhood), śhleṣhma vivardhate (kapha increases). In madhyame (middle age), pittameva tu (pitta increases). Bhūyiṣhṭaṁ (Likewise,) vāyuḥ (vāta) vardhate (increases) vṛddhe (in the elderly). Agnikṣhāravirekaistu (Treatments like agnikarma, or cautery, kṣhāra, or alkalis, and vireka, or purgatives) bālavṛddhau (in both the young and the old) vivarjayet (should be avoided). Tatsādhyeṣhu vikāreṣhu (However, in the diseases curable by these), mṛdvīṁ kuryāt kriyāṁ śhanaiḥ (these treatments can be performed gradually in a mild form).

Principle #2: Age and general usage of medicaments

तत्रोत्तरोत्तरासु वयोवस्थासूत्तरोत्तरा भेषजमात्राविशेषा भवन्ति, ऋते च परिहाणेः; तत्राद्यापेक्षया प्रतिकुर्वीत ॥

सु. सू. ३५।३०

Tatrottarottarāsu vayovasthāsūttarottarā bheṣhaja-mātrā-viśheṣhā bhavanti, ṛte cha parihāṇeḥ; tatrādyāpekṣhayā pratikurvīta ||

Su. Sū. 35/30

The quantity of medicines should be steadily increased throughout the period of middle age, each year up to parihāṇi (around 40 years), when it should start gradually decreasing to the level used in children.

The principle here is that as the individual matures fully and their strength grows to its maximum point, the quantities used for medicine should increase accordingly. Then, as the peak of maturity is passed and strength begins to naturally diminish, the quantities also must be scaled back gradually. In addition to this principle, Suśhruta also provides guidance on restricting intense treatments for the young and old.

CURRENT PRACTICAL APPLICATION

Suśhruta specifically mentions certain intense treatments and lines of management that should be avoided in the two age groups (young and old) because they are not fully mature or susceptible to decay.

While these treatments may not be considered standard in certain cultures and countries today, the intention remains the same. Delicate individuals who are young or old should be always be managed cautiously.

This means preferring and utilizing gentler, less invasive and low risk treatments and protocols wherever they are available. However, in situations where more intense approaches are required, they can be very slowly, gently and gradually introduced and applied.

Care should always be taken to modify and adjust the procedures to reduce their intensity and allow slow acclimatization to the treatment. Signs and symptoms of discomfort, pain, irritation or aversion should always be monitored closely and be taken seriously to attempt to prevent unnecessary complications.

Chapter 10: Review

ADDITIONAL READING

Read and review the references listed below to expand your understanding of the concepts in this chapter. Write down the date that you complete your reading for each. Remember that consistent repetition is the best way to learn. Plan to read each reference at least once now and expect to read it again as you continue your studies.

References marked with (skim) can be read quickly and do not require commentary review.

CLASSICS	1st read	2nd read
Charaka		
Suśhruta		
Aṣhṭāṅga Hṛdaya		
Bhāva Prakāśha		

JOURNALS & CURRENT RESOURCES

QUESTIONS & ANSWERS

Record your questions for this chapter here for further research and discussion.

Question:

Answer:

Question:

Answer:

Question:

Answer:

SELF-ASSESSMENT

1.
   a.
   b.
   c.
   d.
   e.

2.
   a.
   b.
   c.
   d.
   e.

3.
   a.
   b.
   c.
   d.
   e.

4.
   a.
   b.
   c.
   d.
   e.

5.
   a.
   b.
   c.
   d.

6.
   a.
   b.
   c.
   d.
   e.

7.
   a.
   b.
   c.
   d.
   e.

8.
   a.
   b.
   c.
   d.
   e.

9.
   a.
   b.
   c.
   d.
   e.

10.
   a.
   b.
   c.
   d.
   a.

CRITICAL THINKING

1.

2.

3.

4.

5.

References

Made in the USA
Las Vegas, NV
31 August 2022

54451776R00203